To the Vogts:
Afterwards
Bill

Cardiology

Cardiology

The Evolution of the Science and the Art
Second Edition

EDITED BY

RICHARD J. BING, M.D.

RUTGERS UNIVERSITY PRESS
New Brunswick, New Jersey, and London

Library of Congress Cataloging-in-Publication Data

Cardiology : the evolution of the science and the art / edited by
   Richard J. Bing. — 2nd ed.
      p.   cm.
   Includes bibliographical references and index.
   ISBN 0-8135-2627-2 (cloth : alk. paper). — ISBN 0-8135-2628-0
(pbk.)
   1. Cardiology—History.   I. Bing, Richard J., 1909–   .
   [DNLM: 1. Cardiology—history.   2. Physicians biography.   WG 11.1
C267 1999]
   RC666.5.B56   1999
   616.1'2'009—dc21
   DNLM/DLC
   for Library of Congress   98-44410
                                                                          CIP

British Cataloging-in-Publication Data for this book is available from the British Library.

First edition © 1992 by Harwood Academic Publishers GmbH, Poststrasse 22,
7000 Chur, Switzerland

This revised edition copyright © 1999 by Rutgers, The State University
Published by arrangement with Harwood Academic Publishers GmbH

Manufactured in the United States of America

To the memory of Mary Whipple Bing

Contents

Illustrations

Preface

The history of cardiology is but a small window facing into the past of the science and art of medicine. This editor has lived through three phases of cardiology: a purely clinical phase, where bedside diagnosis went hand and hand with therapeutic nihilism; a period that stressed the dynamics of circulation, where some cardiac diseases were explained on a purely hemodynamic basis; and, finally, a time when invasive procedures together with biochemistry, biophysics, and molecular biology became the primary influence. The common denominator in this rapidly changing field has been the human factor. Within this short period of history, human nature changed little although cultural changes left an imprint on personal expression.

Although the language and the venue may have changed, the human element with all its diversity has remained. It is the personality of the artist or scientist that determines the ultimate character of his or her work. Therefore, for a historian, the personality of the artist or scientist must be an essential element of study. The historian can do this by recording the impact of individuals on their time and future and by tracing their fleeting shadows during their own lifetimes. Without the human element, history becomes a colorless recitation of facts. This is even more true when dealing with medical science, which has as its final goal the application of science to human beings. The goals of the physician are primarily humanistic. As Ralph Waldo Emerson wrote in his essay on experience: "As I am so I see; use whatever language we will, we can never say anything but what we are." This applies to the artist and to the scientist, and yes, to all human beings.

Therefore, in writing a history of cardiology we have stressed the source of ideas that have guided cardiology to the present and we have dwelled on the mind and emotions, on the lives of the scientists and physicians, their successes and failures, their struggles and disappointments. We have at the same time attempted to achieve a balance between the scientist and her or his work, even though some chapters recount more facts, while others dwell more on personalities. Personalities loom larger in the more remote past: the perspective of time has illuminated and magnified them. The verdict of history has not yet been rendered on those from the immediate past and erosions of time have not yet differentiated the great innovators from their lesser followers. Therefore portions dealing with more recent developments focus more on scientific facts than on scientists. This is especially the case for the most recent developments in the field of hypertension or molecular genetics. However, emphasis on science may help us project the recent past into the future and uncover the underlying facts of science and medicine. The inclusion of recent findings in some chapters begs the question to when history stops and the present begins. Science is a stream of discovery. From where we stand the present emerges and the past begins its descent. The past without the present is incomplete. Although younger readers may prefer today's knowledge to yesterday's history, age brings an appreciation of the lengthening shadows of the past. It is hoped that we have combined today's knowledge with the patina of the past.

We are grateful to Dr. Claude Lenfant and the National Heart, Lung and Blood Institute, National Institutes of Health, to Medtronic, Inc., Minneapolis, MN, and to Mr. and Mrs. Jensen for their financial support; to Ki-Young Suh, Jennifer I. Cordero, and Y. Kelly Cho for their unselfish devotion in completing this book. We also appreciate the support of the executive director of the Huntington Medical Research Institutes, Dr. William Opel.

R.J. Bing, M.D.

Cardiology

Chapter 1   Cardiac Catheterization

D. BAIM
R.J. BING

THE DEVELOPMENT OF cardiac catheterization over the past fifty years has been staggering. Well over one million such procedures are now performed in the United States each year. Precise anatomic and physiologic cardiac diagnoses are established in less than one hour in a lightly sedated patient who is frequently able to return home six hours after the procedure. Drawing on the techniques developed by Dotter and Gruentzig, another three hundred thousand patients undergo catheter correction of the underlying problem using only percutaneous femoral artery puncture under local anesthesia, rather than open surgical thoracotomy.

Claude Bernard was the first to catheterize the heart in animals, motivated by purely basic physiological inquiries (1, 2). The argument had not been settled at that time whether cellular metabolism takes place in the lung, as proposed by Antoine-Laurent Lavoisier, or in other organs, as suggested by Gustav Magnus. Bernard's studies are described in two volumes, the first, *Chaleur Animale*, and the second, *Physiologie Operatoire*, published in 1876 (1, 2). In his straightforward manner, Bernard conceived an experiment to answer this question. If the temperature in the right and the left ventricles is equal, heat production could not have primarily taken place in the lung. Since Bernard found the temperature of the blood in the left ventricle to be slightly elevated, he concluded that Lavoisier was in error: the body heat is due to cellular metabolism taking place in all tissues. Bernard had considered and discarded the idea of making an open window for direct inspection of the heart or to exteriorize the heart, but preferred insertion of a catheter because the procedure was relatively noninvasive. He used a catheter made of lead to give it the right curvature, a forerunner of the preformed

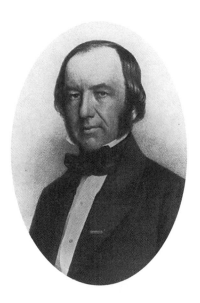

Figure 1.1. Claude Bernard. *(Courtesy of the New York Academy of Medicine)*

catheter of today. Bernard's thinking and writing are characterized by clarity and by directness of approach (3). He was a master at finding ingenious solutions that went straight to the "heart" of the problem and he disliked scientific speculations. As he wrote, "The best philosophical system for the working scientist is not to have any at all!" Bernard was a master of the new science, experimental physiology, and had an unbending devotion to his work despite immense personal difficulties (3; Fig. 1.1).

In 1861 A. Chaveau and Etienne Jules Marey published their work on the measurements of intracardiac pressure (4, 5; Fig. 1.2). Their paper is on the graphic determination of the relationship between the apex beat and the movement of the atrium and ventricles, respectively. By means of pressure tracings they found that "la systole du ventricule et la pulsation cardiaque (choc du coeur) commencent et finissent toute deux simultanement," that is, ventricular systole and apical beat commence and terminate completely simultaneously (Fig. 1.3). Chaveau and Marey also achieved the first recorded simultaneous measurement of pressure in the left ventricle and in the central aorta (4, 5). They defined the influence of the left ventricular systole on the contour of the central aortic pressure curve. Moreover, they were the first to refer to the isometric phase of the left ventricular contraction. Marey set forth the technical procedure in detail: the recording instrument and the graphic tracings (Figs. 1.3 and 1.4). Anticipating

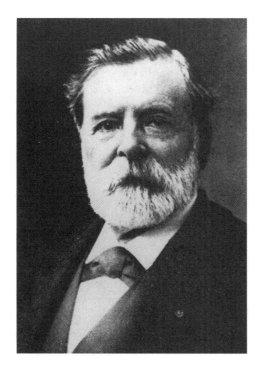

Figure 1.2. Etienne Jules Marey. (Courtesy of the New York Academy of Medicine)

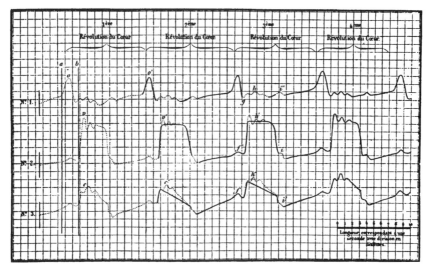

Figure 1.3. Intracavitary tracings of atrial (1), ventricular pressures (2), and apical impulse (3). Time is indicated in the abscissa. (Courtesy of Medtronic, Inc., Minneapolis, MN)

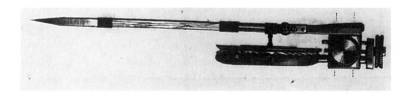

Figure 1.4. Recording device used by Marey (Marey's Capsule). (*Courtesy of Medtronic, Inc., Minneapolis, MN*)

the concerns of later physicians as to the application of catheterization of the heart, Marey wrote in a footnote to his book on the effect of catheterization of the heart of the horse: "One can be reassured of the innocuity of this method by examining the horse, which is scarcely disturbed, walks and eats as usual. In only a few instances is the pulse rate slightly increased, especially at the time of introduction of the catheter within the heart cavities" (6).

Bernard paid tribute to Marey for his development of instruments to graphically record events of the circulation and of biological phenomena. He wrote, "It is true that efforts had been made in the same direction by Herman von Helmholtz, Carl Friedrich , etc., before Marey but they were not amenable to general application and they were doomed to remain personal procedures" (7). He also discussed Marey's work on the relationship of the apical beat to the cardiac cycle. To quote Bernard, "Two opinions existed: An old one which stems from William Harvey and was accepted with a few modifications by an eminent member of your commission, according to which the heart beat results from the contraction of the ventricles; and the other, which is more recent and at first seems simpler and more satisfactory and attributes the phenomenon to the propulsion from the apex of the heart through the surge of blood from the auricular systole. The graphic method provided the answer. An examination of the resultant graphs completely eliminated uncertainty. The relationship between the beat of the heart and the contraction of the ventricle was demonstrated by the synchronous upward movement of the two levers and by the simultaneous elevation in the two curves they recorded" (7).

Bernard's statement, in which he mentions Marey's third book (entitled *La Machine Animale*), is significant. This work deals with Marey's investigation of locomotion of animals on land and in the air, "a subject which only became experimentally approachable with the advent of the ingenious instrument to record events that the eyes of the observer cannot follow." Bernard concluded his recommendation to the academy by writing, "In conclusion it is evident that Marey has accomplished a considerable task with which his name will always be identified" (7).

Marey's investigations on the movements of animals clearly show that he was primarily concerned with the application of physical techniques to physiology. Some have credited Marey with the invention of cinematography, primarily because he advised the brothers Lumière, the acknowledged inventors of cinematography, in the utilization of his methods. However, long before Marey took out a patent on this invention in 1893 and before he communicated his findings to the Academy of Sciences, other patents for similar discoveries were awarded. One in 1888 from England even mentions perforation of films (5).

One of the questions that occupied scientists at that time concerned the movement of horses. What happens when a horse gallops? How many feet are on the ground at any one time? Marey's instrumentation made it possible to state that a galloping horse placed first one then three then two and again one foot on the ground. It is likely that the governor of California, Leland Stanford, who was an enthusiastic horseman saw some of Marey's illustrations (6). He therefore requested Edward Muybridge, an Englishman, who was a land surveyor in California, to repeat Marey's photographic studies. Muybridge accomplished this by placing, in series, twenty-four photographic apparatus that were activated by a galloping horse moving in front of these cameras. Thus, a photographic series originated that demonstrated the movements of the horse in all details. Muybridge came to Paris and delivered a lecture in Marey's laboratory. Marey had closely followed the development of Muybridge's methodology but he considered it inadequate for his own experimentation. For instance, Marey was aware that Muybridge's methods were inadequate for the study of the flight of birds. In order to accomplish this goal, Marey constructed, in 1882, his "photographic gun" (6). The technique for this invention goes back to Pierre Jules Janssen, an astronomer working in Paris, who in 1874 was able to take seventeen rapid pictures of the passage of Venus by the sun. Both investigators, the astronomer and the physiologist, never fought for the patent rights: Janssen was interested in astronomy, Marey in physiology exploration, and for both, the rapid-firing photographic gun was a means to accomplish their goals. Marey was particularly interested in establishing the fundamental conditions for human flight by photographing birds in flight. Finally, he was able to take twenty-four pictures per second of the flight of birds and increased the speed of exposure to 1/1400 of a second.

To summarize, Marey's scientific work originated from an application of engineering skill to physiological goals. It was this combination that made him a unique figure in the history of medicine.

More than fifty years later, Werner Forssmann introduced the era of the clinical application of intracardiac catheterization (Fig. 1.5). Forssmann was born in 1904 in Berlin and died in 1979 after two myocardial infarctions. Forssmann's life, personality, and character are unusual even in the field of science, where

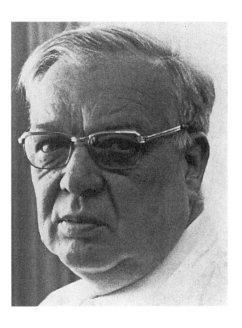

Figure 1.5. Werner Forssmann. *(Courtesy of the New York Academy of Medicine)*

unusual personalities abound. The inspiration for Forssmann's discovery was the work of Marey. In his book, *Experiments on Myself*, Forssmann wrote, "It is strange how an early impression can remain firmly implanted! As a student, I saw the reprint of an old etching in a textbook of physiology. It originated in a paper of Marey's which showed a touching, naive presentation of a man standing before a horse and holding a tube which had been introduced through a jugular vein into the heart of the animal. In the ventricle, the lumen of the tube was closed by a rubber balloon, which transmitted the changes in pressure to a Marey 'tambour' and thence to a pen which described the pressure curves. This picture has excited me to such a degree that it pursued me by day and night. Even today I see exactly as it is even when I close my eyes. The words of these classical French physiologists have convinced me that their experimental studies could be performed in man without danger" (8).

Thus, in the early summer of 1929, Forssmann's plans came to fruition. He presented them to his superior, Professor Schneider, but as he said, his good old chief turned him down because "For this sort of work I cannot permit you to work on any one of my patients. Of course, I think your idea is excellent and that it will contribute much to future work. And possibly the whole thing is completely without danger just as you think in your youthful enthusiasm." He suggested more animal experimentation, but Forssmann said that that was not necessary. "Well then, I will prove that this experiment is without danger and will do it on myself." But that, too, was vetoed by Schneider (8).

Despite these warnings, Forssmann went ahead and persuaded a nurse, Gerda Ditz, to help him. She offered to undergo the heart catheterization herself, but Forssmann, who was determined to do it on himself, tricked her, tying her to the operating table to prevent her from interfering. Then, after local anesthesia of his left antecubital fossa, he inserted a ureteral catheter about 30 cm deep into his vein. He then untied the nurse and asked her to call the nurse in charge of x-rays. Forssmann had to walk down to the basement with the catheter in his heart where a nurse named Eva took pictures showing the catheter in the right ventricle. His chief, Schneider, an understanding and obviously patient physician, told him, "Forssmann, you have done something really great and I want to congratulate you but I believe that your place is not here in this little hospital; you should work in a larger institution," and recommended him through friends to Ferdinand Sauerbruch, the director of the surgical clinic at the University of Berlin. Its main hospital, the Charité, accepted him as a surgical assistant. Schneider advised him not to talk about his work until it had been published. The paper appeared in the *Klinische Wochenschrift* in November 1929 in an article entitled "Die Sondierung des rechten Herzens" (9). It shows a picture of the catheter in the right atrium. But instead of getting praise from Sauerbruch, he got fired. As he wrote, "Late in the evening I was asked to see the Geheimrat. He was well prepared and on his desk lay the *Klinische Wochenschrift* as well as a newspaper and a letter from Unger, who apparently had complained that I had plagiarized his work." He sternly looked at Forssmann for a while in silence and then he yelled: "This is a shameful thing you did and in addition to that you have stolen the priority from one of my most esteemed senior surgeons and why did you not mention that his scientific study was carried out in my department?" Forssmann answered with a short, well-rehearsed lecture on the future of cardiac catheterization. Sauerburch answered with disdain: "That work has no place in surgery. These are purely questions for the internist and physiologist." Forssmann meekly suggested that this work might make it possible for him to "habilitate," that is, to enter the academic career. Sauerbruch answered, "With such circus tricks you never can obtain a position in a decent German clinic. Do you want to be an internist or a surgeon?" Forssmann answered softly, "But I do not know that, Herr Geheimrat. I just am nine months out of medical school and I just do not know what I am good for." That was the last straw. Sauerbruch yelled at him, "For a real surgeon there is only one thing, to operate, to operate, to operate. Get out and leave the clinic immediately." Forssmann writes that rather than submitting to depression, he left the interview elated. Obviously he was relieved and felt justified that he had done the right thing regardless of the prejudice of his "betters" (8).

Soon afterward, Forssmann conceived an even more daring idea: the injection of contrast material into the heart in order to "improve cardiac diagnosis."

First he used the rabbit but soon found that this species was unsuitable and therefore he proceeded to perform his experiments on dogs. The problem was that none of the hospitals to which Forssmann had access had quarters to house dogs for experimental purposes. It was then that his mother came into the breach and offered to care for the animals in her apartment (8). Forssmann injected morphine into the dog to induce basal narcosis, then placed the dog in a sack and drove it to the hospital. Ether narcosis deepened the anesthesia, and under aseptic conditions, the catheter could be introduced through the external jugular vein into the right ventricle. Contrast material was then injected while x-ray pictures were taken. The animal was then returned to his mother's care, where it was kept in the bathtub, a convenient location since the animals were often incontinent. The animal was then replaced by another and the experiments were repeated. Forssmann mentioned that the greatest difficulty was his mother's and grandmother's attachment to the animals. After having taken care of them for a while, they were loath to part with them and according to Forssmann many tears were shed.

The next step was to attempt the injection of contrast material into the human heart. Again, Forssmann accomplished this by self-experimentation. He admits that he had some anxious moments because this was different from simply putting a catheter in his heart: the injection of contrast material meant that a foreign substance was circulating in his blood with unknown consequences. He attempted to see whether he was sensitive to the iodine by "filling a small test tube with the contrast material and pressing the opening for hours against his buccal mucosa." Since there was no reaction he concluded that the inside of the heart was equally tolerant. Thus, after having placed the catheter in his heart he injected the contrast material while pictures were taken. Unfortunately, the technique was not sufficient to obtain clear pictures of the passage of contrast material, but Forssmann found the technique safe since he experienced only slight symptoms such as brief dizziness and transient diminution of vision. Prior to publication, it was arranged that Forssmann would present his findings before the illustrious Surgical Congress of 1931, but his speaking time was cut from eight to four minutes. During his lecture there was little attention and his presentation was accompanied by murmurs of ridicule and snickers of derision. The discouraged Forssmann was consoled by his uncle, a country doctor, with these words: "Don't get angry. Those idiots don't understand what you have in mind. One day you will get the Nobel prize." His uncle had spoken the truth. Despite the local adverse reaction, four weeks after the publication of Forssmann's paper in 1931 (10), O. Klein, in Prague, published a preliminary paper and six months later a definite report on the determination of cardiac output according to Fick's principle (11). This article first described the indirect methods of determining cardiac output, then refers to the work of Forssmann, which made it possible to determine the cardiac output by direct means. Klein performed eighteen catheterizations in man, determining the oxygen and carbon dioxide content of arterial and mixed venous blood and calculated a cardiac output of 4.5 liters/min. He described the procedure as simple and without incident (11).

Despite a few references to Forssmann's work in the literature, it was forgotten after the war, and his whereabouts were unknown. Forssmann owes his resurrection after the war to his English colleagues, but primarily to Sir John MacMichael, who invited him to England. Forssmann never became chairman of a Department of Surgery, a goal that he would have appreciated; he did become honorary professor in several German universities; he made friends with several German medical men, particularly Grosse-Brockhoff, chairman of the Department of Medicine in Duesseldorf. In 1968 I (RJB) met Forssmann and his wife for the first time at a party given by Grosse-Brockhoff. Both were charming people; Forssmann impressed me by his wit and sense of humor.

Forssmann's final years were characterized by research into medical problems not connected with cardiology or science, but with euthanasia, truth at the bedside, and cardiac transplantation (12). He became an opponent of the death penalty; he did consider himself, as he wrote me (RJB), a "medical fossil." In the last letter I received from him in 1978 from Wies-Wambach, nine months before his death, he apologized for not being able to attend a meeting in which I was to talk about cardiac catheterization. He wrote that he had nothing to say about modern cardiology except platitudes, and that he was not willing to talk about the history of cardiology because he realized "how deep I am already in the shadow of the past." He also wrote that it "nauseate[d]" him when his self-experimentation was described as an act of heroism: "This it was not!! I had thought very carefully about whether the method of catheterization would lead to a clinical routine procedure." He had, he wrote, "to rule out the risk to patients, otherwise, it would have been a circus stunt, as I was accused by Sauerbruch and Nissen in their conceit" (12).

H. Schadewaldt, professor of history of medicine at the University of Dusseldorf, wrote in his eulogy of Forssmann, "Men of spirit and zest who love science are most certainly not in need of rules and regulations. The force which pushes them onward lies within themselves, urging them to go forward; they themselves are a law within themselves" (13).

Forssmann shared the Nobel prize with two American scientists, Andre Cournand and Dickinson Richards. Cournand was born in France and Richards was a New Englander. Their cooperation began in 1932. As Cournand wrote, "In 1932, Dickinson Richards, then at Columbia Presbyterian Medical Center and I, Chief Resident of the Chest Service of Bellevue Hospital in New York, agreed on a systemic and comprehensive examination of cardiopulmonary function in normal and diseased man. The lungs, heart, and circulation form a single system for the exchange of respiratory gases between the atmosphere and the tissues of the organism" (14). In 1940 they first attempted to catheterize a patient's heart, but failed because the catheter was obstructed at the level of the axilla. Not long afterward a new opportunity presented itself (14). Homer W. Smith, the renal physiologist, novelist, and professor of physiology at the New York University College of Medicine, was planning to measure cardiac output in hypertensive patients. In a first report published in 1941, Cournand and H.A. Ranges reported the results of the initial catheterization (15). The report emphasized the necessity for a steady state, for simultaneous and prolonged blood and air sampling, the value of the checking provided by comparing results based on application of the Fick principle, the reproducibility of the results, and finally proof that cardiac catheterization was innocuous. New catheters were designed and a new manometer for measurement of pressure was built. Cournand and Richards and their co-workers studied many clinical conditions in humans, including hypertension, circulatory shock, and chronic lung disease. Richards and Cournand made an ideal team. Richards, a great clinician, was a quiet and reserved individual with a keen intellect and compassion for his fellow man (Fig. 1.6). Cournand was a meticulous worker with a passion for accuracy.

Cournand clearly outlined his motivation for catheterization of the heart at that time (16). His interest stemmed from an investigation of the study of ventilation pertaining to perfusion. He was stimulated by "Something important, which could only be revealed in disease: the relationship between alveolar ventilation and perfusion." The lead was given to Cournand and Richards very early in their study on the basis of the application of the Fick principle. This work led them from the study of cardiac output and pulmonary blood flow to a study of the unequal distribution of blood flow.

At Richards' death in 1973, Cournand wrote a moving eulogy (17). He described Richards' background, his New England family, his student days at Yale, his passion for patients, and his dedication to improve the lot of patients at Bellevue Hospital by consistently recommending the building of a new hospital. Richards' editorship with A.P. Fishman of a book, *Circulation of the Blood: Men and Ideas* (18), and a small volume entitled *Medical Priesthoods and Other Essays* (19), are examples of his knowledge of the history of medicine and his passion for truth. His philosophy is best expressed in a letter he wrote to Cournand: "Man's potentiality, or in these days his survival, will depend on his consciousness, more specifically his conscience, more specifically still, the ability of the leaders and their followers to change character, into more merciful beings" (19).

Why was cardiac catheterization developed at the Columbia division of Bellevue? There were two reasons. The main one was that Dickinson Richards was head of the Columbia division of the medical service at Bellevue Hospital, and Bellevue was a progressive inner-city hospital, with medical services run by

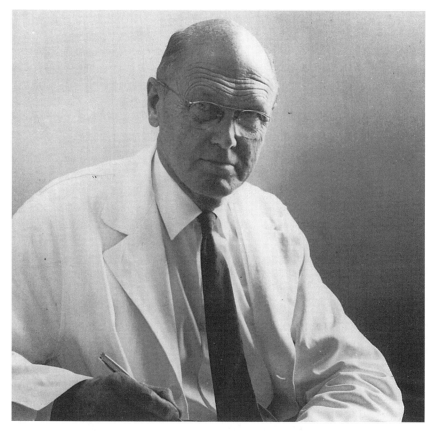

Figure 1.6. Dickinson Richards. *(Courtesy of the New York Academy of Medicine)*

Columbia, New York, and Cornell universities. Richards was the ideal man to promote progressive research. With Tillet as department chairman, and with Homer Smith, chairman of the Department of Physiology, whose name is synonymous with renal physiology, and with Drs. Goldring and Chasis, who applied Smith's methods to the bedside, this was the right environment to accept and execute ideas.

Despite its early purposes as a scientific instrument, the catheter became more and more a diagnostic tool, particularly for selective coronary arteriography and for continuous bedside hemodynamic monitoring with the Swan–Ganz catheter.

The idea for the Swan–Ganz catheter originated with the appreciation of the need to conduct cardiac catheterization in sick patients without fluoroscopy and without moving the critically ill patient (Fig. 1.7). The idea was developed by H.J. Swan while watching the spinnaker on a sailboat; the first suggestion in

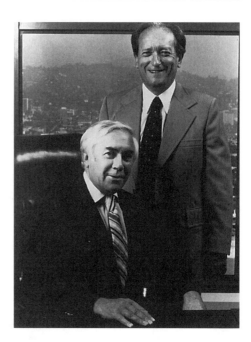

Figure 1.7. William Ganz and Jeremy Swan. (Dr. Ganz is standing.) *(With permission)*

1967 was to place a sail or parachute at the end of a soft catheter and have that device drag the catheter into the pulmonary artery (20). This, Swan writes, was the outcome of a series of coincidences, namely, that he had been director of the cath lab at the Mayo Clinic and that Ron Bradley from London had been a student of his in 1950. Bradley had developed the concept of a very fine soft tubing that sometimes "regrettably and frequently" would spontaneously float into the pulmonary artery; however, the idea of a sail or parachute was technically difficult. The other chance phenomenon that resulted in the introduction of a balloon catheter was Swan's connection with a laboratory that built heart valves. He was able to persuade them to attach a balloon to the catheter (20, 21). William Ganz evaluated it in animal experiments and confirmed the validity of the pulmonary capillary wedge pressure (21, 22). Ganz's outstanding contribution was the incorporation of the measurement of cardiac output by thermodilution, a matter that had occupied him for many years and that further increased the clinical impact of the catheter. As Swan wrote, "Hence, we have effective hemodynamic monitoring today (1980), applied (correctly or incorrectly, rightly or wrongly, efficaciously or harmfully) to approximately two to three million patients per annum."

The study of cardiac metabolism by catheterization was started in 1946, when I (RJB) found that the catheter slipped several times inadvertently into the region of the heart that under the x-ray looked like a portion of the right ventricle but actually was the coronary sinus; when the blood was withdrawn it was much blacker than that obtained from the right ventricle. Others had already observed that the coronary sinus could be catheterized. In 1941, as told by J.H. Comroe, in attempting to catheterize the right ventricle, Cournand obtained a sample of blood with lower oxygen content than right atrial blood (23). Because the fluoroscopic picture showed that the catheter tip was misplaced and was possibly in the coronary sinus (by mere chance), Cournand was concerned with possible damage to the lining of the coronary sinus, and hastily withdrew the catheter (23). Gene Stead had trouble with three patients because the sample of blood from the right heart had a very low oxygen content; he concluded that the catheter must have slipped into the coronary sinus, and discarded the data (23). Sosman, a radiologist in Boston, listed among his "failures and errors" unexpected location of the catheter tip and published in one of his figures an x-ray film showing a catheter tip in the coronary venous sinus (23). In 1947 my (RJB) group at Johns Hopkins Hospital, originally organized to study congenital heart disease, wrote, "When the catheter is in the coronary sinus, it is seen curved upwards to the base of the heart. In the first cases, intubation of these vessels was fortuitous" (24). In the four remaining cases, catheterization of the sinus was carried out deliberately. All our energy was now devoted to the new, rewarding field of coronary blood flow and cardiac metabolism. Fortunately, S. Kety and E.F. Schmidt had devised a method for determining cerebral blood flow using nitrous oxide (N_2O); one was therefore in a position to measure not only the myocardial extraction of foodstuffs by the heart, but also their usage. One of many findings was that the heart in the fasting state preferentially extracted free fatty acids but could also use amino acids and ketones; in human heart failure no changes in utilization of substrates could be detected (25, 26, 27).

In congenital heart disease, it was Cournand's group, particularly with A. Himmelstein and the group of Lewis Dexter at Harvard, and the Johns Hopkins Hospital team of R.J. Bing that defined procedures for the diagnosis of congenital heart disease by intracardiac catheterization (28, 29, 30). Formulas derived from the oxygen content of blood made it possible to calculate regional blood flow such as the effective pulmonary blood flow, the direction and size of the intracardiac shunt, and vascular resistances in the pulmonary and systemic circulation (30). This use of the catheter in congenital heart disease owes its main impetus to the advent of cardiac surgery in the 1940s primarily through the work of Blalock at Hopkins, Robert E. Gross at Harvard, and Clarence Craaford in Stockholm. The fact that children with congenital heart disease · could now be helped by surgery made the catheter an essential tool in clinical diagnosis. The abundance of patients who underwent surgery performed by Blalock provided a wealth of material to study the circulation in these children. The use of the catheter also made possible the recognition and importance of pulmonary hypertension (31) and initiated studies on the adaptation to hypoxia of cyanotic children (32). Every week brought new surprises and new revelations in a field that heretofore had been considered of theoretical importance only (see Chapter 4).

Of great importance was the discovery by Dexter at Harvard that by wedging the catheter into a pulmonary artery, it is possible to record the height of left atrial pressure (29). Without this pioneering study, the work of Ganz and Swan would not have been possible.

Coronary Arteriography

Forssmann had shown that it was safe to inject contrast (radiopaque) material into the human heart (10). But it was a long way from this discovery to satisfactory visualization of the coronary arteries. It was the Swedish school that in the late 1940s pioneered this field, with Stig Radner, B. Broden, J. Karnell, and G. Jonson (33, 34). In 1934 P. Rousthoi in Stockholm published a preliminary report in which he coined the word "angiocardiography" to describe the contrast visualization of the heart (35). His experiments were carried out on rabbits, with catheterization of the root of the aorta from the right carotid artery and the injection of thorotrast. His conclusion was that this procedure would become applicable to humans as well. In 1945 Radner, in Lund, Sweden, based his method on that of Antonio C. Egas Moniz, who soon after Forssmann described a method of visualizing the blood vessels in the brain. The question was how to get the contrast material into the coronary arteries. Radner's technique consisted of perforating the sternum and puncturing, under fluoroscopic control, the ascending aorta. This was then followed by the injection of contrast material, which filled the bulb of the aorta and outlined the coronary arteries (36). In 1947 Radner used a less dramatic procedure by catheterization of the aorta from the radial artery (33). He based his studies on those of G.P. Robb and I. Steinberg, who had rapidly injected intravenously diodrast solution and x-rayed the structures of the cardiovascular system at the point of arrival of the contrast material (37). Radner positioned a catheter in the radial artery and introduced the tip into the ascending aorta under fluoroscopic control. In order to get the opaque substance into the coronary arteries, the injection had to be performed with the catheter inserted far down in the ascending aorta, preferably with the tip close to the semilunar valves (33). Nonselective coronary arteriography was also the method of choice by L. DiGuglielmo and M. Guttadauro (38), of A. Thal (39), and of Charles T. Dotter (40). The latter placed a double lumen catheter into the ascending aorta momentarily occluding that vessel while simultaneously injecting radiopaque material through the other lumen of the catheter. In retrospect, it is astonishing how many investigators continued direct puncture of the aorta, despite the fact that catheterization through a peripheral artery appeared to be safer and simpler.

All this changed with the advent of selective coronary arteriography by F. Mason Sones and E.K. Shirey, and later by Melvin P. Judkins. The paper by Sones was published in *Modern Concepts of Cardiovascular Disease* in 1962, although the procedure had first been carried out in 1958 (41). In his report, Sones mentioned that this procedure was to provide a more objective and precise standard of diagnosis for human coronary artery disease. He noted that a direct (selective) coronary catheterization had been used for deliberate selective pacification of individual coronary arteries in more than 1,020 patients. Rather than publishing extensive papers, Sones prepared a film on coronary arteriography that was distributed by the Committee on Professional Education of the American Heart Association. This film did more to introduce coronary arteriography than any large number of articles could have done.

The first deliberate efforts to perform selective coronary arteriography were made by Sones in 1958. In 1959 a special catheter was fabricated at his request. The history of this epochal discovery is described by Litwak in *Cardiovascular Clinics 1951* and reprinted by Comroe in his book, *The Retrospectroscope* (23). In 1958 Sones and his colleagues at the Cleveland Clinic were studying a young adult and had withdrawn their catheter from the left ventricle into the supravalvular area in preparation for an aortogram. The equipment at that time did not allow them to precisely visualize the catheter tip immediately prior to injection of the contrast material. The contrast material was injected; to Sones' horror, the right artery and its distal branch were clearly visualized. Obviously the catheter had accidentally entered the right coronary orifice when the dye was injected. The patient had remained stable throughout the entire procedure. This fortunate event taught Sones that, contrary to views held at the time concerning electrical instability of the heart, non-oxygen carrying fluid could be injected into a major coronary artery without untoward effects. Sones realized that with proper equipment, he could reduce the coronary artery injectate by tenfold and would then be able to sequentially study the entire coronary circulation of man.

Sones' career began at the University of Maryland with his medical degree and then as a resident at the Henry Ford Hospital in Detroit. He then joined the Cleveland Clinic (Fig. 1.8). Like Forssmann, Sones was an extraordinary personality. Without the work of Sones the efforts in myocardial revascularization would not have been possible. He had a refreshing bluntness that sometimes stunned younger colleagues. When he visited my department (RJB) at Wayne State University in Detroit as part of a project site visit, and one of my younger colleagues presented his studies on coincidence counting in the measuring of coronary blood flow, Sones thoroughly startled the poor fellow with his critical remarks. Once I brought a patient to him, a young woman of twenty-two, who

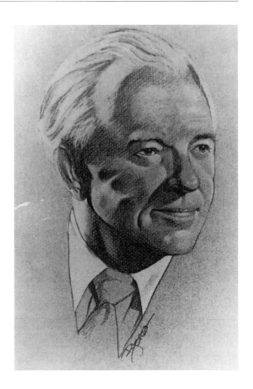

Figure 1.8. F. Mason Sones. (*Courtesy of the* Texas Heart Institute Journal)

had what probably now would be diagnosed as spasm of the coronary arteries (syndrome X), which was at that time considered small vessel disease. To prove his point he performed a myocardial puncture with an unusual amount of skill and courage. He died in 1985 at the age of sixty-six from lung cancer.

A seemingly simple idea was instrumental in making coronary artery visualization more accessible: the percutaneous introduction of a catheter as described in 1952 by Sven I. Seldinger from Sweden (42). He described a method that he considered suitable for aortography via the femoral artery. He writes, "There is a simple method of using a catheter in the same size as the needle and which has been used at Karolinska Sjukhuset since April 1952. The main principle consists in the catheter being introduced over a flexible leader through the puncture hole, after withdrawal of the puncture needle." Sones' technique necessitated incision into the brachial artery and suture of the vessel after the procedure had been terminated, a technique that was beyond the surgical skill of many cardiologists. Judkins, with a group of investigators of similar interests, made selective coronary arteriography possible by the construction and design of preformed catheters (43; Fig. 1.9). These catheters were preformed to enter the left and/or right coronary artery. Judkins described results in one hundred consecutive patients. In each, both coronary arteries were selectively catheterized from the

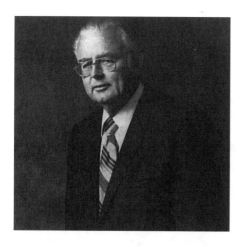

Figure 1.9. Melvin P. Judkins. *(Courtesy of the New York Academy of Medicine)*

femoral artery and contrast injections were filmed by direct serial radiography and cinephotofluorography. Here the Seldinger technique was essential.

Judkins was born in Los Angeles and, after military service as chief of Urology in an American service hospital in Japan, was in family practice for ten years. Following this he took a radiology residency at the University of Oregon Medical Center, followed by fellowships in cardiovascular radiology at the University of Oregon and the University of Lund, Sweden. In 1966 Judkins introduced the method he developed for transfemoral selective coronary arteriography, now known as the Judkins' technique. His efforts grew out of a need to reliably and consistently perform high-quality coronary arteriography in any patient suspected of having ischemic heart disease. Judkins' approach to coronary arteriography was to seek a method of percutaneous catheterization from the large, readily accessible femoral artery to obviate the need for a cutdown and subsequent arterial repair. Up to this time it had been considered virtually impossible to consistently catheterize the coronaries from the femoral approach because of the long distance. Thus, Judkins developed left and right coronary-seeking catheters, each with unique configuration, preshaped to conform to the usual anatomy. The shape of both was unconventional but the configurations were the key to consistent catheterization. When the technique was introduced, the shapes were completely foreign to the thinking of the day; now they are universally accepted.

One of the most important advances in the field of catheterization was made by Andreas Gruentzig (Fig. 1.10). Cardiology, and with it all mankind, owes Gruentzig a tremendous debt of gratitude. He developed a technique for opening obstructed coronary arteries mechanically using a balloon-tipped catheter (44). His work is based on that of Dotter and Judkins. Each had proposed using catheters to dilate an area of hemodynamically important arterial stenosis or to

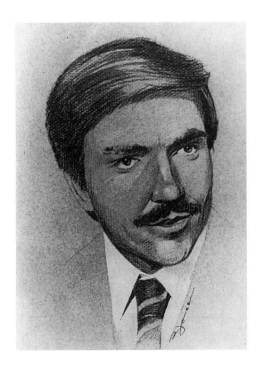

Figure 1.10. Andreas R. Gruentzig.
(*Courtesy of the* Texas Heart Institute
Journal)

recanalize a short arterial occlusion by compressing the soft atheromatous material against the vessel wall. While Dotter used a series of progressively larger
catheters to dilate the vessel lumen, Gruentzig's important addition was the introduction of a double lumen balloon catheter with an inflatable balloon near its
tip whose inflation allowed equal dilation by a much smaller catheter. Thus with
the aid of the balloon, dilatation could be performed to the size of a #9 or #12
French catheter with the introduction of only a #7 catheter. The balloon could
be inflated to predetermined diameter and a pressure of about 4 atmospheres
could be applied to an atherosclerotic plaque with no risk of overdistension of
the vessel.

Gruentzig was born in Dresden, Germany, and studied at the University of
Heidelberg, as well as in England, Switzerland, and Germany. His pioneering work
was done at the University of Zurich, Switzerland, where in 1979 he became
chief of the Department of Cardiology at the university hospital (45). In a symposium in Germany Gruentzig reported his method of angioplasty of the coronary arteries on his first group of forty patients. The technique was successful in
about 60 percent of patients, who showed improved cardiac function. Gruentzig
recalled his own reaction, after he performed the first successful percutaneous
transluminal coronary angioplasty in a thirty-eight-year-old man with 85 percent stenosis in the left anterior descending artery. "I was surprised and the pa-

tient was surprised over how easy it was." Three months after Sones' death on October 27, 1985, Gruentzig and his wife were the unfortunate victims of a plane crash near Atlanta, Georgia.

As with each of the other cardiac catheterization techniques, the acceptance of Gruentzig's percutaneous transluminal coronary angioplasty (PTCA) was at first limited because of skepticism on the part of the medical community and the crude nature of the available catheters. Gruentzig's balloon was a two-lumen device in which one lumen was used for inflating and deflating the balloon, and the other was used for pressure monitoring and contrast injection though a small port terminating ahead of the balloon (46). While there was a short segment of flexible guide wire attached to the tip of the balloon to minimize the chance for subintimal passage of the device, this wire could not be steered or manipulated in any way once the balloon had been introduced into the outer "guiding catheter." The combination of this lack of steering control, the large (1.5 mm) diameter of the deflated balloon, and the low balloon rupture pressure (6 atm or 90 psi), made the device suitable for only a select subgroup of patients with proximal, discrete, subtotal, concentric, and noncalcified lesions of a single vessel. Such patients were estimated to account for no more than 5 percent to 10 percent of the patients with coronary artery disease requiring catheterization, and even with limitation of this technique to such favorable candidates, the success of PTCA in the original (1979–81) NHLBIPTCA Registry was only 65 percent while the incidence of emergency surgery for correction of a PTCA-induced complication was 6 percent (47).

Despite these shortcomings, a number of cardiologists in the United States (Myler, Stertzer, Block, Faxon, Kent, and Simpson, among others) persisted in refining the technique of PTCA. One of the most important contributions was made by John B. Simpson, while a cardiology fellow and junior faculty member at Stanford University in the early 1980s. He felt that a better use of the second lumen of a coaxial dilation catheter would be to carry an independently moveable and shapeable guide wire that would allow improved and safer access to lesions located more distally in the coronary tree (48).

Simpson recalls an interesting moment during the early times of the development of this technique when Charles Dotter came to visit his lab on a grant visit at Stanford University. He was so excited to demonstrate the new catheter device that in his enthusiasm the balloon catheter became overinflated; as Dotter took a very close view of the inflated balloon the balloon ruptured, spraying contrast medium over his glasses and over a very clean coat.

This concept ultimately led to the present precisely steerable guide wires, over which improved balloons with deflated diameters as small as 0.5 mm and rupture pressures as high as 20 atm, can be advanced. These improvements directly contributed to the increased success (85 percent) of PTCA in the second

(1985–86) NHLBI Registry (49), and allowed pioneering cardiologists like Geoffrey Hartzler of Kansas City to extend the technique to patients with increasingly complex multivessel coronary disease (50). In fact, by 1987 more than 250,000 PTCA procedures were being performed annually in the United States, accounting for roughly half of the revascularization (bypass surgery being the other half) (51). In 1998 roughly 500,000 angioplasty procedures are performed annually in nearly 800 of the country's approximately 2,000 cardiac catheterization laboratories, for a variety of indications ranging from stable angina, to unstable angina, to acute myocardial infarction, with worldwide numbers greater than one million per year.

Despite its evident successes, PTCA continued to be faced with four major limitations:

1. difficulty in crossing totally occluded arteries
2. difficulty in dilating rigid (calcified) or markedly elastic (eccentric) lesions
3. difficulty in preventing or reliably reversing abrupt closure of the freshly dilated segment due to excessive local trauma by the balloon
4. restenosis of the dilated segment over subsequent months due to an excessive local healing response

In the late 1980s it became apparent that little progress was being made against these four limitations of PTCA, and a number of physician-inventors began to explore alternative techniques for using the cardiac catheter to enlarge stenotic coronary lumens (52).

This creativity was fostered by an enthusiastic venture capital community that had witnessed the explosive growth of PTCA and the staggering success of companies supplying leading technology. The first of these new approaches to win approval from the Food and Drug Administration (FDA) was also developed by John Simpson. Directional atherectomy (53) uses a cylindrical steel capsule with an oval window on one side to cross the target lesion. As the window is pressed up against the obstructing plaque by a low-pressure balloon mounted on the opposite side of the cylinder, a cup-shaped cutter is advanced inside to shave off the protruding plaque and trap it within the catheter.

The directional coronary atherectomy (DCA) procedure was viewed optimistically at the time of FDA approval in 1990 as a likely replacement for balloon angioplasty. The randomized CAVEAT and CCAT trials conducted in 1991–94 to compare DCA to conventional balloon angioplasty, however, showed little advantage in angiographic restenosis and a suggestion of higher procedural complications. These negative data, combined with the approval of the technically easier technique of stent placement in late 1994, led to precipitous reductions in the number of annual DCA procedures. Only more recently have trials such as the balloon versus optimal atherectomy trial (BOAT) shown that DCA can be used safely to produce higher procedural success with lower restenosis rates than balloon angioplasty. Preliminary data suggest that DCA still has certain "niche" roles in treating ostial or bifurcation lesions, or debulking midvessel lesions prior to stent placement (54).

Other "atherectomy" procedures were also developed in a similar time frame. Rotational atherectomy was conceived by Dave Auth, Ph.D., to use different size burrs coated with microscopic diamond chips to drill through fibrotic or calcified coronary lesions. The burr traveled over a fine guide wire, and was spun at up to 200,000 rpm as it was advanced through the target lesion. Initial problems (sludging of the distal capillary bed with debris creating spasm and local dissection) were overcome by changes in the device (rotational speed, speed of advancement through the lesion), making rotational atherectomy useful in 10 percent to 15 percent of current interventions.

The concept of cutting and removing portions of the obstructive plaque was also behind two other devices: extraction atherectomy and laser atherectomy. The transluminal extraction catheter (TEC) uses low-speed rotation of a sharpened tip combined with vacuum bottle suction through the central lumen of the TEC catheter to try to collect atheromatous material. It has proven to be a better thrombectomy than atherectomy device, and is of only limited use in degenerated saphenous vein grafts. More potent suction thrombectomy devices will likely supplant the use of TEC. Similarly, the concept of using fiber-optic catheters to deliver laser energy to vaporize obstructing plaque received much attention in the early 1990s. Refinements in technique, including using shorter wavelengths (excimer lasers in the near ultraviolet), high energy pulses (instead of continuous output lasers), and avoidance of blood or contrast in the lasing environment (saline flush), overcame some of the problems with dissection seen in the early laser experience. Still, the great capital expense of the lasers themselves (approximately $250,000) and the success of rotational atherectomy have helped to drive this technology almost completely out of the interventional market.

Compared to the mixed blessings of the new atherectomy devices, stents have transformed the area of coronary intervention more than anything since Gruentzig's original balloon catheters. The concept of using metallic endoluminal prostheses (stents) to scaffold the lumen of a blood vessel against elastic recoil and occlusive dissection was advanced by Dotter in the 1970s. The first practical human devices, however, were not implanted until 1984 by Ulrich Sigwart in Switzerland. He utilized the self-expanding metallic braid Wallstent in first peripheral and then coronary arteries. Despite impressive acute angiographic results, there was a disturbingly high (greater than 20 percent) incidence of subacute thrombosis in the weeks following stent placement. A similar fate met the first balloon-expandable slotted-tube stent design developed by Julio Palmaz and refined with the collaboration of Richard Schatz. Despite use of an intensive antithrombotic cocktail, including aspirin, dipyridamole, low-molecular-weight dextran, and heparin, initial Palmaz and Palmaz–Schatz stents implanted in 1988–89 had subacute thrombosis rates of 16 percent, which generally led to major complications (death, myocardial infarction [MI], emergency surgery) in most patients who developed this thrombotic problem. The addition of an uninterrupted switch from intravenous heparin to oral warfarin reduced this thrombotic problem to roughly 3 percent, although it increased the length of stay (to six days) and the incidence of groin hemorrhagic complications (to 10 percent). Still, two randomized trials—STent REStenosis Study (STRESS) and Benestent—showed in 1994 that stenting provided higher acute success, lower residual stenosis, and lower restenosis than conventional balloon angioplasty. Approval of the Palmaz–Schatz stent for elective use in 1994 followed closely the approval in 1993 of the wire coil stent developed by Cesare Gianturco and Gary Roubin for the reversal of abrupt closure due to extensive local dissection following balloon angioplasty. By 1997 these devices had gained in popularity to the extent that roughly half of all coronary interventional procedures were performed with the aid of stents (55).

Investigations by Marie Claude Morice in France and Antonio Colombo in Milan, Italy, showed that if excellent initial expansion of the stent was obtained (monitored by intracoronary ultrasound imaging), the stent thrombosis rates could be reduced to below one percent despite elimination of warfarin (and addition of the antiplatelet agent ticlopidine). This breakthrough and the evident success of stenting using the initial three devices turned an unprecedented wave of medical innovation, engineering expertise, and venture capital toward the development of other improved second-generation stent devices. By 1998 more than twenty different stent designs were in use in Europe, offering easier delivery, better scaffolding of the artery, better access to covered side branches, and a wider range of lengths than the original designs. Stents have also begun to be used as local delivery platforms for drugs, genes, or radiation, in an effort to modify the local healing response that continues to produce restenosis in roughly 20 percent of stents placed.

The history of stenting has been described by Sigwart (56, 57). Formerly it was thought that the word "stent" was derived from the name of a London dentist, Charles Stent, who was the inventor of medical devices, among others a plastic substance that carried his name (Stent's Mass) (56, 57). The material was used in the First World War to stabilize skin transplants. However, the word "stent" has been in existence since the fourteenth century when it was used in the north of England to designate a device used to spread fishing nets across rivers (56, 57).

Like many advances in invasive cardiology and cardiac surgery the use of stents is based on the experimental work of Alexis Carrel, the French surgeon who worked at the Rockefeller Institute in New York. In 1912 Carrel published a paper on stenting, which he called "permanent intubations" (58). He performed experiments in which he inserted glass tubings into the artery of dogs to treat traumatic entry to blood vessels. Carrel's other accomplishments included work on transplantation of organs, including the heart, coronary bypass operations, blood vessel anastomoses, cell cultures, and cultures of whole organs (see Chapter 3). Carrel was an ingenious investigator who left the Rockefeller Institute in New York to return to his native France in 1941 in the mistaken belief that he could help his native country in the difficult war years. He should have realized that dealing with the occupying Nazis was impossible (59). One of the reasons he left the United States was because of difficulties with the director of the Rockefeller Institute and with some faculty members. Some of his co-workers believed that he was less of a scientist and more of a flashy publicity hunter. I (RJB) worked with Carrel and his co-workers, among them flier Charles Lindbergh, as a fellow at the Rockefeller Institute (now Rockefeller University) from 1934 to 1935. I found Carrel to be a scintillating, multifaceted personality who liked to mix science with philosophy and politics. Carrel believed not only in the power of science but also in the metaphysical power of the mind. He also was an admirer of strong personalities. All these features were the outgrowth of an unusual searching and wide-ranging imagination. Carrel's personality could not fit into a mold; he was neither a typical scientist nor a philosopher. He had the admirable ability to see the world around him according to the image he wanted it to be. But he was an ingenious, imaginative scientist (59).

Later experiments on stents were carried out by Cragg and Amplatz and their co-workers in 1982 (60). It was also at this time that Palmaz in San Antonio started work on balloon-expandable stents (61).

Much of the work on stents goes back to the fundamental role of Charles Dotter. He, like Carrel, implanted plastic tubes into blood vessels and finally implanted metal spirals into dog arteries (62, 63). Dotter first experimented with transluminal catheter dilatation but soon found that secondary luminal thrombosis complicated the disease, leaving no lumen to dilate (62). This led to the propagation and trial of coilspring devices (63). This had the advantage that the internally grafted segment of vessels was not removed, incised, or even exposed, thus avoiding trauma to an already diseased vessel. Nitinol was used by Cragg in 1982 and by Dotter in 1983, (60, 63). Nitinol is a specially formulated alloy of nickel and titanium that can be drawn into a wire of precise dimension. It is annealed at 525°C for thirty minutes while being constrained to a desired shape (63).

Sigwart drew attention to the potential benefits of intravascular stenting of coronary arteries in the prevention of occlusion or restenosis after transluminal angioplasty (64). His personal interest began in 1984, when he became frustrated by the acute and long-term results of PTCA, and thought about creating a balloon-expandable tubular structure. After innumerable discussions he settled on a self-expanding tubular mesh made out of fine steel wire, which was later called a "wall stent." The material for this wall stent was already used in coaxial cables, automobile tires, and cardiac catheters. To deploy the self-expanding mesh, he developed a system for frictionless removal of an outer constraining membrane (64).

The initial use of stents after PTCA has an interesting history. Sigwart relates that in a prelunch demonstration before assembled physicians in Lausanne, PTCA was performed in a branch of the left coronary artery of a fifty-one-year-old patient (56, 57). During the lunch hour the patient complained of chest pain while in the intensive care station. Sigwart found complete occlusion of the left coronary artery. After some hesitation, it was decided to implant a stent. The patient immediately became pain-free and the electrocardiogram reverted to normal. As Sigwart wrote, "You can't possibly believe the astonishment of persons in the auditorium when this case was presented following the lunch recess." Later the patient restenosed the right coronary artery and another wall stent was implanted. The patient has been well for eleven years.

In 1984 Palmaz published the first balloon-expandable stent replacement into various arteries (61). As he recalls, "in the early 80s I felt ignored and sometimes scorned for proposing a metallic intravascular implant" (65). He considers himself the originator of the balloon-expandable intravascular stent because he did the early experimental work in this area, publishing the first paper in *Radiology* in 1985 (61). Together with Schatz and others he extended this experience with coronary stents and used them clinically in coronary arteries (53). In his report Schatz and his co-workers described the so-called articulated stent, which has the advantage that it permits simple exchange techniques for delivery and can articulate or flex around curves. Once delivery to the target site is achieved, expansion can be accomplished with a simple balloon inflation. The stent can also be retrieved by withdrawal of the guiding catheter to the femoral sheath before attempting to pull the stent-loaded balloon into the guided catheter. The Palmaz–Schatz stent was, between its approval by the FDA in 1994 and the availability of superior second-generation devices in 1998, one of the most widely used devices in invasive cardiology.

Initially, coronary stenting was not readily accepted by the medical community. The thought that the metallic nature of the stent would accumulate thrombi, which would then precipitate a clotting cascade and result in occlusion was a distinct possibility. The initial rate of stent thrombosis was greater than 20 percent and the median term follow-up of an initial cohort of patients showed an unacceptable mortality rate (55). At this level of complications, stenting was still of value as a "bailout" device to avoid emergency bypass surgery. Elective stenting became possible when the thrombosis rate was reduced to about 3 percent by an acetylsalicylic acid and coumarin regime. The formation of thrombi has now been reduced further (less than one percent) with the recognition that the combination of acetylsalicylic acid and ticlopidin could be substituted for the more difficult earlier regimen involving oral anticoagulants (55).

The overall results of stenting are reported in a recent study by Bauters and co-authors (66). They reported that coronary stenting for an unsatisfactory result after balloon angioplasty of infarct-related lesions considerably reduced restenosis. There occurs a marked reduction of 14 percent to one percent in the rate of occlusion in stented lesions. The authors also deal with a possibility that some of this success is due to therapy with aspirin and ticlopidine, a potent antiplatelet agent. Although this may have contributed to the success, the use of stents plays a major role. Stenting is also now used for saphenous vein grafts, showing that of 191 patients, elective stent placement was associated with an initial success rate of 95 percent and a 35 percent restenosis rate after six months. Seventy percent of patients were event-free. Therefore, stenting of saphenous vein grafts represents marked improvement over balloon angioplasty and is a valid primary therapy for lesions located proximal to or in the body of the graft (55).

These developments in the field of coronary intervention have helped to stimulate the development of catheter-based interventions for other forms of heart disease. Balloon catheter dilatation of congenitally stenotic pulmonic, aortic, and mitral valves by pediatric cardiologists (notably James Lock of Boston's Children's Hospital) was extended to the treatment of rheumatic mitral stenosis in adult patients and to the treatment of calcific aortic stenosis in the elderly (67). Balloon mitral valvuloplasty remains a viable option to surgical commissurotomy or valve replacement (68), but balloon aortic valvuloplasty appears to provide too transient an improvement in the elderly patient to be considered in lieu of surgical aortic valve replacement. Other avenues of catheter therapy in congenital heart disease are impressive. Atrial septal defects can be created using a balloon (Rashkind) or blade-tipped catheter, or closed using a double umbrella device developed James Lock patterned after an earlier device for closure of persistent patent ductus arteriosus (69). Unwanted coronary fistulas or collateral vessels can be closed percutaneously using immobilized coils or detachable balloons. At Boston's Children's Hospital, more than seven hundred interventional catheterization procedures are now performed yearly, providing nonsurgical correction for more than 25 percent of congenital cardiac defects.

With this strong and enthusiastic wave of interventional catheter development has also come a demanding standard for the evaluation of new technology. Tighter oversight by the Food and Drug Administration, the demand by the medical community for randomized trials showing the advantage of these newer techniques over existing medical or surgical options, and increasingly stringent policies of third-party payers will inevitably separate the wheat from the chaff of interventional cardiology.

While the lineage of each of today's commonplace techniques can indeed be traced back to the innovations of our predecessors, we are frequently less cognizant of the blind alleyways they tried and abandoned. Before openly accepting the glowing promise of today's innovations, I (DSB) am always reminded of a talk entitled "The Way We Were" given by Kurt Amplatz at a June 1989 meeting of some of the world's most experienced interventional cardiologists, devoted to examining the results of some of today's investigational techniques. During that talk, Amplatz showed a film from the 1950s about the then promising technique of left heart catheterization via direct cardiac puncture. The statement that more than one hundred cases had been performed, with a mortality of only one percent, made many shift uncomfortably in our seats to think about which of our current techniques would endure, and which would join direct cardiac puncture.

Another new development is invasive electrophysiologic testing combined with therapy in the definition and treatment of arrhythmias. Invasive testing for supraventricular tachycardia, ventricular tachycardia combined with insertion of an automatic defibrillator, cardiac electrosurgery, or catheterization ablations are becoming useful. Because of the relatively high surgical mortality, particularly in patients with poor left ventricular function, insertion of the automatic defibrillator has become increasingly popular. Although there are still complications, the incidence of sudden death is reduced by the insertion of automatic defibrillators. However, there is still some operative mortality, incidence of infection, and incidence of inappropriate shocks. Catheter ablation of ventricular tachycardia foci has still a very limited clinical role (70, 71).

Whatever the future turns taken by cardiac catheterization, a prediction made at a symposium in Leichlingen, Germany, by one of us (RJB) in 1978, nearly the fiftieth anniversary of Forssmann's daring experiments, will undoubtedly ring true: "There is no doubt in my mind that the cardiac catheter has become of lesser importance for physiological methods and of ever greater interest in clinical and diagnostic cardiology" (72). It has, almost exclusively, become a clinical tool, particularly because of the introduction of coronary arteriography, which led to a localization of lesions in the coronary artery; it has also become essential for the development of coronary artery surgery and for the usage of His bundle recording, and most important for the immediate treatment of acute coronary occlusion.

References

1. Bernard, C. Leçons sur la Chaleur Animale, sur les Effets de la Chaleur et sur la Fièvre. Paris, Bailliere, 1876.

2. Bernard, C. Leçons de Physiologie Operatoire. Paris, Bailliere, 1879.
3. Grande, F., and M.B. Visscher (eds.). Claude Bernard and Experimental Medicine. Collected Papers. Cambridge, MA, Schenkman, 1967.
4. Chaveau, A., and E.J. Marey. Determination graphique des rapports du choc du coeur avec les mouvements des oreillettes et des ventricules: experience faite a l'aide a un appareil enregistreur (sphygmographe). C.R. Hebd. Acad. Sci., 53:662, 1861.
5. Exposition and Catalogue on Etienne Jules Marey. Medtronics, France, 1980, pp. 1–70.
6. Snellen, H.A. E.J. Marey and Cardiology. Rotterdam, Kooyker, 1980.
7. Handwritten manuscript by Claude Bernard nominating E.J. Marey for the physiology prize of the Foundation Lecaze by the Institut de France, 1875. St. Julien, Rhone, Musee Claude Bernard.
8. Forssmann, W. Selbstversuch: Erinnerungen eines Chirurgen. Duesseldorf, Drost, 1972.
9. Forssmann, W. Die Sondierung des rechten Herzens. Klin. Wochenschr., 8:2085–2087, 1929.
10. Forssmann, W. Ueber Kontrastdarstellung der Hoehlen des lebenden rechten Herzens und der Lungenschlagader. Muench. Med. Wochenschr., 78:489–492, 1931.
11. Klein, O. Zur Bestimmung des zirkulatorischen Minutenvolumens beim Menschen nach dem Fickschen Prinzip. Muench. Med. Wochenschr., 77:1311–1312, 1930.
12. Personal communication: letter from Werner Forssmann to R.J. Bing. September 26, 1978.
13. Schadewaldt, H. Werner Forssmann. Sonderdruck im Jahrbuch der Universitaet Duesseldorf. Duesseldorf, Triltsch, 1978–80, pp. 35–38.
14. Cournand, A. Cardiac catheterization: development of the technique, its contributions to experimental medicine, and its initial application in man. Acta Med. Scand. (Suppl.), 579:3–32, 1975. Originally: Jiminez Diaz Memorial Lecture, Fundacion Conchite Rabago de Jiminez Diaz, Madrid, 1970, pp. 47–80.
15. Cournand, A., and H.A. Ranges. Catheterization of the right auricle in man. Proc. Soc. Exp. Biol. Med., 46:462–466, 1941.
16. Snellen, H.A. History and Perspectives of Cardiology. Interview with Andre Cournand at Leiden, Holland, November 1979. The Hague, Leiden University Press, 1981, pp. 33–37.
17. Cournand, A. Dickinson Woodruff Richards 1895–1973. Trans. Assoc. Am. Physicians, 86:33–38, 1973.
18. Fishman, A.P., and D.W. Richards (eds.). Circulation of the Blood: Men and Ideas. New York, Oxford University Press, 1964.
19. Richards, D.W. Medical Priesthoods and Other Essays. Connecticut Printers, 1970.
20. Swan, H.J. Personal communication.
21. Swan, H.J., and W. Ganz. Hemodynamic monitoring: a personal and historical perspective. Can. Med. Assoc. J., 121:868–871, 1979.
22. Ganz, W. Personal communication.
23. Comroe, J.H. Retrospectroscope: Insights into Medical Discovery. Menlo Park, CA, Von Gehr, 1977, p. 60.
24. Bing, R.J., L.D. Vandam, F. Gregoire, J.E. Handelsman, W.T. Goodale, and J.E. Eckenhoff. Catheterization of the coronary sinus and the middle cardiac vein in man. Proc. Soc. Exp. Biol. Med., 66:239–240, 1947.
25. Bing, R.J., M.M. Hammon, J.C. Handelsman, S.R. Powers, F.C. Spencer, J.E. Eckenhoff, W.T. Goodale, J.H. Hafkenschiel, and S. Kety. The measurement of coronary blood flow, oxygen consumption, and efficiency of the left ventricle in man. Am. Heart J., 38:1–24, 1949.
26. Bing, R.J. The metabolism of the heart. Harvey Lectures, 50:27–70, 1954–55.
27. Bing, R.J. Cardiac metabolism. Physiol. Rev., 45:171–213, 1965.

28. Himmelstein, A., A. Cournand, and J.S. Baldwin. Cardiac Catheterization in Congenital Heart Disease: A Clinical and Physiological Study in Infants and Children. New York, Commonwealth Fund, 1949.
29. Hellems, H.K., F.W. Haynes, L. Dexter, and T.D. Kinney. Pulmonary capillary pressure in animals estimated by venous and arterial catheterization. Am. J. Physiol., 155:98–105, 1948.
30. Bing, R.J. Physiological methods in the diagnosis of congenital heart disease. Surg. Gyn. Obstet., 88:399–401, 1949.
31. Griswold, H.E., R.J. Bing, J.C. Handelsman, J. Campbell, and E. LeBrun. Physiological studies of congenital heart disease. VII. Pulmonary arterial hypertension in congenital heart disease. Johns Hopkins Hosp. Bull., 84:76–88, 1949.
32. Bing, R.J., L.D. Vandam, J.C. Handelsman, J. Spencer, J. Campbell, and H. Griswold. Physiological studies in congenital heart disease. VI. Adaptations to anoxia in congenital heart disease with cyanosis. Johns Hopkins Hosp. Bull., 83:439–456, 1948.
33. Radner, S. Thoracic aortography by catheterization from the radial artery. Acta Radiol., 29:178–180, 1948.
34. Broden, B., G. Jonsson, and J. Karnell. Thoracic aortography. Acta Radiol., 32:498–508, 1949.
35. Rousthoi, P. Ueber Angiokardiographie. Acta Radiol., 14:419–423, 1933.
36. Radner, S. An attempt at the roentgenologic visualization of coronary blood vessels in man. Acta Radiol., 26:497–502, 1945.
37. Robb, G.P., and I. Steinberg. Visualization of the chambers of the heart, the pulmonary circulation, and the great blood vessels in man. Am. J. Roentgenol., 41:1–17, 1939.
38. DiGuglielmo, L., and M. Guttadauro. Anatomic variations in the coronary arteries. An anteriographic study in living subjects. Acta Radiol., 41:393–397, 1954.
39. Thal, A.P., L.S. Richards, R. Greenspan, and M.J. Murray. Arteriographic studies of the coronary arteries in ischemic heart disease. JAMA, 168:2104–2109, 1958.
40. Dotter, C.T., and L.H. Frische. Visualization of the coronary circulation by occlusive aortography: a practical method. Radiology, 71: 502–523, 1958.
41. Sones, F.M., and E.K. Shirey. Cinecoronary aorteriography. Mod. Concepts Cardiovasc. Dis., 31:735–738, 1962.
42. Seldinger, S.I. Catheter replacement of the needle in percutaneous arteriography: a new technique. Acta Radiol., 39:368–376, 1953.
43. Judkins, M.R. Selective coronary arteriography. Part I: A percutaneous transfemoral technique. Radiology, 89:815–824, 1967.
44. Gruentzig, A.R. Transluminal dilatation of coronary-artery stenosis. Lancet, 1:263, 1978 (letter).
45. Hurst, J.W. Tribute: Andreas Roland Gruentzig (1939–1985): a private perspective. Circulation, 73:606–610, 1986.
46. Gruentzig, A.R., A. Senning, and W.E. Siegenthaler. Nonoperative dilation of coronary artery stenosis—percutaneous transluminal coronary angioplasty. N. Engl. J. Med., 301:61, 1979.
47. Kent, K.M., et al. (eds.). Proceedings of the National Heart, Lung and Blood Institute workshop on the outcome of percutaneous transluminal angioplasty (June 7–8, 1983). Am. J. Cardiol., 53:1C, 1984.
48. Simpson, J.B., D.S. Baim, E.W. Robert, and D.C. Harrison. A new catheter system for coronary angioplasty. Am. J. Cardiol., 49:1216, 1982.
49. Detre, K., et al. Percutaneous transluminal coronary angioplasty in 1985–1986 and 1977–1978. The NHLBI Registry. N. Engl. J. Med., 318:265, 1988.
50. Hartzler, G.O., et al. "High-risk" percutaneous transluminal coronary angioplasty. Am. J. Cardiol., 61:33G, 1988.
51. Baim, D.S., and E.J. Ignatius. Use of percutaneous transluminal coronary angioplasty: results of a current study. Am. J. Cardiol., 61:33G, 1988.

52. Baim, D.S., K. Detre, and K. Kent. Problems in the development of new devices for coronary intervention—possible role for a multicenter registry. J. Am. Coll. Cardiol., 14:1389, 1989.

53. Simpson, J.B., et al. Transluminal atherectomy for occlusive peripheral vascular disease. Am. J. Cardiol., 61:96C, 1988.

54. Baim, D.S., D.E. Cutlip, S.K. Sharman, et al., for the BOAT Investigators. Final results of the balloon versus optimal atherectomy trial (BOAT). Circulation, 97:322–331, 1998.

55. Fischman, D.L., M.B. Leon, D. Baim, et al., for the STRESS Investigators. A randomized comparison of coronary stent placement and balloon angioplasty in the treatment of coronary artery disease. N. Engl. J. Med., 331:496–501, 1994.

56. Sigwart, U. Stents: a mechanical solution for a biological problem? The 1996 Gruntzig Lecture. European Heart Journal, 18:1068–1072, 1997.

57. Sigwart, U. Stents: Die Geschichte eines Schlagworts. Deutsche Gesellschaft fur Kardiologie-Herz-und Kreislaufforschung, 2:20–26, 1997.

58. Carrel, A. Results of the permanent intubation of the thoracic aorta. Surg. Gyn. Obstet., 15:245–248, 1912.

59. Bing, R.J. Evolution in cardiology: triumph and defeat. Persp. in Biol. Med., 34(1): 1–16, 1990.

60. Cragg, A., G. Lund, J. Rysavy, F. Castaneda, W. Castaneda-Zuniga, and K. Amplatz. Nonsurgical placement of arterial endoprostheses: a technique using nitinol wire. Radiology, 147:261–263, 1983.

61. Palmaz J., R. Sibbitt, S. Reuter, F. Tio, and W. Rice. Expandable intraluminal graft: a preliminary study. Radiology, 156:73–77, 1985.

62. Dotter, C.T. Transluminally-placed coilspring endarterial tube grafts: long-term patency in canine popliteal artery. Investigative Radiology, 4:329–332, 1969.

63. Dotter, C.T. Transluminal expandable nitinol coil stent grafting: preliminary report. Radiology, 147:259–260, 1983.

64. Sigwart U., J. Puel, V. Mirkovitch, F. Joffre, and L. Kappenberger. Intravascular stents to prevent occlusion and restenosis after transluminal angioplasty. N. Engl. J. Med., 316:701–706, 1987.

65. Personal communication to RJB.

66. Bauters, C., J. Lablanche, E.V. Belle, R. Niculescu, T. Meurice, E.P. Mc Fadden, and M.E. Bertrand. Effects of coronary stenting on restenosis and occlusion after angioplasty of the culprit vessel in patients with recent myocardial infarction. Circulation, 96:2854–2858, 1997.

67. Letac, B., L.I. Gerber, and R. Koning. Insights on the mechanism of balloon valvuloplasty in aortic stenosis. Am. J. Cardiol., 62:1241, 1988.

68. Palacios, I.F., P.C. Block, G.T. Wilkins, and A.E. Weyman. Follow-up of patients undergoing percutaneous mitral balloon valvotomy: analysis of factors determining restenosis. Circulation, 79:573, 1989.

69. Lock, J.E., J.T. Cockerham, J.F. Keane, et al. Transcatheter umbrella closure of congenital heart defects. Circulation, 75:593, 1987.

70. Scheinman, M.M., T. Evans-Bell, and the Executive Committee of the Percutaneous Cardiac Mapping and Ablation Registry. Catheter ablation of the atrioventricular junction: a report of the Percutaneous Cardiac Mapping and Ablation Registry. Circulation, 70:1024–1029, 1984.

71. Kastor, J.A., L.N. Horowitz, A.H. Harken, et al. Clinical electrophysiology of ventricular tachycardia. N. Engl. J. Med., 304:1004–1020, 1981.

72. Bing, R.J. History of cardiac catheterization. In: History of Cardiology (Beitraege zur Geschichte der Kardiologie), Bluemchen, G. (ed.). Published by the editor, Monheim, 1979, pp. 165–175.

Chapter 2

Echocardiography and the Doppler Method

P. DOUGLAS
R.J. BING

THE PHYSICAL PRINCIPLE underlying echocardiography (ultrasound of the heart) is based on piezoelectricity, that is, electricity created by the transformation of crystals. These crystals act both as transmitter and receiver of sound pulses. These sound pulses are termed ultrasound because their frequency is much higher than audible soundwaves (1–30 MHz). As applied to cardiology, they are aimed at a heart valve or the wall of the heart chambers from which the pulses are then reflected, forming an echo. The time delay between emission and detection of reflected sound is displayed graphically as distance from the transducer. The sound beam can either be recorded as a single line, as in M-mode echocardiography, or as a composite of many lines forming a two-dimensional tomographic image. Ultrasound permits simultaneous visualization of a whole sector of the heart, thus making possible the evaluation of cardiac wall motion and the motion of the heart valves.

Echocardiography enables real-time, noninvasive imaging of all cardiac and vascular structures. Its impact on the practice of cardiology is immense and the indications for its use so broad as to include the diagnosis and evaluation of all forms of cardiovascular disease. The technique has, for example, become invaluable in the assessment of the physiology and pathophysiology of the left ventricle, determining regional wall motion and the proportion of blood ejected by the heart during systole (the ejection fraction).

The simple reflection of sound from the cardiac walls and valves provides much structural information, but does not permit measurement of direction or velocity of blood flow. Doppler ultrasound must be used for such measurements. In this method, an ultrasound beam is directed toward and reflected from blood flow itself. The wavelength of the reflected beam is shifted (Doppler shift) depending on the direction of flow and velocity of the moving cells. Doppler flow measurements together with echocardiography are particularly useful, enabling measurement of velocity and flow across a cardiac valve, together with imaging of the anatomy of the malformation. Thus, the hemodynamics of valvular lesions can be accurately measured. The technique has become an indispensable tool in the evaluation of patients with congenital, valvular, and coronary heart disease. Blood flow determinations can also be used to calculate pressure gradients across a valve to within 10 percent of those obtained by catheterization of the heart. With the new technology of color flow mapping, Doppler flow measurements have been used as a "noninvasive angiogram."

The principle underlying echocardiography and piezoelectricity was discovered by Jacques and Pierre Curie (Fig. 2.1). While the life of Pierre Curie, husband of Marie, is well known, less is known of Jacques Curie. After graduation, he worked with his brother and Friedel in the laboratory of mineralogy at the Sorbonne. As Marie Curie wrote in the biography of her husband:

> Their experiments led the two young physicists to great success: the discovery of the hitherto unknown phenomenon of piezoelectricity, which consists of an electric polarization produced by the compression or the expansion of crystals in the direction of the axis of symmetry; this was by no means a chance discovery. It was the result of much reflection on the symmetry of crystalline matter, which enabled the brothers to foresee the possibilities of such polarization. With an experimental skill rare at their age, the young men succeeded in making a complete study of the new phenomenon, established the conditions of symmetry necessary, and formulated remarkably simple laws (1).

The technical difficulties of this work and the measurement of minute amounts of deformations of the crystal were described by Marie: "Fortunately, they were provided with a small room adjoining the physics laboratory so that they might proceed successfully with their delicate operations. From these theoretical and experimental researches, Pierre and Jacques Curie immediately deduced a practical application in the form of a new apparatus, a piezoelectric quartz electrometer, which measures in absolute terms small quantities of electricity, as well as electric currents of low intensity. This apparatus has since then rendered great service in experiments on radioactivity." This statement is no exaggeration if we think of the wide application of piezoelectricity in the field of cardiology alone.

In a paper published in 1879, entitled "Physique Cristallographique,"

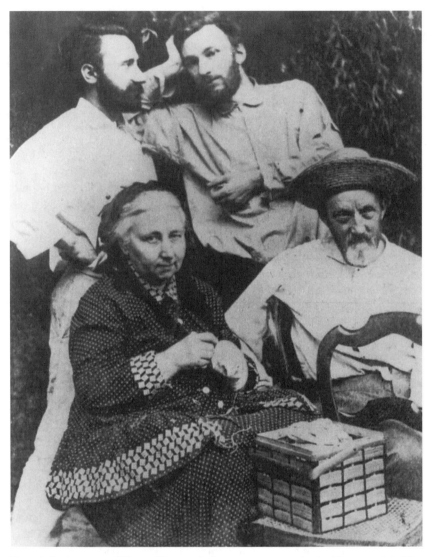

Figure 2.1. Jacques and Pierre Curie with their parents at a picnic. *(Courtesy of the New York Academy of Medicine)*

Jacques and Pierre Curie presented to the French Academy the experimental results leading them to "the conclusion that in nonconductive crystals the surface of the crystal and the production of electricity are related" (2). In a second report, published in 1880, Jacques and Pierre Curie reported "a new way of developing polar electricity in crystals, by putting pressure on the axis of symmetry" (3). In 1881 they described the converse piezoelectric effect: when a voltage was applied

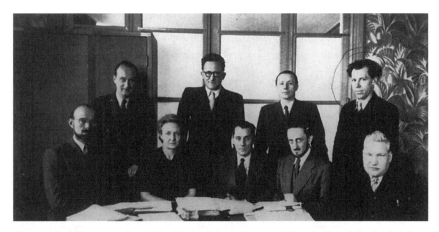

Figure 2.2. The scientific staff of Iréne Joliot-Curie and her husband Frederik Joliot. Jean Langevin is standing at the upper right. (*Courtesy of the Universite Pierre et Marie Curie, Paris, France*)

to the crystal, displacement and compression occurred. This phenomenon was first theoretically predicted by M. Lippmann in 1881 (4).

These pioneering experiments were soon followed by those of other scientists of the late nineteenth century. Lord Kelvin suggested a molecular theory underlying piezoelectric phenomena and produced a mechanical model of piezoelectricity (5). W. Voigt formulated the fundamental piezoelectric principle (6).

The first application of piezoelectricity was made under the duress of World War I. Langevin (Fig. 2.2) at the Curie Institute in Paris in 1917 constructed an ultrasound generator for underwater detection of submarines, thereby originating the modern science and art of ultrasonics. He commented that during these original experiments he felt almost insupportable pain, "as if the bones were heated," when he held his hand underwater near the transmitter. It was also noted that fish died when they swam into the ultrasound beam. Langevin's device consisted of a mosaic of quartz crystals glued between steel plates (7). When a voltage was applied, the crystal expanded and sent out longitudinal waves. Similarly, when a wave struck the crystal, it would cause the quartz to vibrate and generate a voltage that could be detected by vacuum tubes. In 1921 W. Cady, at Wesleyan University in the United States, demonstrated that quartz crystals could be used to control oscillators and that stable oscillators could be obtained in this fashion (7). This was a forerunner of the wide application of crystals to control the frequency of military communication equipment, which now accounts for the use of more than 30 million crystals in a single year.

In 1946 ultrasound was still used only for industrial purposes, for example, to inspect the interior of solid parts (8). F.M. Firestone, at the University of

Michigan, used a quartz crystal that was in contact with the object through a thin film of oil squirted onto the surface. He was the first to measure the reflected rather than transmitted sound waves. As Firestone wrote,

> When an oscillatory voltage is applied between these coatings, the crystal grows thicker and thinner in synchronism with the electrical oscillations. This causes the lower phase of the crystals to vibrate (change shape rapidly) and thereby radiate sound waves through the oil film into the object to be studied. By proper choice of the thickness of the crystal, it will give a thickness resonance and correspondingly increase the strength of the radiated sound waves. This permits determinations of defects in the matter examined.

The first attempt to use ultrasound for medical diagnosis was reported in 1942 by K.T. Dussik (9). In 1950 W.D. Keidel used ultrasound transmitted through the chest to a receiver placed on the back (10). In his article, "On a New Method for the Registration of Volume Changes of the Human Heart," Keidel demonstrated the application of a "field of ultrasound" to register phasic volume changes of the heart. The article was, as could be expected, primarily concerned with technical considerations, but it contained three illustrations comparing ultrasound tracings with phonocardiograms. The technique did record cyclic variations in ultrasound transmission synchronous with the cardiac cycle, but was not sufficiently advanced to obtain quantitative measurements of cardiac volume changes.

The greatest advance in the use of ultrasound in cardiology was made in Lund, Sweden, by Inge Edler and C. Hellmuth Hertz, when they applied the unidimensional ultrasound method to examination of the in vivo human heart in 1954 (11). This also represented a tremendous advance in the use of ultrasound in medicine, as the heart was the first organ visualized by this technique. Hertz, a physicist, and Edler, a cardiologist, later received the Lasker Award in Medicine in 1977 for this work (Figs. 2.3 and 2.4). They obtained echograms with a sound-generating crystal applied to the chest wall in the left precordial area. The echo signal varied with the position of the crystal and the direction of the beam. They moved the crystal back and forth along the axis of the heart and recorded the reflected signal on film. They summarized the results by stating that with the ultrasound method, signals from various parts of the human heart could be obtained in vivo, and that the movement of the structures of the heart could be continuously recorded. One of the most significant advances was the finding that it was possible in the living subject, by means of ultrasound, to produce real-time reflections from identifiable cardiac structures. At first, Edler and Hertz were only able to visualize the posterior left ventricular wall. With improvements in instrumentation, the anterior leaflet of the mitral valve was visualized. They and others originally thought it represented the anterior surface of the left

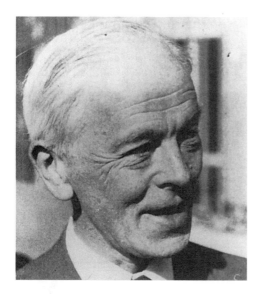

Figure 2.3. Inge Edler. (Courtesy of the New York Academy of Medicine)

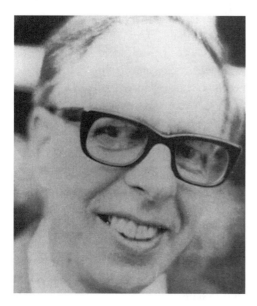

Figure 2.4. Carl Hellmuth Hertz. (Courtesy of the New York Academy of Medicine)

atrium, in part because it was not clear that cardiac valve tissue could actually reflect ultrasound. Thus, several years passed before the origin of this echo was properly identified by anatomic correlation (see below) and its significance was fully appreciated. Once this structure was identified, Edler's work then focused on the abnormal motion pattern of the mitral valve and he was able to identify the restricted movement characteristic of mitral stenosis. The ability to make this diagnosis by ultrasound sparked the interest of a number of other investigators and provided the stimulus for growth of the technique in the late 1950s.

In part because of early difficulty in identifying the site of reflection of cardiac echoes in man, Edler and Hertz based their results on experimental data on animals. In 1953 and 1954, they used the isolated bovine heart suspended in the upright position, creating artificial valve movements by induced phasic left ventricular pressure changes. A sequence of photographs of the manipulated anatomic specimen was then compared frame by frame with the ultrasonic record. The direction of the ultrasonic beam was further verified by needle puncture, giving them the opportunity to define the structures encountered. In this way, Edler and colleagues were able to visualize and identify most of the cardiac structures now recognized by M-mode echocardiography. Through this in vitro work, Hertz and Edler demonstrated the potential for in vivo imaging of wall thickness, thrombi, and cavity and vascular sizes. One of several important observations was that ultrasound was reflected from both internal and external surfaces of the heart, as well as the cardiac valves.

Further work in the 1950s led to in vivo recognition of the tricuspid valve echogram and aortic regurgitation by Edler et al. and of a left atrial tumor and thrombus in 1959 by a German group working under Effert (12). Edler et al. went on to present a movie at the Third European Congress of Cardiology in 1960 demonstrating the echocardiographic appearances of mitral and aortic stenosis, mixed mitral disease, left atrial masses, and exudative pericarditis. Their subsequent review, published in 1961 in the *Acta Medica Scandanavica* (13), remained the most comprehensive available until 1972.

The first echocardiograms were performed in the United States in 1957 by J.J. Wild in an excised heart (14). One of Wild's co-workers, an engineer named John Reid, joined with Claude Joyner at the University of Pennsylvania and reported imaging of the in vivo human heart in 1962 (15). In a presentation to the American Heart Association's National Meeting, Joyner summarized his experience with "echo ultrasound cardiograms" in man. Some 260 patients had been scanned. He described "a characteristic echo . . . which appears to represent motion at the mitral valve" and compared the motion of this echo in normals, and in patients with atrial fibrillation, mitral regurgitation, and mitral stenosis before and after commissurotomy. The authors quickly recognized the usefulness of ultrasound in decision making and assessment of prognosis, publishing a study on the preoperative evaluation of mitral stenosis in 1965 (16).

Harvey Feigenbaum has significantly contributed to the development of echocardiography. His textbook has been used by virtually every cardiology fellow since its publication in 1972 as the first book on the topic (17). Feigenbaum trained scores of academic and clinical cardiologists, helped to found the American Society of Echocardiography in 1975, and continues to contribute substantially to the echocardiographic literature. It is interesting to consider Feigen-baum's early experiences with the technique. In his words, he "became interested in echocardiography in the latter part of 1963, while operating a hemodynamic laboratory and becoming frustrated with the limitations of cardiac catheterization and angiography" (17). Although he was originally intrigued by the prospect of measuring cardiac chamber sizes, his first achievement was the detection of pos-terior pericardial effusions in 1965 (18). While this discovery provided much of the initial impetus for the growth of echocardiography in the United States, it really arose from the limitations of the equipment employed—a borrowed system intended only for echo encephalography. Attention was directed toward the posterior left ventricular wall by default, "principally because our gain settings were low, and this was the only echo that we could reasonably record. We were afraid to turn up the gain because we then recorded so many echoes that we be-came totally confused" (17). Feigenbaum, Popp, and co-workers soon obtained more suitable equipment and rapidly described measurement of posterior wall thickness, pericardial effusion, and left ventricle and right ventricle volumes and stroke volumes (19, 20, 21, 22), proving that left ventricular structure and func-tion could be assessed noninvasively. While these early, pioneering efforts pro-duced remarkable results, they were not always accurate. For example, in 1967 Feigenbaum et al. described a technique for ultrasound measurement of stroke volume (19). In it, the most anterior cardiac echo was incorrectly ascribed to the left ventricular free wall rather the right ventricular free wall since it was not known that the ultrasound beam must first pass through the anteriorly located right ventricle before arriving at the left ventricle, and because septal echoes had not yet been identified. In addition, a posterior wall echo was wrongly attributed to the mitral ring. The difference between these two misidentified structures was taken to be representative of left ventricular diameter. However, rather than measuring systolic and diastolic volumes directly, stroke volume was calculated by multiplying the distance between the left ventricular anterior and posterior echoes by the maximal excursion of the echo ascribed to the mitral ring. By incorporating a measure of left ventricular size and one of systolic function, the method yielded results that correlated closely ($r = 0.97$) with Fick determina-tions of stroke volume.

Two years later a report was published recognizing septal echoes, stating that "A new group of echoes was found" (22). This was not strictly accurate, how-ever, since Hertz and Edler had noted echoes between the tricuspid and mitral valves in the 1950s but had failed to identify them. The previous error in ana-tomic orientation of the cardiac chambers relative to the chest wall was, how-ever, corrected.

The identification of an increasing variety of structures and diseases by echocardiographers in the late 1960s owed much to refinement of image display.

Initial instrumentation provided only a unidimensional oscilloscopic display, to which the element of time was added by delayed exposure of Polaroid film. Strip chart recorders eliminated the need to capture brief echoes and enabled continuous hard copy recordings of the left heart from apex to left atrium (sector scan). Coupled with the introduction of beam focusing, this advance paved the way to more detailed imaging and enabled the use of ultrasound in older patients in whom adequate images could not previously be obtained.

For the first fifteen years, echocardiograms were used primarily to diagnose valvular and pericardial disease by means of M-mode echocardiography. M-mode echocardiography is a unidimensional method of sound waves reflected from cardiac structures—an "ice pick" view. The signal is displayed over time, often on paper, to give a linear recording of the motion of a valve or wall throughout several cardiac cycles. The method was not initially used to address coronary artery disease in part because of the technical limitations noted above. In addition, coronary disease held a much less central position in those early years of coronary care units (first implemented in 1963), selective angiography (1958), and coronary revascularization (1964). Indeed, the first echocardiographic description of the segmental wall motion abnormalities characteristic of acute myocardial infarction appeared as recently as 1971 (23, 24). In one of these early reports, Inoue et al. described a decrease in the amplitude of posterior wall excursion and systolic thickening velocity in coronary artery disease. His "gold standard" for comparison was the apexcardiogram since normal values for these echocardiographic parameters had been defined only one year before, by Kraunz and Kennedy (25).

In 1972 Stefan and Bing published experimental work correlating the appearance of echocardiographic and mechanical evidence of myocardial infarction, confirming the importance of echocardiography in the diagnosis of coronary artery disease (26).

The growth of echocardiography can also be gauged by its acceptance in the area of medical science. Echocardiography was first included as a subtitle in the Index Medicus in 1973. The American Society of Echocardiography was formed in 1975 to "promote, maintain, and pursue excellence in the ultrasonic examination of the heart." Surveys taken by the new organization revealed that 21 percent of Cardiology Departments had echocardiographic equipment in 1975, rising rapidly to 57 percent in 1979 and 65 percent in 1981 (27).

Application to Congenital Heart Disease

Given the limited field of view of M-mode echocardiography and early instrumentation, congenital heart disease generally proved much more difficult to diagnose than mitral stenosis or pericardial effusion. The complexity of congenital heart disease delayed the appreciation of the true usefulness of echocardiography. Early echocardiographic diagnosis relied chiefly on the appearance of right ventricular volume overload in the diagnosis of atrial septal defect and was otherwise limited to detection of an atretic valve or chamber. One of the first reports of direct diagnosis of congenital heart disease was a description of hypoplastic right and left heart syndromes published by Chestler et al. in 1970 (28). Chestler went on to describe a variety of other abnormalities, and along with Lundstrom and the still active Edler, wrote the first reviews on the subject in 1971 (29, 30). In 1972 the first echocardiography text published devoted only ten pages and nine figures to congenital heart disease and cited but twelve references (17). Given this limited experience, it is not surprising that the 1972 edition of Alexander Nadas's classic text *Pediatric Cardiology* devoted thirty-one pages to vector- and phonocardiography, but did not even mention ultrasound (31). The value of echocardiography in young patients was quickly recognized over the next few years, aided by the introduction of two-dimensional imaging. Sahn et al. published the first descriptions of two-dimensional imaging in cyanotic congenital heart disease in 1973 and noted its usefulness in defining great artery and chamber orientation and outflow tract anatomy (32). The second edition of Feigenbaum's text, published in 1976, devoted thirty-eight pages to congenital heart disease and included thirty-three figures, ten of which were two-dimensional echograms (33). More important, even at this early date, echocardiography was already beginning to be considered as a replacement for angiography: "In many situations, catheterization may be eliminated and in others, the catheterization can be markedly limited, thus reducing the risk of the invasive procedure" (33). In many instances, intrauterine echocardiography now furnishes the diagnosis of complicated congenital cardiac malformations before birth.

Two-Dimensional Echocardiography

Two-dimensional echocardiography records reflected sound waves from a pie-shaped slice of the heart, thereby providing information about structures across an entire plane (tomographic imaging). Two-dimensional echocardiograms are recorded on videotape so that cardiac motion may be seen in a real-time format. Two-dimensional echo allows visualization of much more of the heart than does M-mode echo.

In addition to pioneering work with M-mode echocardiography, Wild and Reid built the first two-dimensional scanner in 1952 (34). Using this single crystal, mechanical "echoscope," they first directed their attention to tissue characterization of human breast malignancy and later, in 1957, obtained cross-sectional images of the excised human heart, including recordings of a myocardial scar, the left coronary artery, and the aorta (14). Other investigators were experimenting with similar equipment, including Howrey and Bliss in 1952 (35). Japanese investigators played an important role in developing the technique, with in vivo, human two-dimensional echocardiography first described in Japan in 1962 by Nagayama et al. at Kagoshira University (36). The technique was further refined by other investigators in Japan during the next ten years (37, 38). The technique was variously termed "ultrasonic cardiokymography" and "ultrasonotonography" to reflect its unique ability to provide cross-sectional images. Ebina et al. first began clinical studies in 1965 with a mechanically rotating single crystal device and published a large series in 1967 (37). The transducer used was extremely bulky as it contained its own water bath within which the transducer moved. Ebina instituted the significant advancement of a simultaneously displayed electrocardiogram, providing a reference for timing during the cardiac cycle, and noted that the motion of cardiac contraction occurred most prominently in the minor rather than the major axis.

N. Bom, a Dutch engineer, described the first practical real-time multiscan ultrasonograph in 1971 (39), and published his experience with a series of 150 patients in 1973 (40). This machine provided rapid electronic activation of an array of crystals, thereby achieving accurate reproduction of cardiac motion. Prototype instruments were built nearly simultaneously in the United States at the National Institute of Health (41), Indiana University (42), and Duke University (43), by McDicken in Scotland (44), and elsewhere. Hertz was a pioneer with this method as well as with M-mode and noted some of the problems common to these early scanners—limited frame rate and bulky transducers (45). Engineers and cardiologists were soon debating the relative merits of linear or phased array and mechanical techniques (46) and commercially made systems rapidly became available. Two-dimensional echocardiography represented a tremendous advance over the unidimensional M-mode technique, to the extent that M-mode strip chart recording has been rendered an anachronism in many clinical laboratories. Two-dimensional imaging continues to improve with refinements in instrumentation, especially transducers, image acquisition and processing techniques, hormone imaging, new crystals, and so on.

In the late 1990s a number of significant achievements at every level of image acquisition have contributed to a spectacular improvement in ultrasound's capabilities. These include the introduction of new ceramic materials in transducers, automated border detection based on radiofrequency signals, wholly digital processing, and image reconstruction from harmonic analysis of the reflected signal. Many additional improvements are proprietary—developed and used by only one ultrasound system manufacturer.

New Views on Echocardiography

Several new methods have recently arisen using gastroscope- and catheter-mounted two-dimensional transducers such that echocardiography now is capable of imaging previously inaccessible or unresolvable cardiac anatomy. One of these, transesophageal echocardiography, was first attempted in man nearly simultaneously by Japanese and American investigators in the mid-1970s (47, 48, 49, 50, 51). Impetus for these developments came from the difficulty of obtaining adequate images in obese or barrel-chested patients or those with chronic lung disease, and, for the Japanese, in the specific hope that the anterior left ventricular free wall could be better visualized (48). In addition to the discomfort of swallowing the transducer, the vibrations created by some early mechanical probes were severe enough to limit examinations. Refinements eliminated this problem and instrumentation progressed rapidly, from a rigid M-mode transducer, to one mounted on a flexible shaft, to mechanical and then phased array, steerable two-dimensional systems. Introduction of the currently available phased array systems was slower, since such instrumentation was thought to be too bulky. In fact, Hisanaga et al., the first to use a mechanical two-dimensional system, stated in 1980 that phased array was "probably not suited for transesophageal scanning because of the proximity of the esophageal transducer to cardiac structures and because of the difficulty of swallowing a linear array of transducers with many coaxial cables" (49). Nevertheless, phased array systems have proven to be eminently feasible. The ability to angle as well as rotate the transducer and pulsed Doppler accompanied the availability of the first commercially made probe in 1987. Subsequent additions of color Doppler and multiplane capabilities, along with miniaturized probes for pediatric applications and nasally inserted probes for long-term monitoring, have only extended the capabilities of this technique.

Most initial studies were performed in the awake patient, but widespread acceptance of the new methodology in the United States followed clear demonstration of its usefulness as a monitoring, as well as diagnostic, tool during cardiac and vascular surgery. Anesthesiologists and, to a lesser extent, surgeons have therefore played an important role in popularizing transesophageal echo and demonstrating its value in detecting regional and global left ventricular dysfunction, as well as assessing the adequacy of valve repairs and of corrections of congenital abnormalities (52, 53, 54, 55, 56). These new indications have taken echo out of the hands of radiologists and cardiologists for the first time, and promise substantial further development.

In a very short time, transesophageal echo became widely available in both academic and community hospitals. The technique has proven very useful in the evaluation of prosthetic valves, endocarditis, cardiac masses and clots, aortic dissection, and septal defects (57). These current indications for its use were accurately predicted by Hisanaga et al., who in 1980, in the first report on the use of a mechanical two-dimensional probe, noted that detection of left atrial thrombus, wall motion abnormalities, and atrioventricular valve abnormalities should be counted among the potential uses of transesophageal echo, and that for visualization of the atrial septum, the "transesophageal view is essential—it cannot be replaced by other views" (49). Indeed, in a remarkably short time, this technique has become an essential part of the echocardiographer's, surgeon's, and anesthesiologist's armamentarium.

Intravascular and intracardiac echocardiography are other new approaches to cardiac ultrasound imaging. Following early work by Martin and Watkins in 1980 (58), Paul Yock and David Linker, Americans from the University of California at San Francisco, working with Norwegian investigators from the University of Trondheim, published the first reports of clinically useful intravascular echocardiography (59). Many catheters are currently approved for routine use, and several companies are conducting clinical trials of improved models as this is a very active area of investigation. The high-frequency (20 and 30 MHz) miniaturized transducers currently available are mounted on catheters and can be used to visualize arteries and veins, limited only by the size of the catheter. They are capable of providing high-resolution images of peripheral arteries as well as coronary vessels, and may prove immensely useful in characterizing local vessel and plaque anatomy, as well as guiding interventional procedures. This technique holds great promise in providing "direct vision" guidance of new interventional techniques including angioplasty, atherectomy, stent placement, laser angioplasty, and so on. Other potential applications of this new technique include diagnosis of vascular pathology, determination of vessel lumen size, wall and plaque architecture, and vascular distensibility. Intravascular methods are also being investigated for use in the pulmonary and peripheral circulations (60). Application of lower-frequency catheters to intracardiac use has proven valuable in guiding transseptal punctures and electrophysiologic procedures such as ablation (61, 62).

Another very active area of research is that of three-dimensional echocardiography, which reduces the spatial and geometric assumptions inherent in any tomographic technique. There are many approaches to three-dimensional echo, but most require some sort of image registration in space with off-line reconstruction—a tedious process hampering clinical acceptance, but one that is potentially capable of tremendous quantitative accuracy. Newer approaches rely on rotating transducers within their housing and volumetric imaging. These are, however, still in their infancy and appear unable as yet to offer quantitative information needed for accurate calculation of left ventricular size, mass, and function (63, 64).

A third promising area of research is that of contrast echocardiography. Although this technique has long been a mainstay of the research laboratory, the introduction of albunex in 1996 marked the beginning of the clinical application of this method. Current indications include cavity opacification and enhancement of Doppler signals. Many second- and third-generation contrast agents are

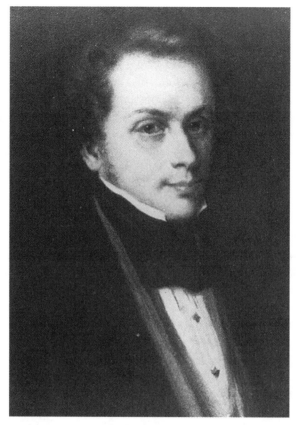

Figure 2.5. Christian Johann Doppler. *(With permission from the Christian Doppler Institute, Salzburg, Austria)*

under development, and promise to introduce perfusion imaging into the world of cardiac ultrasound. This will be an extraordinary advance, as the only methods currently available to obtain such information are radioisotope (nucelotide)-based (65, 66).

Application of the Doppler Principle to Cardiology

In 1842 Christian Johann Doppler called attention to the fact that "the color of luminous bodies, just like the pitch of a sounding body, changes with motion of the body to and from the observer." Doppler was born in Salzburg, Austria, on November 19, 1803, and died in Venice, Italy, on March 17, 1853 (Fig. 2.5). The son of a noted master stonemason in Salzburg, Doppler showed exceptional gifts for this craft. But his poor health led his father to plan a career in business for him. Doppler's mathematical abilities were soon recognized by the astronomer Simon Stampfer, who suggested that Doppler attend the Polytechnic Institute in Vienna. Doppler found this experience dull and returned to Salzburg in 1825, where he pursued his studies privately. After finishing the high school course in philosophy in a short time and after tutoring in mathematics and physics, in 1829 he moved to Vienna, where he was employed for three years as a mathematical assistant. In Vienna, he wrote his first paper on mathematics and electricity. In 1835 he was on the verge of emigrating to America, going as far as selling his possessions and reaching Munich, when he was informed that he had obtained a position as professor of mathematics and accounting at a secondary school in Prague. In 1841 he became full professor of elementary mathematics and practical geometry at the technical academy in Prague; it was here that he enunciated his famous principle. In 1847 Doppler moved to a mining academy in Schemnitz, Bohemia, as a professor of mathematics and physics. In 1848 he returned to Vienna where, in 1850, he became professor of experimental physics at the Royal Imperial University of Vienna. In 1853 he sought a cure for a lung ailment, probably tuberculosis, dying during a trip to Venice (67).

It is a fascinating facet of Doppler's life that he gave private instruction to a twenty-year-old Augustinian monk, Johann Gregor Mendel, who failed the oral examination in physics. As Doppler wrote, "his essay (Mendel's) makes it clear the candidate is formally well educated, but in the physical sciences, he has not progressed beyond the elementary stage." Mendel finally passed the course to become the founder of modern genetics.

Doppler was interested in applying his principle first to astronomy. In his article published in 1842, "Ueber das farbige Licht der Doppelsterne und einiger anderen Gestirne des Himmels," he argued that all stars emitted white light and that the color of some of the stars was due to their motion toward us or away from us (68). This was an erroneous conclusion: the approach of a star would simply produce a slight shift, and no change in color would take place. But the principle is correct: an apparent shift in the frequency of waves received by an observer depends on the relative motion between the observer and the source of the waves. This principle applied to all wave phenomena. The most spectacular application was in astronomy. In 1929 E.P. Hubble examined the frequency shift of light from distant galaxies. He found that the light was red-shifted (its frequency decreased) as he looked at the increasingly distant galaxies; he thus verified that the galaxies are receding from us with relative velocities that increase in the proportion to the distance. This knowledge led to the concept of an origin of the universe, commonly referred to as the "Big Bang."

Buys Ballot, a Dutch student who was working on his doctorate at the University of Utrecht, did not believe Doppler's theory. He was able to persuade the Dutch government to place at his disposal the railroad between Utrecht and

Amsterdam, together with a locomotive capable of obtaining a speed of fifty miles per hour and a flat-car (69). In the winter of 1845, Ballot had horn-players posted along the track and on the railway car. But it was so cold that the musicians were unable to blow their instruments. In June of the same year, the experiment was repeated involving teams of musicians with previously calibrated instruments, musically trained observers, and Ballot himself riding on the foot plate of the locomotive. It was observed that as the locomotive passed the players stationed on each side of the track, the note blown by the musicians on the train was perceived one-half a tone higher as it approached and one-half a tone lower as it receded. Thus, the Doppler effect for sound waves was confirmed in a curious way.

Doppler's concept also encountered criticism from Petzval (67). Petzval's opposition to Doppler's theory was based partly on its simplicity: "Without the application of differential equations, it is not possible to enter the realms of great science." In addition, Petzval confused two completely different situations: one in which there is relative movement between the sound source and the listener, and the other in which the medium is in motion, but the sound source and listener are stationary. In this latter case, the Doppler principle agrees that there would be no change in tone. In the bitter controversy between Petzval and Doppler, the latter was backed by his pupils von Ettingshausen and Mach.

At the time of the unveiling of the bust of Doppler in the colonnades of Vienna University in 1901, Egon von Oppolzer referred to the argument between Petzval and Doppler:

> His opponent bandied with such expressions as "great science" and "small science" in the Academy of Sciences, being of the opinion that great truths could not be found in a few lines and through an equation with only one unknown, and that at least one differential equation is necessary—and in this way he believes to have shown the incorrectness of the Doppler principle. Whoever probes somewhat deeper will find in these attacks, not a purely scientific motive, but a more personal goal. It is the old contradiction between genius and talent, which must lead to a struggle when, on the side of the talent there is no understanding of intuitive action and individual brilliance. For Doppler surveying his principle, it is of clear certainty, and for him—a true natural researcher—the attack on a law which has already been confirmed through experiments is completely incomprehensible (67).

The potential usefulness of the Doppler principle in cardiovascular diagnosis was first recognized in 1954 by Kalmus, who devised an intravascular acoustic flowmeter that measured the differences in frequency between sound transmitted across upstream and downstream flow (70). Doppler's principle was first utilized in cardiology by S. Satomura in 1956 (71) to detect cardiac motion and time the opening and closing of the cardiac valves. He used a continuous ultrasound beam transmitted through the chest wall to the heart and reflected from the heart structures, which underwent a frequency shift, or Doppler effect, of the transmitted sound whose magnitude and direction was based on the speed and direction of movement of the heart. The frequency of the reflected sound was proportional to the velocity of components of the target. Satomura noted the superiority of this method over conventional phonocardiography, but did not appreciate that sound could be reflected from blood cells as well as cardiac structures—that flow could be detected. Indeed, he mentions "Doppler heart noises" as occurring only in diseased hearts "when the reflecting object of the ultrasound, such as the ventricular wall, suffers an irregular vibration of small amplitude" (72). Nevertheless, the ability of this application of Doppler's theory to detect valve motion was subsequently found to be of value in measuring isovolumic relaxation time, and therefore diastolic function in a variety of disease states (73).

Simultaneously, an appreciation of the potential value of Doppler-based ultrasound measurements of blood flow velocity in the aorta was gained in animal experiments that used a pair of implanted crystals to record velocity shifts in sound transmitted obliquely across flow (74). This method was adapted to use in man by measurement of the frequency shift of reflected, rather than transmitted, sound. Once the velocity of blood flow in the ascending aorta could be recorded, the technique was adapted for measurement of cardiac output (75, 76, 77). Appreciation of the difficulties involved and of potential sources of error have contributed to the failure of Doppler measurements of cardiac output to be included in routine clinical practice. However, the concept of measurement of volume flow by integration of the Doppler velocity curve is routinely applied in the echocardiographic laboratory for calculation of pulmonary to systemic flow ratios in cardiac shunts and the aortic valve area, among other uses. Early on, investigators noted that the pattern of flow in the ascending aorta was characteristically altered in some disease states. Joyner and colleagues noted diastolic flow reversal in aortic regurgitation in 1970 (78), and midsystolic notching in idiopathic hypertrophic subaortic stenosis in 1971 (79).

By far the most important development in cardiac Doppler analysis was that of range-gating, or pulsed wave Doppler, by Baker et al. at the University of Washington in 1970 (80). This method allows localization of flow velocity measurements to specific valves and chambers. It is based on the principle that blood flow in a small area within the heart can be recorded by the use of intermittent pulses of transmitted sound. The receiver then "listens" for reflected sound only at the end of the time interval required for the pulse to travel from the transducer to the area of interest and back. Sound reflected from both nearer and more distant structures is thereby excluded. Coupled with localization of the signal, the ability of the technique to distinguish between laminar and turbulent flow enabled accurate identification of cardiac murmurs. Baker et al. correctly noted its potential usefulness in murmur localization, determination of orifice size from jet diameter, and measurement of pulmonary flow. Unfortunately, the concept of murmur localization caused confusion between the new Doppler technique and the then currently popular, and far less useful, electronic stethoscopy.

The development of pulsed Doppler resulted from a close collaboration between industry and academia, which benefited both. Baker's group worked closely with Astengo and colleagues at Advanced Technologies Laboratory (ATL) in the initial development of the pulsed wave Doppler technique. The first commercial system was introduced in 1975 by ATL, a mere two years after publication of the first report of its use in man. Industry contributed further with the introduction of fast Fourier analysis of the pulsed Doppler signal by Gessert and Taylor at Honeywell. This allowed linear signal processing and two-dimensional visualization of the area from which flow velocity was recorded.

Soon after the introduction of pulsed Doppler, Holen et al. (81) demonstrated the correlation between measured Doppler flow velocities and pressure gradients, forming the basis for assessments of valvular and vascular stenosis, prosthetic valves, and estimation of chamber pressures using regurgitant or shunt jet velocities. Two years later, in 1976, Holen et al. (82) and Hatle et al. (83) simultaneously published methods for estimating mitral orifice area. Publication of methods for calculation of mitral valve area by the pressure half time method, and measurement of pulmonary artery pressure and aortic stenosis gradients soon followed (84, 85, 86). The ability to quantify stenosis by continuous wave methods, and detect turbulent flow due to regurgitation or shunts by pulsed methods, combined to make Doppler an immensely important and widely adopted addition to the echocardiographic laboratory in the early 1980s.

Another group at the University of Washington, Brandestini and colleagues, developed a multigated or multichannel Doppler system, which allowed determination of velocity in several areas of interest simultaneously (87). This digitally processed system displayed velocity by color coding superimposed on a conventional M-mode echocardiogram. The first report of its clinical use in abstract form in 1982 (88) coincided with a preliminary report by Bommer et al. at the University of California at Davis, of "real time, two-dimensional color flow Doppler" (89). The Japanese investigators Kitabatake, Namekawa, et al. (90, 91) were also developing "blood-flow imaging" based on color-coded blood flow mapping on two-dimensional echoes, including the development of the autocorrelation method capable of the rapid data analysis required (91). Indeed, the first book on color Doppler and the first commercially available machine were introduced in 1982 (92), both from Japan.

Current instrumentation allows for superimposition of color-coded velocity on the tomographic image. While, in theory, color Doppler's ability to detect flow is identical to that of pulsed Doppler, the display format substantially enhances both the sensitivity and specificity of the technique. Small or eccentric jets are more easily detected and the origin of abnormal flow more easily identified. Color Doppler is also extremely useful for describing the direction of a jet, so that the continuous wave beam may be more accurately oriented to high velocity flow. Finally, color flow substantially decreases the time necessary to perform the echo-cardiographic exam.

A new application of Doppler has been introduced by several manufacturers, called Doppler tissue imaging. This technique allows direct assessment of the velocity of small regions of the myocardium during both contraction and relaxation. Although primarily a research tool, its promise in the clinical laboratory is substantial (93, 94, 95).

It has taken nearly 150 years for the clinical importance of Doppler's effect to be widely appreciated in cardiac diagnosis, and almost a hundred years for the Curies' early experiments with piezoelectricity to be applied to cardiac imaging in routine practice. The developments that have enabled translation of their work into useable format occurred in the 1950s and 1960s for both Doppler and conventional imaging echocardiography—long before the clinical significance of this work was appreciated by most cardiologists. The development of echocardiography has been a truly international effort, with major contributions by investigators in Europe, Japan, and the United States, and has frequently depended on contributions from industrial as well as academic research. Few techniques have so profoundly altered the approach to cardiovascular diagnosis. Ultrasound, at its best, can provide information not otherwise obtainable by the physical examination, or invasive pressure monitoring and angiography combined. In the future, given the rapid changes in the structure and financing of health care, diagnostic techniques such as echocardiography will have to be judged useful, not only by physicians, but also by administrators. The use of echocardiography must be justified by its impact on patient diagnosis, of course, but also on treatment strategies and overall health outcomes. And it will have to do this in a cost-effective manner, better and less expensively than other competing techniques (96). Given the power of echocardiography, its portability, and the promise of developing techniques, it is likely to be a valuable part of the physician's armamentarium for years to come.

References

1. Curie, M., and P. Curie. New York, Macmillan, 1923.
2. Curie, J., and P. Curie. Physique cristallographique sur l'électricité polaire dans les hemièdres à faces inclines. C.R. Hebd. Sci., 9:383–387, 1880.
3. Curie, J., and P. Curie. Lois du dégagement de l'électricite par pression dans l'arme-dine. C.R. Hebd. Sci., 92:186–188, 1881.
4. Lippman, M. Principes de la conservation de l'électricité. Ann. Chim. Phys., 145, 1881.

5. Kelvin, L. On the piezoelectric property of quartz. Philos. Mag., 36:1–99, 1890.

6. Voight, W. Lehrbuch der Kristallphysik. Leipzig, Teubner, 1910.

7. Cady, W.G. Piezoelectricity. New York, Dover, 1964.

8. Firestone, F.M. The supersonic reflectoscope, an instrument for inspecting solid parts by means of sound waves. J. Acoust. Soc. Am., 17:287–299, 1946.

9. Dussik, K.T. Ueber die Moeglichkeit hochfrequente mechanische Schwindungen als diagnostiches Hilfsmittel zu verwenden. Z. Gesamte Neurol. Psychiatr., 174:153–165, 1942.

10. Keidel, W.D. Ueber eine Methode zur Registrierung der Volumenaenderungen des Herzens am Menschen. Z. Kreislauff., 39:257–271, 1950.

11. Edler, I., and C.H. Hertz. Use of ultrasonic reflectoscope for continuous recording of movements of heart walls. Kungl. Fysiogr. Sallsk. (Lund.) Forhandl., 24:5–40, 1954.

12. Effert, S., and E. Domanig. The diagnosis of intra-atrial tumor and thrombi by the ultrasonic echo method. Germ. Med. Mth., 4:1, 1959.

13. Edler, I., A. Gustafson, T. Karlefors, and B. Christensson. Ultrasound cardiography. Acta Med. Scand., 170 (Suppl. 370):67–82, 1961.

14. Wild, J.J., H.D. Crawford, and J.M. Reid. Visualization of the excised human heart by means of reflected ultrasound or echography. Am. Heart J., 54:903–906, 1957.

15. Joyner, C.R., J.M. Reid, and J.P. Bond. Reflected ultrasound in the assessment of mitral valve disease. Circulation, 27:503–511, 1963.

16. Joyner, C.R., and J.M. Reid. Ultrasound cardiogram in the selection of patients for mitral valve surgery. Ann. N.Y. Acad. Sci., 118:512–524, 1965.

17. Feigenbaum, H., and S. Chang. Echocardiograph. Philadelphia, Lea & Febiger, 1972.

18. Feigenbaum, H., J.A. Waldhausen, and L.P. Hyde. Ultrasound diagnosis of pericardial effusion. JAMA, 191:711–717, 1965.

19. Feigenbaum, H., A. Zaky, and W.K. Nasser. Use of ultrasound to measure left ventricular stroke volume. Circulation, 35:1092–1099, 1967.

20. Feigenbaum, H., R.L. Popp, J.N. Chip, and C.L. Haine. Left ventricular wall thickness measured by ultrasound. Arch. Int. Med., 121:391–395, 1968.

21. Feigenbaum, H., S.B. Wolfe, R.L. Popp, C.L. Haine, and H.T. Dodge. Correlation of ultrasound with angiocardiography in measuring left ventricular diastolic volume. Am. J. Cardiol., 23:111, 1969.

22. Popp, R.L., S.B. Wolfe, T. Hirata, and H. Feigenbaum. Estimation of right and left ventricular size by ultrasound. A study of the echoes from the interventricular septum. Am. J. Cardiol., 24:523–530, 1969.

23. Inoue, K., H. Smulyan, S. Mookherjee, and R.H. Eich. Ultrasonic measurement of left ventricular wall motion in acute myocardial infarction. Circulation, 43:778–785, 1971.

24. Ratchin, R.A., C.E. Rackley, and R.O. Russell. Serial evaluation of left ventricular volumes and posterior wall movement in the acute phase of myocardial infarction using diagnostic ultrasound (abstr.). Am. J. Cardiol., 29:286, 1972.

25. Kraunz, R.F., and J.W. Kennedy. Ultrasonic determination of left ventricular wall motion in normal man. Am. Heart J., 79:36–43, 1970.

26. Stefan, G., and R.J. Bing. Echocardiographic findings in experimental myocardial infarction of the posterior left ventricular wall. Am. J. Cardiol., 30:629–639, 1972.

27. American Society of Echocardiography White Paper: Echocardiography: 1986 and Beyond, March, ASE.

28. Chestler, E., H.S. Jaffe, and R. Vecht. Ultrasound cardiography in single ventricle and hypoplastic left and right heart syndromes. Circulation, 42:123–129, 1970.

29. Chestler, E., H.S. Jaffe, W. Beck, and V. Schrire. Echocardiography in the diagnosis of congenital heart disease. Pediat. Clin. N. Amer., 18:1163–1190, 1971.

30. Lundstrom, N.R., and I. Edler. Ultrasoundcardiography in infants and children. Acta Paediat. Scand., 60:117–128, 1971.

31. Nadas, A.S., and D.C. Fyler. Pediatric Cardiology. Philadelphia, W.B. Saunders Company, 3rd ed., 1972.
32. Sahn, D.J., R. Terry, R. O'Rourke, G. Leopold, and W.F. Friedman. Multiple crystal cross-sectional echocardiography in the diagnosis of cyanotic congenital heart disease. Circulation, 50:230–238, 1974.
33. Feigenbaum., H. Echocardiography. Lea & Febiger, 2nd ed., 1976.
34. Wild, J.J., and J.M. Reid. Application of echo-ranging techniques to the determination of the structure of biological tissues. Science, 115: 226–230, 1952.
35. Howrey, D.H., and W.R. Bliss. Ultrasonic visualization of soft tissue structure of the body. J. Lab. Clin. Med., 40:579–592, 1952.
36. Nagayama, T., S. Nakamura, K. Hayakawa, and Y. Komo. Ultrasonic cardiokymogram. Acta Med. Univ. Kagoshima, 4:229, 1962.
37. Ebina, T., S. Oka, M. Tanaka, S. Kosaka, Y. Terasawa, K. Unno, D. Kikuchi, and R. Uchida. The ultrasono-tomography of the heart and great vessels in living human subjects by means of the ultrasonic reflection technique. Jap. Heart J., 8:331–353, 1967.
38. Uchida, R., Y. Hagiwara, and T. Irie. Electroscanning ultrasonic diagnostic equipment. Jap. Med. Elec., 58, 1971–72.
39. Bom, N., C.T. Lancee, J. Honkoop, and P.C. Hugenholtz. Ultrasonic viewer for cross-sectional analyses of moving cardiac structures. Bio-Medical Eng., 6:500, 1971.
40. Bom, N., C.T. Lancee, G. VanZwieten, F.E. Kloster, and J. Roelandt. Multiscan echocardiography. I. Technical description. Circulation, 48:1066–1074, 1973.
41. Griffith, J.M., and W.L. Henry. A sector scanner for real time two-dimensional echocardiography. Circulation, 49:1147–1152, 1974.
42. Eggleton, R.C., J.C. Dillion, H.C. Feigenbaum, K.W. Johnston, and S. Chang. Visualization of cardiac dynamics with real time B-mode ultrasonic scanner (abstr.). Circulation (Suppl. III), 49/50:27, 1974.
43. Von Ramm, O.T., and F.L. Thurstone. Cardiac imaging using a phased array ultrasound system. I. System design. Circulation, 53(2):258, 1976.
44. McDicken, W.M., K. Bruff, and J. Patton. An ultrasonic instrument for rapid B-scanning of the heart. Ultrasonics, 12:269–272, 1974.
45. Hertz, C.H., and K. Lundstrom. A fast ultrasonic scanning system for heart investigation. 3rd International Conference on Medical Physics. Gottenburg, Sweden, August 1972.
46. Eggleton, R.C., and K.W. Johnston. Real time mechanical scanning system compared with array techniques. IEEE, Proceedings in Sonics and Ultrasonics, Catalog No. 74-CH 0896-1, p. 16, 1974.
47. Frazin, L., J.V. Talano, L. Stephanides, H.S. Loeb, L. Kopel, and R. Gunnar. Esophageal echocardiography. Circulation, 54:102–108, 1976.
48. Matsuzaki, M., Y. Matsuda, Y. Ikee, Y. Takahashi, T. Saskai, Y. Toma, K. Ishida, T. Yorozu, T. Kumada, and R. Kusukawa. Esophageal echocardiography of left ventricular anterior wall motion in patients with coronary artery disease. Circulation, 63:1085–1092, 1981.
49. Hisanaga, K., A. Hisanaga, N. Hibi, K. Nishimura, and T. Kambe. High speed rotating scanner for transesophageal cross-sectional echocardiography. Am. J. Cardiol., 46:837–842, 1980.
50. Hisanaga, K., A. Hisanaga, K. Nagata, and Y. Ichie. Transesophageal cross-sectional echocardiography. Am. Heart J., 100:605–609, 1980.
51. Hisanaga K, A. Hisanaga, Y. Ichie, K. Nishimura, N. Hibi, Y. Fukui, and T. Kambe. Transesophageal pulsed Doppler echocardiography (abstr.). Lancet, 1:53–54, 1979.
52. Schlueter, M., B.A. Langenstein, J.A. Polster, et al. Transesophageal cross-sectional

echocardiography with a phased array transducer system. Technique and initial clinical results. Br. Heart J., 48:67–72, 1982.

53. Kremer, P., M. Cahalan, P. Beaupre, N.S. Schiller, and P. Hanrath. Intra-operative myocardial ischemia detected by transesophageal two-dimensional echocardiography (abstr.). Circulation, 68 (Suppl. III):332, 1983.

54. Pandian, N.G., M. England, J. Hudson, et al. Continuous monitoring of cardiac function by two-dimensional echocardiography using precordial and esophageal transducers. Ultrasonic Imaging, 6:225, 1984.

55. Topol, E.J., J.L. Weiss, P.A. Guzman, et al. Immediate improvement of dysfunctional myocardial segments after coronary revascularization: detection by intraoperative transesophageal echocardiography. J. Am. Coll. Cardiol., 4:1123–1134, 1984.

56. Spotnitz, H.M., C.Y.H. Young, A.J. Spotnitz, et al. Intra-operative left ventricular performance evaluated by two-dimensional ultra-sound. Circulation, 62:329, 1980.

57. Seward, J.B., B.K. Khandheria, J.K. Oh, M.D. Abel, R.W. Hughes Jr., W.D. Edwards, B.A. Nichols, W.K. Freeman, and A.J. Tajik. Transesophageal echocardiography: technique, anatomic correlation, implementation, and clinical applications. Mayo Clin. Proc., 63:649–680, 1988.

58. Martin, R.W., and D.W. Watkins. An ultrasonic catheter for intravascular measurement of blood flow: technical details. IEEE Trans. Sonics Ultrasound, 27:277–278, 1980.

59. Yock, P.G., E.L. Johnson, and D.T. Linker. Intravascular ultrasound: development and clinical potential. Am. J. Cardiac Imaging, 2:185–193, 1988.

60. Pandian, N.G., A. Weintraub, A. Kreis, S.L. Schwartz, M.A. Konstam, and D.N. Salem. Intracardiac, intravascular, two-dimensional, high-frequency ultrasound imaging of pulmonary artery and its branches in humans and animals. Circulation, 81: 2007–2012, 1990.

61. Chu, E., A.P. Fitzpatrick, M.C. Chin, K. Sudhir, P.B. Yock, and M.D. Lesh. Radiofrequency catheter ablation guided by intracardiac echocardiography. Circulation, 89: 1301–1305, 1994.

62. Chu, E., J.M. Kalman, M.A. Kwasman, J.C. Jue, P.J. Fitzgerald, L.M. Epstein, N.B. Schiller, P.G. Yock, and M.D. Lesh. Intracardiac echocardiography during radiofrequency catheter ablation of cardiac arrhythmias in humans. J. Am. Coll. Cardiol., 24:1351–1357, 1994.

63. Roelandt, J.R. Three-dimensional echocardiography: new views from old windows. Br. Heart J., 74:4–6, 1995.

64. Belohlavek, M., D.A. Foley, T.C. Gerber, T.M. Kinter, J.F. Greenleaf, and J.B. Seward. Three- and four-dimensional cardiovascular ultrasound imaging: a new era for echocardiography. Mayo Clin. Proc., 68:221–240, 1993.

65. DeMaria, A.N. (guest ed.). A new generation of ultrasound contrast agents for echocardiography. Clin. Cardiol., 20 (Suppl I), 1997.

66. Kaul, S. Myocardial contrast echocardiography: fifteen years of research and development. Circulation, 96:3745–3760, 1997.

67. Eden, A. Christian Doppler, thinker and benefactor. Salzburg, Austria, The Christian Doppler Institute for Science and Technology, 1988.

68. Doppler, C. Ueber das farbige Licht der Doppelsterne und einiger anderen Gesterne des Himmels. Abhandl. Koenigl. Boehmisch. Gesellsch. Wissensch., 2:465–482, 1842.

69. Doppler, J.C. Dictionary of Scientific Biography, 4:167, 1971.

70. Kalmus, H.P. Electronic flowmeter system. Rev. Sci. Instr., 25:201–206, 1954.

71. Satomura, S. Studies on cardiac function test by ultrasonic Doppler method (abstr.). Jpn. Circ. J., 20:227–228, 1956.

72. Satomura, S. Ultrasonic Doppler method for the inspection of cardiac function. J. Acoustical Soc. Am., 29:1181–1185, 1957.

73. Yoshida, T., M. Mori, Y. Nimura, G. Hikita, S. Takagishi, K. Nakanishi, and S. Satomura. Analysis of heart motion with the ultrasonic Doppler method and its clinical application. Am. Heart J., 61:61–75, 1961.

74. Franklin, D.L., R.M. Ellis, and R.F. Rushmer. Aortic blood flow in dogs during treadmill exercise. J. Appl. Phys., 14:809, 1959.

75. Light, L.H. Transcutaneous observation of blood velocity in the ascending aorta in man. Biol. Cardiol., 26:214, 1969.

76. Light, L.H., G. Gross, and P.L. Hansen. Non-invasive measurement of blood velocity in the major thoracic vessels. Proc. Roy. Soc. Med., 67:142–143, 1974.

77. Huntsman, L.L., E. Gams, C.C. Johnson, and E. Fairbanks. Transcutaneous determination of aortic blood flow velocities in man. Am. Heart J., 89:605–612, 1975.

78. Thompson, P.D., R.G. Mennel, H. Mac Vaugh, and C.R. Joyner. The evaluation of aortic insufficiency in humans with a transcutaneous Doppler velocity probe (abstr.). Ann. Intern. Med., 72:781, 1970.

79. Joyner, C.R., Jr., F.S. Harrison Jr., and J.W. Gruber. Diagnosis of hypertrophic subaortic stenosis with a Doppler velocity flow detector. Ann. Intern. Med., 74:692–696, 1971.

80. Baker, D.W. Pulsed ultrasonic Doppler blood-flow sensing. IEEE Trans. Sonic Ultrasonics, SU-17:3, 1970.

81. Holen, J., R. Aaslid, K. Landmark, and S. Simonsen. Determination of pressure gradient in mitral stenosis with a noninvasive ultrasound Doppler technique. Acta Med. Scand., 199:455–460, 1976.

82. Holen, J., and S. Nitter-Hauge. Evaluation of obstructive characteristics of mitral disc valve implants with ultrasound Doppler techniques. Acta Med. Scand., 201:429–434, 1977.

83. Hatle, L., A. Brubakk, A. Tromsdal, and B. Angelsen. Noninvasive assessment of pressure drop in mitral stenosis by Doppler ultrasound. Br. Heart J., 40:131–140, 1978.

84. Hatle, L. Noninvasive assessment and differentiation of left ventricular outflow obstruction by Doppler ultrasound. Circulation, 64:381–387, 1981.

85. Hatle, L., B.A.J. Angelsen, and A. Tromsdal. Noninvasive estimation of pulmonary artery systolic pressure with Doppler ultrasound. Br. Heart J., 45:157–165, 1981.

86. Hatle, L., B.A.J. Angelsen, and A. Tromsdal. Noninvasive assessment of atrioventricular pressure halftime by Doppler ultrasound. Circulation, 60:1096–1104, 1979.

87. Brandestini, M.A., M.K. Eyer, and J.G. Stevenson. M/Q-mode echocardiography: the synthesis of conventional echo with digital multigate Doppler. In: Echocardiology, Lancee, C.T. (ed.). The Hague, Martinus Nijhoff, 1979.

88. Stevenson, G., I. Kawabori, and M. Brandestini. Color-coded Doppler visualization of flow within ventricular septal defects: implications for peak pulmonary artery pressure (abstr.). Am. J. Cardiol., 49:944, 1982.

89. Bommer, J., and L. Miller. Real-time two-dimensional color-flow Doppler: enhanced Doppler flow imaging in the diagnosis of cardiovascular disease (abstr.). Am. J. Cardiol., 49:944, 1982.

90. Kitabatake, K., M. Inoue, M. Asao, et al. Non-invasive visualization of intracardiac blood flow in human heart using computer-aided pulsed Doppler technique. Clinical Hemorrheology, 1:85, 1982.

91. Namekawa, K., C. Kasai, M. Tsukamoto, and A. Koyano. Imaging of blood flow using auto-correlation techniques. Ultrasound Med. Biol., 8:Suppl. 2203–2208, 1982.

92. Omoto, R. Color Atlas of Real-Time Two-Dimensional Doppler Echocardiography. Tokyo, Shindan-to-Chiryo, 1st ed., 1984; 2nd ed., 1987.

93. Sutherland, G.R., M.J. Stewart, K.W.E. Groundstroem, et al. Color Doppler myocardial imaging: a new technique for the assessment of myocardial function. J. Am. Soc. Echocardiogr., 23:1441–1458, 1994.

94. Miyatake, K., M. Yamagishi, N. Tanaka, et al. New method for evaluating left ventricular wall motion by color-coded tissue Doppler imaging: in vitro and in vivo studies. J. Am. Coll. Cardiol., 25:717–724, 1995.

95. Gorscan, J., V.K. Gulati, W.A. Mandarino, and W.E. Katz. Color-coded measures of myocardial velocity throughout the cardiac cycle by tissue Doppler imaging to quantify regional left ventricular function. Am. Heart J., 131:1203–1213, 1996.

96. Douglas, P.S. Justifying echocardiography: the role of outcomes research in evaluating a diagnostic test. J. Amer. Soc. Echocardiogr., 9:577–581, 1996.

Chapter 3

Cardiopulmonary Bypass, Perfusion of the Heart, and Cardiac Metabolism

R. DEWALL
R.J. BING

Perfusion of the Heart and Cardiac Metabolism

Perfusion systems of several different types are used in medicine and physiology: cardiopulmonary bypass; perfusion of isolated hearts (Langendorff and supported heart preparation); perfusion of isolated organs (Carrel–Lindbergh system); and heart-lung preparation.

In cardiopulmonary bypass, the whole body is perfused with the exclusion of the heart and lungs. But even here there is the exception that the bronchial arteries continue to provide blood flow to the bronchi and pulmonary tissues to be aspirated by the surgeon from the opened heart and returned to the perfusion system. Normally, the bronchial blood flow represents 2 percent or less of the cardiac output.

In perfusion of the heart in vitro, the perfusion fluid either enters the aorta and coronary arteries by gravity (Langendorff preparation) or is pumped into the left atrium; the left ventricle then ejects against a variable resistance (supported heart preparation). In perfusion of an isolated organ, a pumping system directs perfusion fluid into that organ, which is maintained in vitro. Pulsation rate and pressures are adjustable and sterility can be observed (e.g., Carrel–Lindbergh perfusion system). In the heart-lung preparation of Starling, the heart pumps blood through the lung for oxygenation, and the perfusate is returned to the heart.

The Langendorff preparation was first described in 1885 (1). Langendorff himself devised several variations. In 1903 in the *Munich Medical Journal* he defended the priority of his discovery against the American workers Martin, Applegarth, and Porter (2). "I feel obliged, even though it goes against my grain to fight for priorities, to defend my publications in the most decisive terms and to protest against giving credit to authors who neither deserve nor claim it." He gave credit to Martin, who attempted to nourish the isolated mammalian heart through an isolated blood supply. But Martin, so said Langendorff, did not work with the completely isolated heart. Langendorff stated, "In Martin's case, coronary flow depended on activity of the left ventricle." He continued: "It is therefore not permissible, as it has happened, to write of the method of Martin *and* Langendorff, particularly since independent of Martin and without knowledge of his publication I was able to finally conclude my procedure" (2). The Martin whom Langendorff quotes was none else then Professor H. Newel Martin, who was the first professor of biology of the Johns Hopkins University (3). Martin developed his perfusion model in 1882 (3). He was a brilliant but erratic investigator, who had been recommended by Thomas Huxley to the professorship of biology at Johns Hopkins. Unfortunately, Martin was not chosen by the Johns Hopkins board of directors; he became an alcoholic suffering from peripheral neuritis. He was treated by William Osler, who was well aware that the source of his condition was chronic alcoholism. He died in the fall of 1895 of a sudden hemorrhage possibly due to esophageal varices (3).

Major controversies toward the end of the nineteenth century and in the early twentieth century concerned oxygen usage by the heart, the importance of glucose and lactic acid in cardiac metabolism, and particularly the role of inorganic material in the initiation and maintenance of cardiac rhythm. It was the time of Clark in Edinburgh (4), Loewi in Graz (5), Langendorff in Rostock (1), Lussana in Bologna (6), Howell in Baltimore (7), Ringer in London (8), Vernon in Oxford (9), Starling in London (10), Martin in Baltimore (11), Evans and Locke from London (12, 13), Rohde from Heidelberg (14), and many others, all of them perfusing isolated hearts.

In 1883 Ringer profitted from his mistake in his experimental setup by discovering the effect of electrolytes on the heart: "I discovered that saline solution which I had used had not been prepared with distilled water, but with pipe water supplied by the New River Water Company. This water contains minute traces of various inorganic substances. I at once tested the action of saline solution made with distilled water and found that I did not get the effects described in the paper referred to. It is obvious therefore that the effects I had obtained are due to some of the inorganic constituents of the pipe water" (15). Ringer then analyzed the water supplied by the New Water Company and found that it contained considerable quantities of calcium, potassium, magnesium, sodium, and chloride (15). Ringer also found that compounds can be mutually antagonistic and that a toxic dose of calcium chloride can be antagonized by a toxic dose of potassium chloride and vice versa (16).

It is astonishing that there was some question as to the use of oxygen by the heart. Kronecker reported the results of his pupil McGuire, who found that "oxygen was not essential for the nutrition of the heart" (17, 18). Possibly, Kronecker accepted the results of his pupil McGuire at face value without checking them.

Perfusion of the heart was the only method for the study of cardiac metabolism at the beginning of the twentieth century. Tigerstedt summarized these studies in his *Physiology of Circulation* (19). The twelfth chapter in his book is entitled "The Chemical Conditions for the Beating Heart." The first portions of this chapter are devoted to the perfusion and metabolism of the heart of cold-blooded animals. The remainder deals with the perfusion and metabolism of warm-blooded animals. Both sections review the subject thoroughly. Without perfusion of the isolated heart, none of the early studies on cardiac metabolism would have been possible. Many of the findings on the isolated perfused heart were later confirmed on the human heart in situ (20). Utilization of "fat" by the perfused frog heart is one example. On the occasion of Tigerstedt's one hundredth birthday, Liljestrand wrote an article summarizing his life and accomplishments (21). Tigerstedt served as professor of physiology at the Karolinska Institute in Stockholm and in the same capacity in Helsingfors, in his native Finland. Aside from his general interest in the circulation, Tigerstedt was particularly interested in the kidney. This led to the discovery of renin, arrived at by extracting kidney homogenates with saline and injecting the extract into rabbits. He determined that the resulting elevation in blood pressure was derived from the renal cortex. Tigerstedt and Bergman pointed out that the newly discovered substance, which they called renin, may be active in producing cardiac hypertrophy in patients with renal disease. Tigerstedt's name should be prominently mentioned whenever the history of hypertension and cardiac metabolism is discussed (see Chapter 12).

The Carrel–Lindbergh system maintains an organ outside the body at any desired "pulse rate" and perfusion pressure (22). How did Charles A. Lindbergh, who was the first to fly over the Atlantic Ocean, become interested in a subject that appears to be far removed from his chosen field of aviation (Fig. 3.1)? Like many factors that redirect our lives, the occasion here was one that came about by chance. In 1929 Lindbergh's wife's oldest sister was found to have rheumatic heart disease. When an operation of the heart was ruled out by the physician because "The heart could not be stopped long enough for surgeons to work on it," Lindbergh asked why a mechanical pump could not be substituted until the arrested heart could be repaired (23, 24). Lindbergh therefore made up his mind to design a pump capable of circulating blood through the body while the heart was being repaired. This farsighted idea was discouraged by Alexis Carrel of the Rockefeller Institute, who, well aware of the extreme difficulties of oxygenating the blood in such a system, believed that it was easier and more promising to design a pump for the "culture" of whole organs. Carrel, an ingenious surgeon, had

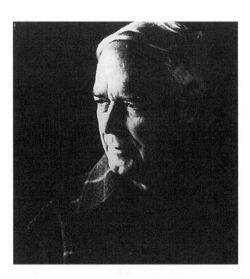

Figure 3.1. Charles Lindbergh. *(Courtesy of Richard J. Bing)*

previously worked on a new method of suturing blood vessels and on the culture of cells introduced by Ross Harrison. Carrel now was interested in extending his ideas to studying the interplay between perfusion fluid and organ in sterile perfusion experiments lasting days or weeks. By using artificial fluids, Carrel felt that he could examine individually and separately the influence of each constituent of the perfusate on the integrity and behavior of the isolated organ that was being perfused. Actually, this was a big step into the future, as the past thirty years have demonstrated. During my (RJB) years of cooperation with Lindbergh and Carrel, I never heard them refer to the original idea of Lindbergh—that of devising a pump for cardiopulmonary bypass. Lindbergh had been way ahead of his time!

Starling, a distinguished professor of physiology at University College, London, used the heart-lung preparation to study the relation between muscle fiber and length and strength of contraction—the basis of the subsequent Starling's law (10). Previous work by Otto Frank, a well-trained mathematician and physicist, also dealt with the relationship between length of muscle fibers and strength of contraction (25).

Frank used a small, simple, yet elegant preparation of the whole frog heart, perfused with diluted ox blood. He was able to fill or empty the heart chambers and make continuous records throughout the cardiac cycle of pressures in various parts of the systems, volumes in the heart chamber (filling), and volume output. Frank wrote, "I discovered the following law concerning the dependence of the form of the isometric pressure curve on the initial tension: the peaks (maxima) of the isometric pressure curve rise with increasing initial length (filling). I call this part of the family of curves the first part. Beyond a certain level of filling, the pressure peaks decline (second part of the family of curves)." Starling expressed his final conclusion in a similar vein: "The law of the heart is therefore the same as that of skeleton muscle, namely that the mechanical energy set free on passage from the resting to the contracted states depends on the area of chemically active surface, i.e., on the length of the muscle fiber. This simple formula serves to explain the whole behavior of the isolated mammalian heart" (10). The law of the heart is now referred to as the Frank–Starling law.

The heart-lung preparation represented a milestone in the development of our knowledge of cardiac metabolism. In a seminal paper in *Recent Advances in Physiology* (1939), Evans wrote a chapter on the metabolism of cardiac muscle, in which he described the gaseous metabolism of heart muscle, oxygen usage of the mammalian heart, mechanical efficiency of the heart, the influence of diastolic volume on myocardial oxygen usage, influences of heart rate, and foremost, myocardial usage of foodstuffs such as fat and carbohydrates (12). He also added a paragraph on the changes in cardiac metabolism during lack of oxygen. Most of the work described was done on the heart-lung preparation. Evans presented formulas on the mechanical efficiency of the heart and he demonstrated the influence of Starling's law of the heart on the oxygen utilization of the heart. He found a connection between diastolic volume and myocardial oxygen utilization. He predicted that the heart uses "fat." He determined that glucose utilization by the heart was a function of glucose concentration in the blood, and confirmed that the heart utilizes lactic acid.

These studies represented the basis for future work by Bing on metabolism of the human heart as carried out by coronary sinus catheterization, and still further gave impetus to other biochemical observations on the human heart (20).

Cardiopulmonary Bypass

Many inspired contributors advanced the development of heart surgery and heart-lung bypass techniques. The work in both areas served to build the foundation of successful open heart surgery that we know today.

Successful cardiopulmonary bypass became a reality in the early 1950s. While it seemed a new idea at the time, the foundations were in fact prepared over many preceding decades. The success of open heart surgery required resolution of two primary problems: the first was developing the perfusion equipment and understanding how to use it; the second was integrating the knowledge of cardiac surgical problems with an understanding of cardiopulmonary bypass techniques. Unfortunately, in the early days of bypass surgery, difficulties were experienced initiating successful open heart surgical programs (26–29). These continued to exist for two decades or more after the beginnings of open heart surgery (30–31).

Problems in the design of an effective cardiopulmonary bypass machine are manifold. Cardiopulmonary bypass is accompanied by means of a device, a heart-lung machine or pump-operator. A heart-lung machine is used to support a patient's total blood circulatory system, freeing the body's need for its own heart and lung function. This permits the opening of the patient's heart for surgical repairs. Due to the anatomic relationship of heart to lungs, circulation must be diverted for surgical repair of the heart.

Two basic components comprise the heart-lung machine. The first is the pump (heart substitute) that serves to maintain the patient's circulation through the pump-oxygenator circuit. The second is the oxygenator (lung substitute) that adds oxygen and removes excess carbon dioxide from the blood. In the development of pump-oxygenator systems, providing a suitable blood pump was easily accomplished, as serviceable pumps had been in existence for decades.

All oxygenators have a common theme: a respiratory gas mixture must be placed in close relationship to blood. The reaction time between hemoglobin and oxygen is less than one-hundredth of a second (32, 33). The limiting factor in the oxygenation of blood is the passage of the respiratory gas through the alveolar membrane (lung tissue), through the blood plasma, and through the red blood cell wall to reach the hemoglobin within the red blood cell.

For oxygenation, the blood must be delivered from a pool (the pulmonary artery in the human case) or from a reservoir or collecting chamber (artificial oxygenator) and spread in a thin film to minimize the distance through which the respiratory gasses must diffuse to reach the hemoglobin within the red blood cell. In the biologic sense, this is the thin film created by passage of blood through the pulmonary capillaries. In mechanical oxygenators, the blood must be distributed in a thin film. This filming is accomplished by pouring the blood to cover a large two-dimensional surface, such as spreading it over a screen or casting it in a thin film over bubbles of respiratory gas. More recent oxygenator innovations pass the blood through gas-permeable, tiny plastic tubes that mimic the normal lung.

Another necessary factor in oxygenator function is the respiratory gas to which the blood is exposed. The normal air we breathe is composed of approximately 78 percent nitrogen and 21 percent oxygen with the balance made up of lesser gasses. Water vapor (humidity) in the respiratory gas is of lesser importance for the oxygenating process. As hemoglobin absorbs oxygen, carbon dioxide is released.

The respiratory gas is generally exposed to the blood film at one atmosphere of pressure—760 mm Hg at sea level. The oxygenation process depends on the altitude at which the oxygenator is expected to function. For example, Denver's altitude of 5,000 feet affects the oxygenation process differently than altitudes at sea level. For example, people may even experience high-altitude mountain sickness due to the low atmospheric pressure at higher altitudes (34). Conversely, if the respiratory gas and blood film were exposed to more than one atmosphere of pressure, the thickness of the blood film could be increased, and the time of exposure decreased—similar to the effects an individual experiences when exposed to a hyperbaric situation such as deep-sea scuba diving.

For the development of successful extracorporeal circulation, it was necessary to have a mechanism to keep the blood from clotting outside the body in a mechanical pump-oxygenating system. The essential component required was an anticoagulant the body would tolerate.

ANTICOAGULATION

The success of extracorporeal circulation depends on proper anticoagulation. In early studies (35, 36, 37), defibrination was the method used to prevent blood from clotting. In 1903 Brodie introduced hirudine, a leach extract, and sodium citrate as anticoagulants (38). None of the agents was suitable for cardiopulmonary bypass activities in laboratory experiments seeking animal survival.

The discovery of heparin by Jay McLean was necessary to enable practical extracorporeal circulation (39). In 1915 McLean arrived at Johns Hopkins University as a second-year medical student. He immediately began working in the laboratory of William Henry Howell (40, 41), who was investigating which body tissues contained clot-promoting agents. McLean stated in his primary paper that he was assigned to "determine, if possible, whether the thromboplastic effect (of tissue extracts) may be attributed to an impurity, or as a property of cephalin itself" (39). In addition he wrote, "The cuorin (from ox heart) on the contrary when purified by repeated precipitation in alcohol at 60 degrees, has no thromboplastic effect, indeed it possesses an anticoagulation power." This was McLean's only reference to a natural anticoagulant that he incidentally observed while working on other substances. McLean did not use the term "heparin" for his newly discovered agent. After this primary effort in the study of blood-clotting mechanisms, his attention was directed to other areas, and he left Howell's laboratory.

Following McLean's departure, Howell and his associates continued work on the purification of the newly discovered anticoagulant and named the substance heparin since the extract was derived from the liver (40, 41). Commercial-, but not clinical-, grade heparin was first available in 1922 through the Baltimore firm of Hynson, Westcott, and Dunning (42).

In 1929 the development of heparin moved from Baltimore to the Toronto laboratories of Charles H. Best, of insulin fame (42). Best, working at the Connaught Laboratories, experienced difficulties with blood clotting in glass cannulas. He persuaded two organic chemists, Arthur Charles and David Scott, to pursue the purification of heparin. Their work was published in 1937 (43), and purified heparin became available by 1937. It was from Toronto that John Gibbon was able to obtain a supply of heparin for his first animal survivor (44).

While the availability of heparin was necessary for the development of ex-

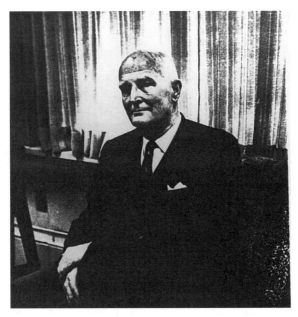

Figure 3.2. John H. Gibbon Jr. *(Courtesy of the New York Academy of Medicine)*

tracorporeal circulation, the practical applicability of heparin was enhanced by the observation in 1937 that protamine was a heparin antagonist (45). This discovery permitted a time-limited application of heparin, desirable for successful extracorporeal circulation.

During the 1930s heparin purification was achieved in Denmark (46) and Sweden (47, 48, 49). Craaford's familiarity with heparin in Sweden in 1937 (50) laid the foundation for Björk's successful perfusion experiments in 1948 (51).

INSTRUMENTATION

As early as 1812 Le Gallois wrote, "If one could at least substitute for the heart a kind of injection of arterial blood, either natural or artificially made, one would succeed easily in maintaining alive indefinitely, any part of the body whatsoever" (47). Dozens of systems for pumping and oxygenation of blood outside the body have been described since 1812.

John Gibbon's work ushered in the modern era of extracorporeal circulation that was made possible by the availability of heparin.

JOHN GIBBON

John Gibbon, a fourth-generation physician, was born in 1903 (Fig. 3.2). He seriously considered dropping out of medical school after the first semester because he was unhappy with the heavy load of memorization that normally accompanies the first two years of medical school. Gibbon had developed an interest in poetry and had actually considered becoming a poet. As he wrote,

> During my days at Princeton, I entertained the idea of becoming a poet. The courses I enjoyed most were advanced composition and two courses in 16th Century French—one poetry, the other prose. And I loved English poetry. But my father pointed out, like thousands of fathers before him, that poetry is a rather uncertain mode of livelihood. I was also smitten with painting, and to this day I put in considerable time in front of the easel. However, bowing to the goddess of necessity, I enrolled at Jefferson Medical College in Philadelphia, where my father was a professor of surgery. The first year of medical school was frankly, boring as hell—all the needless memorization. But when I told my father that I liked (sic) to quit he replied that he did not care if I did not wind up practicing medicine, but that when a person starts something, he should finish it. I agreed to continue and after that things got interesting anyway (53).

Gibbon noted that his passion for research stemmed from his internship at Pennsylvania Hospital. At that time, he was comparing the effects of potassium chloride with those of sodium chloride in the diet of a hypertensive patient who did not know which kind of salt was being served to him. Gibbon was supposed to keep track of the patient's blood pressure. "What the results were I cannot recall, but I do remember my excitement at realizing that such controlled experimentation could add to the store of human knowledge" (53, 54).

Gibbon served on the surgical service of Edward D. Churchill at the Massachusetts General Hospital, Harvard Medical School, from 1930 to 1931. During 1931 Churchill operated on a female patient to remove her gallbladder. The operation seemed to go well, but several days later all the signs and symptoms of a pulmonary embolism developed. In 1931 the only possible cure for a pulmonary embolism was the Trendelenburg operation, which involved rapidly opening the patient's chest, localizing the thrombus in the pulmonary artery, and incising the artery and removing the thrombus. Unfortunately, rapid was not fast enough, and the mortality rate of the Trendelenburg operation was forbidding. For these reasons, Churchill decided to wait until the patient appeared to be in the last stages of the disease before attempting to remove the embolus. Gibbon observed the patient's vital signs all night. After ten hours, her blood pressure began to decrease and her condition became critical. Churchill was able to remove the embolus and clamp the incision in the pulmonary artery in six and one-half minutes, but the patient died (53, 54).

Assisting Churchill and waiting with the mortally ill patient during this stressful night, Gibbon began to think about some sort of device that might prevent a fatal outcome for those patients with pulmonary embolisms. As he said later, "The thought occurred to me that the patient's life might be saved if some of the blue blood in her veins could be continuously withdrawn into an extracorporeal blood circuit, exposed to an atmosphere of oxygen and then returned to the patient by way of a systemic artery in the central direction" (53, 54). The same thought occurred to Lindbergh (22), but Gibbon was surgically trained and, therefore, better qualified for the difficult task of devising a treatment for pulmonary embolism.

Mary Hopkins, Gibbon's wife and a trained surgical technician, aided his endeavor. Although Gibbon worked on various problems, he never abandoned the idea of developing a heart-lung bypass. He often mentioned his ideas to his surgical colleagues, but was rarely met with an enthusiastic response. He said, "Nobody encourages me." When Gibbon approached the head of the Department of Medicine at the Massachusetts General Hospital concerning his ideas of making a heart-lung bypass, he was strongly advised to spend his time on more promising projects if he wanted to succeed in academic medicine (54).

Churchill, while skeptical of Gibbon's ideas, agreed to grant him a year-long fellowship. He also provided him with a laboratory and money to hire a technician, who was Gibbon's wife. In 1934 Gibbon and his wife studied the possibility of building a heart-lung machine. As Gibbon writes, "So my wife and I, now with two children, returned to Boston in the autumn of 1934 to spend a year working on the first temporary artificial heart-lung blood circuit" (53).

At that time, Gibbon's research took some bizarre forms. He writes,

> My wife and I experimented on ourselves and on friends. For instance, to find out how vasoconstriction and vasodilatation in the extremities could be caused by a slight shift in body temperature, we used to sit in the bathroom with thermal couplers attached to our toes and with our hands and forearms immersed in hot water. Also, and I know this sounds odd, my wife would stick a highly sensitive thermometer into my rectum, after which I would swallow a stomach tube. We then poured ice water down the tube and measured the effect of this on temperature. We also tried such things as injecting an ice-cold solution into a vein of my forearm (53).

After his year of research in Boston, Gibbon returned to Philadelphia, where he noted that he learned a great deal about research techniques through his association with Eugene Landis. He writes, "It was this man (Landis) who gave me unwavering encouragement in what had by now become a principal ambition, to build an extracorporeal-blood circuit capable of temporarily taking over the cardiorespiratory functions" (54, 55).

Gibbon first used a Dale–Schuster finger-cot pump (56, 57). Gibbon added the internal valves that he had constructed from solid rubber stoppers. The blood oxygenator was the main problem. In systematic fashion, Gibbon read the literature and consulted engineers, but engineers dealt with fluids other than blood and did not consider the relationship of oxygen to hemoglobin. Blood foaming also became an obstacle. Blood foam cannot be returned to the systemic circulation and must be removed from the oxygenator. Gibbon decided to use cats as experimental animals since they were small and less expensive than dogs. The cats' size fit the technical resources available at the time. Of all the oxygenator models he tried, Gibbon decided that a revolving vertical cylinder with blood distributed over the interior surface by centrifugal force would be the most effective approach. Such a model was built after the method Hooker devised in 1915 (58). The problem with this system was hemolysis and the difficulty preserving a thin film of blood on the interior surface of the revolving cylinder.

Gibbon initially primed his pump with saline solution and gum acacia, the latter to give it more colloidal-osmotic pressure. In the beginning, the animals survived only for the immediate period following the procedure. By reducing the priming volume, the traumatic effect of extracorporeal circulation on the blood, such as hemolysis, was reduced.

Later, the finger-cot pump was replaced by a roller pump and primed with donor cat blood. Using this approach, Gibbon was able to occlude the pulmonary artery of cats for at least ten minutes, followed by survival of the cats for several hours.

Issekutz introduced the roller pump in 1927 (59), and DeBakey modified it in 1934 (60). A roller pump uses a flexible hollow conduit placed within a rigid circular channel. The ingress and egress of the conduit are connected by long tubes to conduct fluids from patient to pump-oxygenator and back. The conduit is stroked within its channel by a roller attached to the end of a bar. The end of the bar opposite the roller is attached to a motorized axle located at the center of the circle defined by the arc of the channel. The bar is driven in one direction with the roller adjusted to nearly occlude the flexible conduit, forcing fluid through the conduit. The roller bar's speed of rotation governs the fluid's rate of flow. The roller-pump principle served as the major pumping mechanism for heart-lung machines during the first several decades of open heart surgery.

Gibbon's work on the heart-lung machine was interrupted by four years of Army service beginning in 1942. In 1946 he returned to Philadelphia as professor of surgery and head of Surgical Research at the Jefferson Medical College (53, 54). An important development occurred. Executives of International Business Machines (IBM) offered to help modify Gibbon's prewar apparatus. Both IBM and Gibbon agreed that neither party would profit commercially from the arrangement. The engineers from IBM transformed Gibbon's prewar apparatus into an elaborate machine that was completed in 1949. The new instrumentation permitted the use of dogs, which introduced other problems, including particulate embolization that necessitated use of a filter placed between the arterial pump of the extracorporeal circuit and the arterial cannula of the recipient dog.

The first clinical use of the Gibbon heart-lung machine occurred in April 1952. Unfortunately, this patient was misdiagnosed (as atrial septal defect, not found at the operation), and the baby died soon after. An autopsy revealed that the child had a patent ductus arteriosus. Success was achieved on May 6, 1953, when the second intracardiac procedure using a heart-lung machine was accomplished. This time an atrial septal defect was found and successfully repaired. The procedure progressed without complications (53). This was the first successful surgical correction of an intracardiac defect using a heart-lung machine, and marked the beginning of a new era in cardiac surgery.

Gibbon's records show that the patient was connected to the heart-lung apparatus for a total of forty-five minutes. For twenty-seven of those minutes, her cardiorespiratory functions were maintained by the machine alone. With the patient's atrium opened, Gibbon closed the defect using a continuous silk suture. Cecilia, the patient, recovered uneventfully. Later, cardiac catheterization showed that the defect had been completely closed.

The publicity surrounding that operation disturbed the patient at first; later she shed her shyness and in 1963 made appearances as the American Heart Association's National Queen. Gibbon writes, "For me the experience was emotionally draining. In fact, I think that operation was the only time in my career that I did not personally dictate or write the operative procedure. I guess the tension of the event was too much to relive immediately afterwards" (53).

Gibbon attempted intracardiac surgical repair of congenital heart defects in two children, but the results were not encouraging. He continued experimental work on dogs for several years. His article on the repair of an atrial septal defect was published in 1954 (61); it was the last paper from Gibbon's research laboratory.

THE SWEDISH INFLUENCE

Efforts to purify heparin took place in Denmark (46) and Sweden (47, 48, 49) simultaneously with the developments in Toronto. Craaford, from the Karolinska Institutet in Stockholm, wrote in 1936 of his experience with the clinical use of heparin as a postoperative treatment for the prevention of thrombosis (50). Craaford influenced the work of Björk (51) at the Karolinska who, in 1948, published his work involving a rotating-disc oxygenator that resulted in successful animal perfusion.

The rotating-disc oxygenator, as described by Björk, was formed of many metallic discs, separated by thin spacers and mounted on a centrally located axle. The disc assembly, contained in a horizontal glass cylinder, rotated on its central axis in a pool of venous blood several centimeters deep. A thin film of blood collected on each rotating disc and was elevated into a respiratory gas mixture. Venous blood was pumped into one end of the rotating-disc oxygenator. The thin film of blood on each rotating disc absorbed oxygen as it released its excess carbon dioxide. Becoming oxygenated as it flowed through the oxygenator reservoir, the blood was then pumped out the opposite end as arterialized blood.

Melrose developed some variations in the geometry of the Björk system, reporting them in 1953 (62).

Fredrick Cross, who received his surgical education at the University of Minnesota in Owen Wangensteen's department, adapted the Björk rotating-disc oxygenator concept (63), improving its design and efficiency to accomplish important clinical success. The Cross concept achieved acceptance in many of the world's open heart surgical centers. Cross's adaptation employed 60 to 120 plastic-coated, stainless-steel discs, 12 cm in diameter. Flow rates could be increased or decreased depending on the number of discs used; likewise, the rotational speed of the discs could be altered. There was a practical limit to the rotational speed used, as foaming could develop at higher rates of speed. The Cross system had three basic advantages: it worked well, it was simple to use, and it was relatively inexpensive. The disadvantages included its being labor-intensive and requiring a large priming volume. The rotating-disc systems were constructed of a great many parts, and all blood proteins had to be cleaned after each use; then the system needed reassembly. This preparation was burdensome.

A variation of the disc-filming technique was developed and used by Craaford in 1957 (64). It consisted of six cylinders rotating in a basin of venous blood while being exposed to a respiratory gas. At higher flow rates this system was inefficient, and, as a consequence, incorporated a bubbling device on the venous inlet as a preoxygenator. The Craaford cylinder system achieved some regional popularity in Europe. It had the same advantages and disadvantages as the Cross disc oxygenator.

UNIVERSITY OF MINNESOTA CONTRIBUTIONS

The pacesetting and driving spirit for the development of open heart surgery occurred at Minneapolis and Rochester, Minnesota, following World War II, due to the cooperation of gifted men. First of all, Owen H. Wangensteen headed the Department of Surgery at the university from 1930 to 1967. Wangensteen was characterized by Lillehei as follows:

> Wangensteen was a truly visionary surgeon. His lifelong recognition of the relevance of basic science, and the insight to be derived from research in the training of young surgeons created the milieu and opportunities for great achievements by many of his pupils. Proverbial was Dr. Wangensteen's ability to spot talent and capabilities in his younger men whose aptitudes were not all obvious to others, often not even them-

selves, and then he would proceed to develop those assets by blending his material assistance with intellectual stimulation and encouragement (65).

Maurice Visscher, a renowned cardiovascular physiologist, was also on the faculty of the university, serving as chairman of the Department of Physiology from 1936 to 1968. Working together these two educators were great inspirational leaders for several decades (66).

During the late 1940s Clarence Dennis at the University of Minnesota became interested in the development of cardiopulmonary bypass. His experience was in both physiology and surgery. Dennis continued pump-oxygenator studies at the Downstate Medical Center of the State University of New York where he was chairman of Surgery. While still in Minnesota, Dennis tried various ideas on oxygenators and ultimately developed a filming system in which venous blood was delivered to the center of multiple, 50 cm diameter rotating circular screens (67). The Dennis screen oxygenator was used as cardiopulmonary support during the repair of a child's atrial septal defect on April 5, 1951 (68). Unfortunately, due to technical considerations, the patient died. Later, Dennis and his group concluded that air embolization was a major problem. Perfusion rates approximating normal cardiac output were used by Dennis (69).

On September 2, 1952, at the University of Minnesota Hospital, F. John Lewis became the first person to close an intracardiac defect under direct vision using inflow stasis and moderate hypothermia (70) without circulatory support. Lewis and Bigelow's work (71) described much of the physiology of hypothermia that would later be used with hypothermic perfusions.

CONTROLLED CROSS-CIRCULATION

In 1897 Theodor Billroth noted that the limits of surgery stopped at the walls of the heart since it would never be possible to perform surgery on such a vital organ (72). Billroth's admonition seemed to hold true into the early 1950s. Progress toward successful open heart surgery appeared stalled due to a number of unsuccessful attempts with the perfusion systems available at that time. A feeling prevailed that a sick human heart would never tolerate surgical intervention with the necessary cutting and sewing required to the heart muscle (73).

Lillehei distanced himself from these gloomy prospects by pursuing new ideas to overcome the obstacles. Years later, John Kirklin of the Mayo Clinic characterized Lillehei as "one of the most talented cardiac surgeons ever to work in this field" (73). In the same forum, Denton Cooley of the Texas Heart Institute observed that Lillehei was "a talented investigator and pioneer surgeon who provided the can opener for the largest picnic thoracic surgeons will ever know" (73). Lillehei thoroughly earned these and many more accolades that came to him over the years (see Chapter 11).

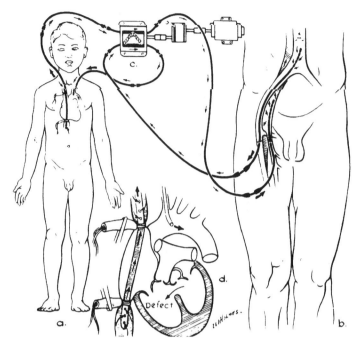

Figure 3.3. Cross-circulation arrangement used by C. Walton Lillehei.
(*Courtesy of the* Journal of the American Medical Association 75:928–945,
copyright 1957)

With the new awareness that successful cardiopulmonary bypass aided open
heart surgery and was possible with reduced perfusion rates, C.W. Lillehei and
two surgical fellows, Morley Cohen and Herbert Warden, envisioned a solution
to the problems of extracorporeal circulation. A small portion of a donor animal's arterial blood supply could be withdrawn through a precisely regulated pump.
This blood was perfused (pumped) to a smaller animal while simultaneously returning from the smaller animal an equal amount. Open heart surgery could then
be accomplished on the smaller animal while its blood flow and metabolic needs
were supplied by the larger animal. After dozens of successful laboratory experiments, controlled cross-circulation was deemed safe for clinical application (74,
75, 76). The key to its success was the precise regulation of blood exchange between the donor and recipient through well-calibrated pumps (Fig. 3.3).

    Clinical application of controlled cross-circulation raised some ethical
problems, uppermost being the donor risks. These risks included: potential problems of a general anesthetic, mixing blood from two individuals in spite of its
being well matched, and the possibility of a pumping mishap. Against these donor
risks, the alternative was the inevitable early death of the patient if left un-

treated. Before proceeding with the clinical application, all of these considerations were reviewed with Dr. Wangensteen and other members of the surgical department. Also of great importance to the project was the approval and participation of the pediatric Cardiology Department, particularly Paul Adams and Raymond Anderson (77).

In 1954, with all concerned parties in concurrence, the first successful correction of a ventricular septal defect was accomplished on March 26, 1954. Over the next sixteen months forty-five patients had surgical corrections of congenital heart defects with the aid of controlled cross-circulation. One nonfatal donor complication was followed by complete recovery (73).

Successful open heart surgery by Lillehei and his associates immediately attracted world attention that stimulated renewed interest in the use of extracorporeal circulation at the world's major heart centers.

In 1955, a year following his initial success, Lillehei presented a paper on the first total repair of tetralogy of Fallot defects (78). Alfred Blalock in a discussion of this paper said,

> I must say that I never thought I would live to see the day when this
> type of operative procedure could be performed. It is my guess that the
> ultimate answer will be the artificial heart-lung as developed by our pres-
> ident, Dr. Gibbon, and as it is being used now by more and more people.
> Dr. Gibbon has used it successfully for intracardiac surgery. I have heard
> that Dr. Kirklin of the Mayo Clinic, has now used it successfully in clos-
> ing several ventricular septal defects (78).

Clarence Dennis and his associates' interest in extracorporeal circulation filtered down to the medical students on the surgical services at the University of Minnesota. Richard DeWall was among these students. Finishing medical school in 1952, DeWall spent a year of internship in the U.S. Public Health Service in New York before returning to general practice in Minnesota.

DeWall was interested in laboratory medicine and expressed this interest to Richard Varco, the head of heart surgery at the University under Wangensteen. Varco offered DeWall an opportunity to work in C.W. Lillehei's laboratory, where Lillehei and his personnel were in the midst of experiments with controlled cross-circulation. DeWall was hired as an animal attendant and began work in Lillehei's laboratory on March 1, 1954, the month of the first clinical controlled cross-circulation operations. DeWall had the benefit of Wangensteen's educational philosophy of giving young aspirants the chance to prove themselves.

The controlled cross-circulation experiments on dogs served as an excellent learning experience in perfusion physiology. DeWall gained significant experience in laboratory methods and perfusion physiology due to Lillehei, Cohen, and Warden's shared knowledge. DeWall served as the perfusionist for most of

the clinical controlled cross-circulation operations. The donor for the operations provided an excellent physiologic oxygenator as well as continuously maintaining metabolic and blood homeostasis of both donor and patient. From the
beginning, Lillehei had recognized the obvious disadvantages of using donors,
namely, donor risk and size limitation of the patient. Thus, during the early course
of cross-circulation clinical activities, Lillehei asked DeWall if he would be interested in directing his efforts toward the development of an oxygenator system
to replace the donor. In early 1954 no generally recognized oxygenator existed.
DeWall accepted the challenge.

BUBBLE OXYGENATORS

Clark and associates' work (79) in 1950 marked the opening of the modern era
of the bubble oxygenator. In their system, venous blood was bubbled by oxygen
introduced through a microporous glass filter that produced pin-head-sized bubbles. Clark introduced silicone defoaming agents to bubble-oxygenator design.
The silicone agents removed excess bubbles from the blood and coated surfaces
the blood might contact. Silicone-coated surfaces were gentler to blood than glass
or metal surfaces. The Clark system was tested clinically by Helmsworth (80, 81)
with disappointing clinical results, possibly due to air embolism. Other bubble
systems described at this time did not advance the application of perfusion systems. Bubble systems for extracorporeal oxygenation remained suspect.

DeWall decided to pursue concepts not previously studied in oxygenator
systems. Since a hyperbaric approach had not been investigated, this seemed a
logical course to follow. For materials, Lillehei suggested that DeWall explore
the use of a large-bore polyvinyl hose. The hose was inexpensive, used in the
food processing industry, and readily available. Polyvinyl proved to be more compatible to blood than metal or glass containers. DeWall's hyperbaric concept involved exposing a thick film of venous blood to three atmospheres of oxygen
pressure. He anticipated that a thick blood film would be easier to manage than
spreading a thin layer over a large area. The arterial venous oxygen difference is
six volumes percent (82). Six volumes percent of oxygen could be transferred
to blood plasma in the absence of hemoglobin; at three atmospheres pressure, it
would supply the total oxygen requirement to oxygenate normal venous blood
without elaborate filming or bubbling techniques.

The hyperbaric apparatus used a four-foot polyvinyl hose. Venous blood
streamed down the hose, which was placed in a helical coil on its vertical axis.
The lower quarter of the tube, filled with blood, served as a reservoir. Halfway
down the hose, an oxygen inlet put oxygen into the system under three atmospheres pressure. At the top of the helix, a valve regulated pressure within the
tube. Exposed to the high oxygen pressure, blood flowing down the tube became
arterialized and accumulated in the reservoir. However, bubbles developed in the

reservoir blood and in the blood after decompression. It was then observed that bubbles remaining in the reservoir of the helix would layer on top of the oxygenated blood, becoming trapped, and would not be evacuated with the arterialized blood.

Previous oxygenator literature indicated problems with bubble or foam formation. Using these observations, DeWall decided to accept bubbles and learn how to master them. In reviewing methods for the oxygenation of blood, the direct introduction of oxygen into the venous blood seemed the simplest and most economical approach to blood oxygenation. It also appeared that if the bubbles were kept large, there would still be sufficient blood gas interface for the exchange of oxygen and carbon dioxide; yet the coalescence and removal of the bubbles could be simplified.

Clark's bubble oxygenator used a microporous glass filter for oxygen dispersion, causing the formation of bubbles, 1 mm or less in size, which were difficult to remove from the arterialized blood. Such small bubbles also did not adequately transfer the excess carbon dioxide from the blood into the respiratory gas mixture for elimination from the system (79). DeWall chose to make a gas-dispersion system forming large bubbles, 5 mm to 10 mm in diameter. This was accomplished by means of twenty-two multiple-size hypodermic needles inserted through a rubber stopper and placed at the bottom of a 1.5 inch diameter polyvinyl hose. The length of the tube carrying the bubble mixture was altered depending on the time desired for the blood-oxygen contact and the expected perfusion rate. Venous blood was introduced over the top of the oxygen-dispersion needles. With these variables, the size of the oxygenator could be changed depending on the patient's size and optimize the amount of blood necessary for priming the system.

Silicone, as described by Clark (79), was used to coat the top of the bubble chamber. The blood's contact with the silicone-coated surfaces served to coalesce the flowing bubble mass, but it did not eliminate all of the smallest bubbles. The blood was arterialized by the bubble contact and after the bubbles were eliminated, the arterialized blood was introduced from the oxygenation hose into the top of a vertically positioned coiled (helix) hose, 1 inch in diameter and 150 inches to 250 inches long. The hose length varied with individual patient needs. About this time, Norman Shumway, working with F.J. Lewis at the University of Minnesota, confirmed that larger bubbles dispersed more easily than small, foam-sized bubbles (83).

A safe blood debubbling system evolved using information from DeWall's hyperbaric-oxygenator experiments, which demonstrated that bubbles could be removed from a bubble blood mixture by being trapped in a helically coiled hose. It was apparent that blood containing bubbles had a lesser density than blood free of bubbles. Blood containing bubbles from a blood, respiratory-gas mixing chamber, as described above, flowed into the top of a coiled-hose helix 18 inches high filled with blood. This blood was continuously removed from the bottom end of the hose through a blood filter and returned to the patient. As the mixed blood progressed down the tube, lighter bubbled blood layered above normal blood, becoming trapped against the upper wall of the hose and thus allowing heavier, bubble-free blood to slide beneath. Hydrostatic pressure increased as the blood passed down the tube. The bubbles in bubble-containing blood coalesced under increasing hydrostatic pressure as the blood flowed down the tube. The coalesced bubbles released their excess oxygen and carbon dioxide, which passed up and out of the tube.

DeWall, with the encouragement, support, and input of Lillehei, had the helical-reservoir blood oxygenator ready for use in open heart surgery by Lillehei and his team within nine months after starting the project (84, 85).

The simple, disposable helical-reservoir oxygenator was first used May 13, 1955 (85, 86), on a small child with a ventricular septal defect. Dr. Lillehei was the operating surgeon. The appeal of the helical-reservoir system was that it was efficient, heat-sterilized, easy to assemble, inexpensive, disposable after a one-time use, and had no moving parts. The system fulfilled its purpose when used by knowledgeable surgeons.

A number of surgical groups were unsuccessful at that time using the helical-reservoir system (as well as other systems) and, in the process, condemned it (22, 23, 24). Their lack of success could be attributed to two factors. First, success in the early days of open heart surgery required the union of two disciplines, under-standing of perfusion physiology and competence with the perfusion equipment. Second, surgical acumen was needed in the new surgical specialty of open heart surgery. As the helical-reservoir oxygenator appeared to be a jerry-built appara-tus, some observers thought they could improve on it without understanding the principles involved. They were unwilling to spend the time and effort in research laboratories and teaching clinics to learn their craft.

The helical-reservoir pump oxygenator system came into wide use in the United States and abroad (87, 88, 89, 90). The pump used with the helical-reser-voir system was a finger-cam pump (Sigmamoter Inc., Middleport, N.Y.), readily available at the time as a laboratory pump for fluids. This was also the pump used for all controlled cross-circulation circulation experiments and clinical cases. The principle of this pump was that a flexible conduit was placed between a compression plate and serially compressed by metal fingers. Each finger's base was adapted to a cam shaft, activating each finger a few degrees out of phase with the preceding finger. In this manner, fluid (blood) was pushed in one direction.

The inexpensive, disposable helical-reservoir, bubble-oxygenator system soon evolved into commercially available units constructed with polyvinyl sheet ma-terial (91). Thorough animal laboratory work tested the commercial design and animal safety preceded the approval of this oxygenator's manufacture for clinical application. The commercial oxygenators had one especially important characteristic. They were constructed using set measurements that eliminated the tendency for inquiring yet often unprepared minds to tinker with design.

The Rygg–Kvisgaard oxygenator system (92), similar in many respects to the plastic-sheet oxygenator (91), became popular toward the end of the 1950s, especially in Europe. In the early 1960s a disposable rigid-bubble oxygenator made of polycarbonate (92, 93) became available. Several manufacturers provided such rigid, simple systems that replaced the use of filming oxygenators. Bubble-oxygenator systems remained in general use until the introduction of membrane oxygenators in the early 1980s.

Three comprehensive books were published in 1960, 1962, and 1981, reflecting the status of extracorporeal circulation, its related physiology, and equipment (22, 94, 95).

Mayo Clinic Contributions

In 1948 John Kirklin developed his interest in congenital heart disease while working with children at the Boston Children's Hospital during a six-month tutelage following his surgical residency at the Mayo Clinic.

Upon returning to the Mayo Clinic from Boston, Kirklin mentioned that his renewed interest in intracardiac surgery had been stimulated by an operation on a patient with pulmonary valvular stenosis. The autopsy on the patient who died two days later revealed that the patient suffered from a severe secondary subvalvular obstruction that thwarted the attempt to relieve the right ventricular obstruction by a closed valvotomy. Kirklin studied the autopsy specimen with Jesse Edwards, a cardiac pathologist, and Earl Wood, a cardiac physiologist, and concluded that an open technique would have been necessary for successful surgery (96).

Kirklin and his associates decided to develop an extracorporeal circulatory system of the Gibbon–IBM type (97). After two and one-half years of intensive work in Mayo's engineering shops and animal laboratories, a Mayo–Gibbon pump-oxygenator was produced (98, 99). At the Mayo Clinic on March 22, 1955, one year after Lillehei's success in Minneapolis with controlled cross-circulation, Kirklin successfully repaired a child's ventricular septal defect using the Mayo–Gibbon heart-lung machine (100).

Kirklin developed a thorough knowledge of the pathophysiology and surgical problems represented by congenital heart disease. This, combined with diligent effort in the research laboratories in perfecting their heart-lung machine, enabled him and his team to be masters of open heart surgery early on. Kirklin effectively coordinated two new and difficult disciplines, as Lillehei had done. Following his first success, Kirklin soon operated on seven other patients,

promptly reporting these cases (96, 100). This clinical success immediately attracted worldwide attention.

The Mayo–Gibbon pump-oxygenator was costly to produce and expensive
to maintain and clean. Consequently, it never achieved widespread usage once the
simple, inexpensive, and disposable systems became available in the late 1950s.

For the first two years of open heart surgery, only two centers in the world
performed these operations: the University of Minnesota, Minneapolis, and the
Mayo Clinic in Rochester. The fact that the two cities were only ninety miles
apart made it convenient for heart surgeons from all over the world to visit both
places on the same trip. At the University of Minnesota, they saw what appeared
to be simple techniques, using a primitive-appearing apparatus. Although ap-
pealing, due to affordability and seemingly easy duplication, was it too simple?
Could it be trusted? At the Mayo Clinic, they saw a beautifully engineered and
sophisticated Mayo–Gibbon machine with its gleaming, stainless-steel appearance, but it was very costly. This presented a real dilemma for most visitors.

MEMBRANE OXYGENATORS

Original concepts usually undergo refinements and continuous improvement.
Such was the case with pump-oxygenator systems. The first successful oxygenators had employed a direct exposure of a respiratory gas to blood filmed over
discs, screens, or bubbles. If an ideal oxygenator had been possible, it would have
separated the blood from the respiratory gas by means of a membrane. Efficient
and well understood gas-permeable membranes were not available during most
of the 1950s. The belief that blood-membrane-gas interface creates less blood
trauma than direct blood-gas interface rationalized the pursuit of a membrane
oxygenator.

Clowes experienced difficulties with bubble oxygenators (21); consequently,
he directed his attention from 1955 to 1960 to the development of a membrane
oxygenator system. The gas permeability of a number of membranes was one of
the studies that he reported in 1960 (94). Galletti expanded this list of potentially suitable membranes (22). Clowes developed a parallel-plate oxygenator
using two membranes, polyethylene and ethylcellulose. The parallel-plate concept involved layering multiple sheets of membrane, 0.5 m^2 in size, which were
supported and sealed at the edges by a frame. Venous blood and respiratory gas
were directed into alternate layers of the membrane plates and removed from the
opposite end. The oxygenator was positioned on its horizontal axis. The Clowes
membrane oxygenator worked clinically (94), but it was cumbersome to manage
and difficult to assemble. It could not compete with the simplicity of filmers
and bubblers. Clowes' work helped lay the foundation for future membrane-
oxygenator development.

Bramson initiated the next stage in membrane oxygenation in 1965, summarizing his work in 1981 (95). The Bramson membrane oxygenator used a reinforced silicone rubber membrane that was more efficient than the membranes available to Clowes. The Bramson oxygenator was a parallel-plate design in a circular, rather than rectangular shape and accessed by a complicated manifold introduced into its core. The membranes, however, were disposable in this system and the apparatus required arduous hand assembly.

By 1980 the stage was set and the time right for an efficient, commercially produced membrane oxygenator. Such systems could provide circulatory support for days at a time. Filmers and bubblers had been unable to do this because of their destructive impact on blood when used over long periods of time.

Three configurations evolved. One geometry employed the use of hollow fibers or tiny tubes as small as 200 microns in diameter, grouped in parallel. Venous blood was directed through the tubes with the respiratory gas outside. De-Wall described such an oxygenator in 1958 (101), but this work predated the availability of materials and technology for commercial development. In the 1980s systems built to the hollow-fiber configuration became available. A second type of membrane oxygenator, made available in the 1980s, was a parallel-plate oxygenator with the plates folded like accordion bellows. The third design took the form of a large sheet of reinforced silicone rubber. The sheet was rolled into a spiral with separate pathways for the venous blood and respiratory gas, as described by Kolobow (102). Membrane-oxygenator history and performance are found in several books relating to extracorporeal circulation (22, 94, 95, 103).

Membrane oxygenators are now used in most perfusions in the United States. A partial list of membrane-oxygenator manufacturers includes: Bentley, Bos-CM40 Capillary Membrane Oxygenator, American Bentley-American Hospital Supply; Cobe Membrane Lung (CML EXCEL) Cobe Labs, Lakewood, CO (Parallel Plate, folded membrane); and Sci-Med Spiral Membrane Oxygenator, Minneapolis, MN. One can expect technology and perfusion equipment to be refined and further developed in the future.

HEMODILUTION

Extracorporeal circulation implies blood circulation by means of an apparatus outside the body. To begin circulation, the apparatus must be primed, or filled with a fluid. In the early days of open heart surgery, surgeons only considered blood as the priming fluid. Due to preservatives used, stored blood was highly acidic; it also lost its ability to clot. Because of this, fresh blood, drawn the day of surgery and preserved in a nonacidic heparin mixture, was the standard priming fluid of the times. The blood volume required for priming was up to 1,800 cc for bubble oxygenators and 3,000 cc for film oxygenators (90).

In addition, surgical blood loss had to be replaced. The blood-banking system became severely strained. Early in the morning prior to surgery, blood types between donors and patients had to be matched. Using many different blood sources increased the risk of hepatitis. Logistic problems limited the number of patients that could be accommodated for surgery. By the late 1950s the introduction of low-prime, commercially available bubble-oxygenator systems (91, 92, 93, and others) began to replace the filming systems.

In 1961 Foote, Trede, and Maloney recommended the use of standard ACD (acid-citrate-dextrose) preserved-bank blood as acceptable for priming an extracorporeal circuit (104). They showed that the natural body-blood buffer system compensated for the acid state of the bank blood. The use of ordinary, stored bank blood as a prime for perfusion systems eased procurement problems; however, surgeons continued to search for alternative priming solutions.

Hemodilution is the dilution of blood with nonblood agents. Cooley (105, 106), Zuhdi (107), and Greer (108) introduced a major movement using hemodilution techniques for priming an extracorporeal circuit. Cooley's discovery of hemodilution resulted from emergency surgery on a patient with a pulmonary embolism. Since there was insufficient time to obtain blood for a prime, he used 5% dextrose and water in place of a blood prime. The patient did well in spite of a significant dilution of blood. These surgeons noted the patient's exceptional recovery following perfusions using a hemodilution prime.

The patient's hematocrit was reduced from the normal value of 40% to 20% to 25% following a perfusion using hemodilution prime. Because of hemodilution, the patient's urinary output during the operation was excellent. With such good urinary output during the perfusion, circulating blood volume dropped. To compensate for this drop, an additional amount of diluting solution was returned to the oxygenator system, to equal the urinary loss. When the procedure ended, the pump-oxygenator contents were returned to the patient, as needed.

Surgeons continued to investigate a variety of priming solutions (109, 110). They hoped to find a perfusate more physiologic than 5% dextrose and water. Some tried adding blood plasma and albumin, thinking their greater osmotic pressure would be advantageous. These agents, however, were expensive and still carried the hepatitis risk. Many groups added a variety of electrolytes and buffers to priming solutions. The hope was to offset the hyponatremia caused by the nonelectrolyte containing 5% dextrose in water. Today, balanced electrolyte solutions, commercially prepared, serve as priming agents.

Hemodilution techniques, combined with improved perfusion equipment, have reduced blood needs for the average open heart surgical case by over 50 percent. In some circumstances, open heart surgical procedures can be accomplished totally without using blood.

HYPOTHERMIA

Decreasing a patient's temperature (hypothermia) is an important adjunct to open heart surgery. A body's metabolic rate increases or decreases with temperature, as does the rate of all chemical reactions. A person with a normal body temperature can tolerate about four minutes of complete circulatory arrest without experiencing cerebral damage. As the body temperature decreases, the brain can tolerate longer periods of time without blood flow.

In 1950 Bigelow (71) wrote of his experiments using moderate hypothermia in dogs. This work studied the animals' physiologic responses to a body temperature drop of 8° to 10°F. Bigelow accomplished this by wrapping the subject in temperature-controlling blankets that could cool or warm. The experiments' purpose was to develop techniques permitting surgery inside a dog's heart for up to eight minutes with temporary inflow occlusion and circulatory arrest. Inflow occlusion involved the blockage of blood flow to the heart. No extracorporeal circulatory support was used.

Lewis (70) also studied the effects of moderate hypothermia and applied it clinically, becoming the first surgeon to repair a defect inside the heart under direct vision. This occurred on September 2, 1952, when he repaired an atrial septal defect in a five-year-old child.

Unfortunately, the repair of some intracardiac defects requires more than eight minutes, and some defects can only be approached by an incision through the ventricle. The heart can tolerate an incision through the atrium at temperatures of moderate hypothermia without disturbing heart function. However, at such temperatures, the ventricle becomes irritable from an incision and fibrillates, or loses an effective beat. Operating at moderate hypothermic temperatures requires that the patient maintain a regular heart beat even if slower than normal. The cold, fibrillating heart is difficult to restart, compromising the patient's recovery. These factors limited the usefulness of moderate hypothermia for open heart surgery. Without an extracorporeal circulation method to rewarm the patient, transventricular surgery is hazardous.

During the earliest open heart operations, attempts were made to maintain body temperatures at normo-thermic levels by placing the patient on heated blankets. Cool operating rooms and large surfaces of the exposed open chests caused significant heat loss, and, as a consequence, heating elements were incorporated into extracorporeal circulatory circuits. Adverse metabolic changes in the patient that resulted from increasingly long and difficult operations became apparent. The lessons of moderate hypothermia, which reduced metabolic demands and resulted from lowered body temperatures, led to the introduction of combined blood cooling and warming systems to extracorporeal blood-circulation circuits. This occurred by the late 1950s and has since been incorporated into all extracorporeal blood circuits.

METABOLIC HOMEOSTASIS

General anesthesia compromises a patient's metabolic normalcy. Extracorporeal circulation contributes to this compromise and interferes with normal cardiovascular reflexes. A patient's survival depends on maintaining a normal metabolic balance; therefore, an extracorporeal circulation system must be monitored for the patient's metabolic responses during perfusion. In the early years of perfusion-supported surgery, blood samples were removed from the circuit for periodic checks of hematocrit, oxygen content, acid-base balance, and electrolyte values. Additional constituents of the blood were also occasionally tested.

Anesthesia, hypothermia, extracorporeal circulation, and duration of the surgery can cause many rapid changes in the important metabolic factors in the blood, making intermittent spot checks inadequate. From the beginning of open heart surgery, efforts have been directed toward the development of rapid monitoring systems of metabolic balance. Many systems, now incorporated directly in the extracorporeal blood circuit, monitor data continuously for the patient's safety.

Advances in the treatment of heart disease during the past twenty years would not have been possible without the cardiopulmonary bypass. It took many years of hard work before its first clinical use. Many years later it became generally available throughout the world. Each individual step (anticoagulation, oxygenators, hemodilution, metabolic homeostasis, azygos flow principle) had its own tortuous road to success. It is to be expected that this development will continue, making open heart surgery even more accessible and successful.

The success with cardiopulmonary bypass has opened the door to modern cardiac surgery. This has been made possible by courageous pioneers, some of them, like Gibbon, with little scientific training, but with persistence and imagination. It is encouraging that advances in medicine can still be made by imaginative, hands-on physicians. But much remains to be done. There are as yet no useful blood substitutes; this would be a major advance in trauma and military surgery and would avoid the dire complications of blood contaminated with hepatitis and AIDS virus.

References

1. Langendorff, O. Untersuchungen uberlebender Saeugetierherzen. Arch. Gesamten Physiol., 61:291–338, 1895.
2. Langendorff, O. Geschichtliche Bemerkungen zur Methode des Uberlebenden Warmblueterherzens. Muench. Med. Wochenschr., 50(1):508–509, 1903.
3. Fye, B.H. Newell Martin—A remarkable career destroyed by neurasthenia and alcoholism. Journal of the History of Medicine and Applied Sciences, 40:133–166, 1985.
4. Clark, A.J. The action of ions and lipoids upon the frog's heart. J. Physiol., 47:66–107, 1913.
5. Loewi, O., and O. Weselko. Ueber den Kohlehydratumsatz des isolierten Herzens normaler und diabetischer Tiere. Pfluegers Arch. Gesamte Physiol., 158:155–188, 1914.
6. Lussana, F. Action de l'Alanine sur le coeur isole de tortue. Arch. Int. Physiol., 9:393–406, 1910.

7. Howell, W.H. On the relation of the blood to the automaticity and sequence of the heart beat. Am. J. Physiol., 2:47–81, 1899.
8. Ringer, S. Concerning the influence exerted by each of the constituents of the blood on the contraction of the ventricle. J. Physiol., 3:380–393, 1882.
9. Vernon, H.N. The respiration of the tortoise heart in relation to functional activity. J. Physiol., 40:295–316, 1910.
10. Starling, E.H. The Linacre Lecture on the Development of the Heart Given at Cambridge, 1915. London, Longmans, Green, 1918.
11. Martin, H., and E.C. Applegarth. On the temperature limits of the vitality of the mammalian heart. Studies from the Biology Laboratory, Johns Hopkins University, 4:285, 1890.
12. Evans, C.A. The metabolism of the cardiac muscle. Recent Advances in Physiology. London, Churchill, 6th ed., 1939, pp. 157–215.
13. Locke, F.S., and O. Rosenheim. The disappearance of dextrose when perfused through the isolated mammalian heart. J. Physiol., 31:xiv, 1904.
14. Rohde, E. Stoffwechseluntersuchungen am ueberlebenden Warmblueterherzens: zur Physiologie des Herzstoffwechsels. Hoppe-Seyler's Z. Physiol. Chem., 68:181–235, 1910.
15. Ringer, S. A further contribution regarding the influence of the different constituents of the blood on the contraction of the heart. J. Physiol., 4:29–42, 1883.
16. Ringer, S. On the mutual antagonism between lime and potash salts in toxic doses. J. Physiol., 5:247–254, 1884.
17. Kronecker, H. Ueber die Speisung des Froschherzen (Meeting of the Physiol. Soc., Berlin). Arch. Anat. Physiol., p. 21, 1878.
18. Bing, R.J. The course of science and cardiac metabolism. Circulation Research, 38:151–155, 1976.
19. Tigerstedt, R.A. Physiologie des Kreislaufes. Berlin, DeGreyter, 2nd ed., 1921, vol. 1, p. 334.
20. Bing, R.J. The metabolism of the heart. Harvey Lectures, 50:27–70, 1954–55.
21. Liljestrand, G. Zum hundertsten Geburtstage Robert Tigerstedts. Acta Physiol. Scand., 31:9–29, 1954.
22. Carrel, A., and C. Lindbergh. The Culture of Organs. New York, Hoeber, 1938.
23. Bing, R.J. Lindbergh and the biological sciences. Texas Heart Inst. J., 14:231, 1987.
24. Malinin, T.I. Surgery and Life: The Extraordinary Career of Alexis Carrel. New York, Harcourt, Brace, Jovanovitch, 1979.
25. Frank, O. Zur Dynamik des Herzmuskels. Z. Biol., 14:370–439, 1895.
26. Clowes, G.H.A., Jr., W.E. Neville, A. Hopkins, J. Anzola, and F.A. Simeone. Factors contributing to success or failure in the use of a pump-oxygenator for complete bypass of the heart and lungs. Experimental and Clinical Surg., 36:557–559, 1954.
27. Galletti, P.M., and G.H. Brecher (eds). Heart-Lung Bypass: Principles and Techniques of Extracorporeal Circulation. New York, Grune & Stratton, 1962.
28. Diesh, G., S.A. Flynn, D. Marable, D.G. Mulder, K.J. Schmutzer, W.P. Longmire Jr., and J.V. Maloney Jr. Comparison of low flow (azygos) and high flow principles of extracorporeal circulation employing a bubble oxygenator. Surg., 42:67, 1957.
29. Abrams, L.D., F. Ashton, E.J. Charles, A.L. D'Abreu, J. Fejfar, E.J. Hamley, W.A. Hudson, R.E. Lee, R. Lightwood, and E.T. Matthews. Total cardiopulmonary bypass in the laboratory. Lancet, 2:239, 1958.
30. Showstack, J.A., K.E. Rosenfeld, D.W. Garnick, H.S. Luft, R.W. Schaffarzick, and J. Fowles. Association of volume with outcome of coronary artery bypass graft surgery. Scheduled vs. nonscheduled operations. JAMA, 257(6):785 and 257(18):2438, 1987.
31. Kaiser, G.C. Institutional variation of coronary artery bypass graft surgery: emphasis on myocardial protection. Circulation, 65:85–89, 1982.

32. Hartridge, H., and F.J.W. Roughton. The kinetics of haemoglobin II. The velocity with which oxygen dissociates from its combination with haemoglobin. Proc. Roy. Soc., 104:395, 1923.
33. Hartridge, H., and F.J.W. Roughton. The rate of distribution of dissolved gases between the red blood corpuscle and its fluid environment. J. Physiol., 62:232–242, 1927.
34. Houston, C.S. Going Higher, The Story of Man and Altitude. Little, Brown, 1987.
35. DeWall, R.A., T.B. Grage, A.S. McFee, and M.A. Chiechi. Theme and variations on blood oxygenators. I. Bubble oxygenators. Surg., 50:931–940, 1962.
36. DeWall, R.A., T.B. Grage, A.S. McFee, and M.A. Chiechi. Theme and variations on blood oxygenators. II. Film oxygenators. Surg., 51:251, 1962.
37. DeWall, R.A., and T.B. Grage. The evolution of blood bubble oxygenators. In: Congenital Heart Disease. F.A. David Co., Philadelphia, 1962, pp. 133–148.
38. Brodie, T.G. The perfusion of surviving organs. J. Physiol., 29:266–275, 1903.
39. McLean, J. The thromboplastic action of cephalin. Am. J. Physiol., 41:250–257, 1916.
40. Howell, W.H., and E. Holt. Two new factors in blood coagulation, heparin and pro-antithrombin. Am. J. Physiol., 47:328, 1918.
41. Fry, W.B. Heparin: the contributions of William Henry Howell. Circulation, 69: 1198, 1984.
42. Baird, J. Presidential address: "Give us the tools . . ." The story of heparin as told by sketches from the lives of William Howell, Jay McLean, Charles Best and Gordon Murry. J. Vasc. Surg., 11:4, 1990.
43. Charles, A.F., and D.A. Scott. Studies on heparin: IV. Observations on the chemistry of heparin. Biochem. J., 30: 1926, 1936.
44. Gibbon, J.H., Jr. Artificial maintenance of circulation during experimental occlusion of pulmonary artery. Arch. Surg., 34:1105–1131, 1937.
45. Chargaff, E., and K. Olson. Studies on the chemistry of blood coagulation, studies on the action of heparin and other anticoagulants. The influence of protamine on the anticoagulant effect in vivo. J. Biol. Chem., 122:153–167, 1937.
46. Schmitz, F., and A. Fisher. Ueber die chemiche Natur des Heparins: II. Die Reindarstellung des Heparins. Ztschr. f. Physiol. Chem., 216:264–273, 1933.
47. Jorpes, J.E. The chemistry of heparin. Biochem. J., 29:1817, 1936. 1) On heparin, its chemical nature and properties. 427–433.
48. Jorpes, J.E. Heparin: Its Chemistry, Physiology and Application in Medicine. London, Oxford Press, 1939, pp. 218–229.
49. Jorpes, J.E. The origin and physiology of heparin: the specific therapy in thrombosis. Ann. Intern. Med., 27:361–370, 1947.
50. Craaford, C. Preliminary report on post-operative treatment with heparin as a preventative of thrombosis. Acta Chir. Scand., 29:1817, 1937.
51. Björk, V.O. Brain perfusions in dogs with artificially oxygenated blood. Acta Chir. Scand., 96:1–122, 1948.
52. Le Gallois, J.J.C. (1770–1814) Quoted and illustrated by Griffenhagen, G.B., and C.H. Hughes. In: The History of the Mechanical Heart. Smithsonian Report for 1955, pp. 339–356. Publication #4241.
53. Gibbon, J.H., Jr. Medicine's living history. Medical World News, 13:47, 1972.
54. Gibbon, J.H., Jr. The development of the heart-lung apparatus. Rev. Surg., 27:231, 1970.
55. Hill, J.D., and J.H. Gibbon Jr. The development of the first successful heart-lung machine. Ann. Thorac. Surg., 34:337–341, 1982.
56. Finnegan, M.O. The development of the heart-lung for intracardiac surgery 1930–1957. Thesis (B.A.) Princeton, NJ, Princeton University, 1983.
57. Dale, H.H., and E.H. Schuster. A double perfusion pump. J. Physiol., 64:356–364, 1928.

58. Hooker, D.R. The perfusion of the mammalian medulla: the effect of calcium and of potassium on the respiratory and cardiac centers. Am. J. Physiol., 38:200–208, 1915.

59. Issekutz, V.B. Beitraege zur Wirkung des Insulins. Biochem. Ztschr., 183:283, 1927.

60. DeBakey, M.E. Simple continuous-flow blood transfusion instrument. New Orleans M. & S.J., 87:386–389, 1934.

61. Gibbon, J.H., Jr. Application of a mechanical heart and lung apparatus to cardiac surgery. Minn. Med., 37:171, 1954.

62. Melrose, D.G. A mechanical heart-lung for use in man. Brit. Med. J., 2:57, 1953.

63. Cross, F.S., R.M. Berne, U. Horose, E.B. Kay, and R.D. Jones. Evaluation of rotating disc type of reservoir-oxygenator. Proc. Soc. Exper. Biol. and Med., 93:210, 1956.

64. Craaford, C., B. Norberg, and A. Senning. Clinical studies in extracorporeal circulation with a heart-lung machine. Acta Chir. Scand., 112:220, 1957.

65. Lillehei, C.W. A personalized history of extracorporeal circulation. Trans. Am. Soc. Artif. Int. Org., 28:5, 1982.

66. Wangesnsteen, O.H., and S.D. Wangensteen. The Rise of Surgery. Minneapolis, University of Minnesota Press, 1978.

67. Karlson, K.E., C. Dennis, D. Westover, and D. Sanderson. Pump oxygenator to support the heart and lungs for brief periods. I. Evaluation of oxygenator techniques. Surg., 29:678, 1951.

68. Dennis, C., D.S. Spreng Jr., G.E. Nelson, K.E. Karlson, R.M. Nelson, J.V. Thomas, W.P. Eder, and R.L. Varco. Development of a pump oxygenator to replace the heart and lungs. An apparatus applicable to human patients and applied to 1 case. Ann. Surg., 134:709, 1951.

69. Newman, M.H., J.H. Stuckey, B.S. Levowitz, L.A. Young, C. Dennis, C. Fries, E.J. Gorayeb, M. Zuhdi, K. Karlson, S. Adler, and M. Gliedman. Complete and partial perfusion of animal and human subjects with the pump-oxygenator. Surg., 38:30, 1955.

70. Lewis, F.J., and M. Taufic. Closure of atrial septal defects with aid of hypothermia: experimental accomplishments and the report of one successful case. Surg., 33:52, 1953.

71. Bigelow, W.G., J.C. Callahan, and J.A. Hopps. General hypothermia for experimental intracardiac surgery. Ann. Surg., 132:531, 1950.

72. Billroth, T. Cited by Löwenbach, G. Beitrag zur Kenntniss der Geschwuelste der submaxillar-speicheldruese. Virchow's Arch. (Path. Anat.), 150:73–111, 1897.

73. Lillehei, C.W., R.L. Varco, M. Cohen, H.E. Warden, C. Patton, and J.H. Moller. The first open heart repairs of ventricular septal defect, atrio-ventricular communis, and tetraology of Fallot using extracorporeal circulation by cross circulation: a thirty year follow-up. Ann. Thorac. Surg., 41:4, 1986.

74. Warden, H.E., M. Cohen, R.C. Read, and C.W. Lillehei. Controlled cross circulation for open intracardiac surgery. J. Thorac. Surg., 28:33, 1954.

75. Warden, H.E., M. Cohen, R.A. DeWall, E. Schultz, J.J. Buckely, R.C. Read, and C.W. Lillehei. Experimental closure of intraventricular septal defects and further physiological studies on controlled cross circulation. Surgical Forum, American College of Surgeons, 1954. Philadelphia, W.B. Saunders Co., 1955, pp. 22–26.

76. Lillehei, C.W., M. Cohen, H.W. Warden, and R.I. Varco. The direct vision intracardiac correction of congenital anomalies by controlled cross circulation. Surgery, 38: 11, 1955.

77. Adams, P., R.L. Anderson, C.W. Lillehei, and N. Meyne. Reversibility of pulmonary hypertension following closure of ventricular septal defects. AMA Am. Dis. Child, 98:558, 1955.

78. Lillehei, C.W., M. Cohen, J.E. Warden, R.C. Read, J.B. Aust, and R.L. Varco. Direct vision intracardiac surgical correction of the tetralogy of Fallot, pentalogy of Fallot, and pulmonary atresia defects. Report of first ten cases. Ann. Surg., 142:418, 1955.

79. Clark, L.C., Jr., F. Gollan, and B. Vishwa. The oxygenization of blood by gas disper-sion. Science, 111:85, 1950.
80. Helmsworth, J.A., L.C. Clark Jr., S. Kaplan, R.T. Sherman, and T. Largen. Artificial oxygenization and circulation during complete bypass of the heart. J. Thorac. Surg., 34:117, 1952.
81. Helmsworth, J.A., L.C. Clark Jr., S. Kaplan, and R.T. Sherman. An oxygenator pump for use in total by-pass of the heart and lungs. J. Thorac. Surg., 26:617, 1953.
82. Gibbs, E.L., W.G. Lennox, L.F. Nims, and F.A. Gibbs. Arterial and cerebral venous blood: arterial-venous differences in man. J. Biol. Chem., 144:325, 1942.
83. Shumway, N.E., M.L. Gliedman, and F.J. Lewis. A mechanical pump oxygenator for successful cardiopulmonary by-pass surgery. Surgery 40:831, 1956.
84. Lillehei, C.W., R.A. DeWall, V.L. Gott, and R.L. Varco. The direct vision correction of calcific aortic stenosis by means of a pump-oxygenator and retrograde coronary sinus perfusion. Dis. Chest., 30:133, 1956.
85. DeWall, R.A., H.E. Warden, R.C. Read, V.L. Gott, N.R. Ziegler, R.L. Varco, and C.W. Lillehei. A simple expendable artificial oxygenator for open heart surgery. Surg. Clin. N. Amer. Philadelphia, W.B. Saunders Co., pp. 1025–1034, 1956.
86. Lillehei, C.W., R.A. DeWall, R.C. Read, H.E. Warden, and R.L. Varco. Direct vision intracardiac surgery in man using a simple disposable artificial oxygenator. Dis. Chest. 29:1–8, 1956.
87. Cooley, D.A., B.A. Belmont, J.R. Latson, and J.R. Pierce. Bubble diffusion oxygena-tor for cardiopulmonary bypass. J. Thorac. Surg., 35:131, 1958.
88. Cooley, D.A., H.A. Collins, J.W. Giacobine, G.C. Morris Jr., L.R. Soltero-Harring-ton, and F.J. Harberg. The pump oxygenator in cardiovascular surgery: observations based upon 450 cases. Amer. Surgeon, 24:870, 1958.
89. Dubost, C., G. Nahas, C. Lenfant, J. Pasetcq, J. Guery, J. Rauanet, M. Weiss, and R. Heim de Balsac. Chirurgie a coeur ouvert sous circulation extracorporeal: Ensem-ble pompe-oxygenateur de Lillehei-DeWall. Pouman-Coeur, 12:641, 1956.
90. Dubost, C., R. Heim der Balsac, R.A. DeWall, C. Lenfant, J. Guery, J. Passelcq, M. Weiss, and J. Rounet. Extracorporeal circulation and heart surgery. Brit. Heart J., 19:67, 1957.
91. Gott, V.L., R.A. DeWall, M. Paneth, M. Zuhdi, W. Weirich, R.L. Varco, and C.W. Lillehei. A self contained disposable oxygenator of plastic sheet for intracardiac sur-gery. Thorax, 12:1, 1957.
92. Rygg, I.H., and E. Kvisgaard. A disposable polyethylene oxygenator system applied in a heart-lung machine. Acta Chir. Scand., 112:433, 1956.
93. DeWall, R.A., H. Najafi, D.J. Bentley, and T. Roden. A hard shell temperature con-trolling disposable blood oxygenator. JAMA, 197:1065, 1966.
94. Allen, J.G. (ed.). Extracorporeal Circulation. Charles C. Thomas, Publisher, Spring-field, IL. Second printing, 1960.
95. Ionescu, M.I. (ed.). Techniques in Extracorporeal Circulation. London, Butter-worths, 2nd ed., 1981.
96. Kirklin, J.W. Open heart surgery at the Mayo Clinic. The 25th anniversary. Mayo Clin. Proc., 55:339, 1980.
97. Miller, B.J., J.H. Gibbon Jr., and C. Fineberg. An improved mechanical heart and lung apparatus: its use during open cardiotomy in experimental animals. Med. Clin. North Am., pp. 1603–1624, 1953.
98. Donald, D.E., H.G. Harshbarger, P.S. Hetzel, R.T. Patric, E.H. Wood, and J.W. Kirk-lin. Experience with a heart-lung bypass (Gibbon type) in the experimental labora-tory: preliminary report. Proc. Meet. Mayo Clin., 30:113, 1955.
99. Jones, R.E., D.E. Donald, H.J.C. Swan, H.G. Harshbarger, J.W. Kirklin, and E.H. Wood. Apparatus of Gibbon type for mechanical bypass of the heart and lungs: pre-liminary report. Proc. Staff Meet. Mayo Clinic, 30:105, 1955.

100. Kirklin, J.W., J.W. DeShane, R.T. Patric, D.E. Donald, P.S. Hetzel, H.G. Harsh-barger, and E.H. Wood. Intracardiac surgery with the aid of a mechanical pump oxygenator (Gibbon type): Report of eight cases. Proc. Staff Meet. Mayo Clin., 30:201, 1955.

101. DeWall patent—Capillary oxygenator #2, 972, 349, 1958.

102. Kolobow, T., and W.M. Zapol. Partial and total extracorporeal respiratory gas exchange with the spiral membrane lung. Bartlett, R.H., P.A. Drinker, and P.M. Galletti (eds.). Mechanical Devices for Cardiopulmonary Assistance, vol. 6, p. 112, S. Karger, Basel, 1971.

103. Austin, B.A., and D.L. Harner. The heart-lung machine. Phoenix Medical Communications. Phoenix, AZ, 1986.

104. Foote, A.V., M. Trede, and J.V. Maloney Jr. An experimental and clinical study of the use of acid-citrate-dextrose (ACD) blood for extracorporeal circulation. J. Thorac. Cardio. Surg., 42:93, 1961.

105. Cooley, D.A., A.C. Beall Jr., and J.K. Alexander. Acute massive pulmonary embolism: successful treatment using temporary cardiopulmonary bypass. JAMA, 177:283, 1961.

106. Cooley, D.A., A.C. Beall Jr., and P. Grondid. open heart operations with disposable oxygenators, dextrose prime and normothermia. Surg., 51:713, 1962.

107. Zuhdi, N., B. McCollough, J. Carey, C. Krieger, and A. Greer. Hypothermic perfusion for open heart surgical procedure. J. Int. Col. Surg., 35:379, 1961.

108. Greer, A.E., J.M. Carey, and N. Zuhdi. Haemodilution principle of hypothermic perfusion: a concept obviating blood priming. J. Thorac. Cardiovasc. Surg., 43:640, 1966.

109. Long, D.E., V.B. Todd, R.A. Indeglia, R.L. Varco, and C.W. Lillehei. Clinical use of dextran-40 in extracorporeal circulation. A summary of 5 years experience. Transfusion, 6:401, 166.

110. Vasko, K.A., A.M. Riley, and R.A. DeWall. Poloxalkol (Pluronic F-68): a priming solution for cardiopulmonary bypass. Trans. Am. Soc. Art. Int. Org., 28:526, 1972.

Chapter 4 Congenital Heart Disease

A. NADAS
R.J. BING

THE SIXTEENTH AND seventeenth centuries were exciting eras in the anatomical sciences. Anatomists were then what molecular biologists are today—heroes on the frontiers of medical science. One man stands out as a pioneer in the field of anatomy, Niels Stensen of Copenhagen (Fig. 4.1). Stensen, a wide-ranging, restless, and inquisitive intellect, became the victim of his own restless genius and of his attempt to reconcile it with the world about him. In 1671 Stensen (also referred as to Steensen, or as Steno) described the cardiopathology of a stillborn fetus with a cardiac malformation that now bears Fallot's name (1). Erik Warburg published a Danish translation of the original report (2). An excellent biography of Stensen was published in Danish in 1979 (3). In 1913 William S. Miller wrote a thorough history of Stensen in English, followed by F.A. Willius in 1948 (4, 5).

The stillborn fetus described by Stensen was a boy with a cleft plate, which was ascribed to the mother's predilection for rabbit meat. The sternum was made of cartilage and was split in the middle. Other congenital malformations were apparently present. Stensen first believed that the embryo was male, since there was a very prominent clitoris; external genitalia and the presence of a uterus, however, suggested that the fetus was a female. Stensen was particularly impressed by the unusual heart. On the first glance, the pulmonary artery appeared to be much smaller than the aorta. "As I opened the pulmonary artery from the right ventricle, it was immediately clear that the canal which leads from the pulmonary artery to the aorta and which is quite evident in every embryo, was not to be found. When I subsequently opened the right ventricle, the probe passed along the septum into the aorta, and with the same ease into the left ventricle. Therefore, the right ventricle had three openings, one from the atrium, and two into

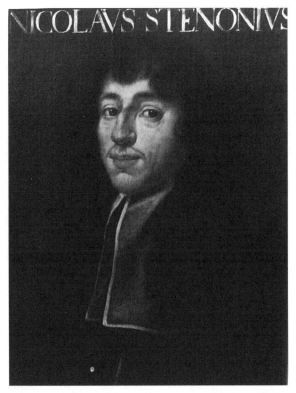

Figure 4.1. Niels Stensen. *(Courtesy of the New York Academy of Medicine)*

the large arteries. The aorta had a common origin in both ventricles." Stensen also speculated on the physiological consequences of this anatomical malformation. "The blood must pass equally into both arteries from the right ventricle" (6). He was not certain whether the blood originating in the right ventricle was shunted first into the pulmonary artery and then through a canal (ductus) into the aorta, or whether the aorta received the blood primarily from the right ventricle. He emphasized that in this embryo, the patent ductus arteriosus, or so he called it the "canal," was closed. He compared this to the normal newborn in which the ductus first conducted blood from the pulmonary artery to the aorta.

Stensen was born in 1638 to Steen Pedersen, who was a goldsmith in Copenhagen. Since his father died early and his mother married again, he lived with his grandparents. He was a sickly child and had a lot of contact with older people and little companionship with children of his own age. The conversations to which he listened were largely concerned with religious matters and he apparently heard a great deal of Martin Luther's teachings (4). In 1656, at the age of eighteen, Stensen entered the University of Copenhagen and selected a mentor, Thomas Bartholin, as was customary at that time. Bartholin was an outstanding anatomist at the time and brought to the University of Copenhagen a fame that extended all over Europe. Stensen not only studied anatomy under Bartholin, but also pursued mathematics and languages—Hebrew, French, German, and later Italian. It has been said that he was able to make such progress in Hebrew that in later life he could easily read the Bible in that language.

These were difficult times for Denmark. The country was at war with Sweden; in 1658 the Swedes invaded Denmark and besieged Copenhagen. Stensen was assigned to a regiment composed of students, who were to repair the fortifications and repel the attacks of the foe. Despite this, Stensen found time to attend lectures and perform anatomical dissections with Bartholin. During this period, Stensen also read the great books of his time, such as Descartes, Kepler, and Galileo.

In 1659 Stensen traveled to Amsterdam with a letter of recommendation to Gerhard Blasius. Blasius had taught medicine in Copenhagen and was a friend of Bartholin. In Amsterdam, Stensen discovered the salivary duct, which now bears his name, Stensen's duct or the duct of Steno. As is often the case then as it is now, the fight for priority was a bitter one. A controversy arose between Stensen and Blasius concerning who was responsible for this discovery. Blasius was enraged that Stensen should claim the discovery which he claimed for himself. He called Stensen a liar, a blasphemer, and a malevolent person inflated with envy. Stensen replied in a letter to Bartholin that "Blasius had never looked for the salivary duct; for he does not give to it either the proper point of beginning or ending, and assigns to the parotid gland so unworthy a function, that of furnishing warmth for the ear, that were I not right in having shown him the duct, I should be tempted to assert that he had never seen it" (4).

This bitter experience with Blasius was enough to cut short Stensen's stay in Amsterdam. In 1661 he moved to Leiden to work with the great anatomist, Sylvius. But the controversy followed him. Blasius still claimed the discovery for himself and wrote a letter to Bartholin, who answered, "Your conscience will tell you who is right in this matter. . . . Farewell and control yourself."

In 1664 Stensen returned to Copenhagen, where he published his revolutionary concept of the heart as a muscle. "The heart has been considered the seat of natural warmth, as the throne of the soul and even as the soul itself. Some have greeted the heart as the sun, others as the king: but if you examine it more closely, one finds it to be nothing more than a muscle." This simple statement caused consternation and controversy (4). The celebrated Swiss physiologist, Haller, writing in 1774, pronounced Stensen's publication a "golden book which contains the rich seed for new discovery." De Hedoville wrote in 1665, "This simple observation overthrew a system to which medicine clung most tenaciously." It is noteworthy that while in Leiden, Stensen met the philosopher Spinoza, who had been excommunicated by his local synagogue and had fled to Leiden. Stensen and Spinoza remained lifelong friends (3).

Since no position was available in Copenhagen, Stensen returned to Holland in 1664 and thence to Paris, where he obtained his doctor's degree. A lecture that he gave in Paris on the structure of the brain attracted much attention. Stensen wrote:

> All you can say is that you find these two different substances, the one
> gray, the one white in the brain; that the white substance is continued
> into the nerves which are distinguished through the entire body; that
> the gray substance serves in some places as an envelope for the white, in
> other places it separates the white fibers from each other (3, 4).

From France, Stensen traveled to Italy and, in 1666, he journeyed to Florence, which became of pivotal importance in his life. In Florence, even at the end of the seventeenth century, the court of the Medici was still the central focus for scientists and artists. Through the influence of his friends, particularly Viviani, the pupil and companion of Galileo, he was appointed personal physician to the Grand Duke, who bestowed on him a pension and a residence. He also received an appointment at the hospital Santa Maria Nuova, which had been founded in 1288 by Portinari, the father of Dante's Beatrice and which still exists today. It was in Florence that Stensen, a Lutheran, converted to Catholicism. This was not in line with his previous philosophy. His friends were either Lutherans or Calvinists—such as Glauber, Borch, Thevenot, Sylvius, Willis (one of the founders of the Royal Society), Lister, and Croone—a pantheist like Spinoza. The fact that he was Lutheran in a high position at a Catholic institute may have contributed to his conversion; later the position was reversed when as a Catholic he occupied a position at the Lutheran Institutes, the University of Copenhagen (2–5).

In Florence, Stensen received a letter from the Danish king offering him a professorship at Copenhagen. His inaugural address is worth quoting:

> What one sees is beautiful; more beautiful is what one knows; but by far
> the most beautiful things are beyond our knowledge. For who can con-
> template the wonderful structure of the human organism without asking
> the question: who is its author?

The stay in Copenhagen was not to be a long one. Again he became involved in a controversy, possibly because of his position as a Catholic professor in a Lutheran university. In May 1674 he resigned his position and returned to Florence, where he took charge of the education of the son of the Grand Duke Cosimo III. In 1675 Stensen became a priest and the pope consecrated him bishop of Titiopolis. He then went to Braunschweig, where the pope appointed him "Apostolic Vicar for the Northern Missions." He moved to Schwerin, in northern Germany, where he died in 1686 at the age of forty-eight. The end of this saga came when the Grand Duke of Tuscany, hearing of his death, sent for his body and had it transported to Florence, where he was entombed with the Grand Dukes in the cathedral of San Lorenzo.

Stensen also was an outstanding geologist. He was prophetic in his concepts of formation of mountains, citing examples of local earth crust formation, showing how individual strata might remain horizontal, be tilted or even thrown into a perpendicular position, or be bent in the form of arches. Mountains, he said, might also originate from the upward action of the volcanic forces on the earth's crust (2–5).

Stensen was one of the least known but brilliant and imaginative scientists of the baroque era.

In 1777, more than one hundred years later, after Stensen's report, Sandifort described the same cardiac malformation, which he called "a very rare disease of the heart." This Dutch physician was born in Dortrecht in 1742, and received his doctor of medicine degree from Frederik Bernhard Albinus. His life and his description of what was later called the tetralogy of Fallot has been reported in detail by Lydia Russell Bennett (7). The report by Sandifort, when compared to Stensen's, illustrates the progress made in medicine over a hundred-year span. While Stensen was primarily concerned with basic anatomic features, Sandifort was also interested in the clinical symptoms. While Stensen observed the cardiac pathologic anatomy of an embryo, Sandifort's observations were based on a patient who lived until childhood, giving him the opportunity to observe the clinical progress. Following the teachings of Boerhaave, Sandifort took very careful clinical records. Like Stensen, Sandifort taught in Leiden, where he founded the Leiden Museum of Pathology, became president of the College of Surgeons, and was made president of the College of Pharmacology (7). One of Sandifort's statements is particularly noteworthy: "Oh, how difficult it is to cure diseases within the breast! Oh, how much more difficult to recognize them, and to give sure diagnosis about them!" (7).

Sandifort's description of the cardiac malformation that bears Fallot's name was made in the *Observationes Anatomico-Pathologicae*, written from 1777 until 1781. Book 1, Chapter 1, of the *Observationes* is entitled "Concerning a very rare disease of the heart." In describing this malformation, he followed the example of the great Leiden physician, Boerhaave, who became the spiritual father of Viennese medicine, which flourished during the nineteenth century. The chapter has twenty-three pages and numerous beautiful illustrations. Sandifort had the opportunity to describe the clinical symptoms as well as the pathological findings in a child whom he called "Blue Boy." He describes the child as being normal during the first year of life, but during the second year "the beginnings of terrible symptoms appeared, which afterward sorely burdened the poor child. In fact, a bluish color of the fingers, even the nails, not continuous, but now more and now less evident, attracted the attention of the parents, particularly when it could be ascribed to no tightness of clothing." The symptoms that he described in this child were "catarrh," blue color of the lips and tongue that often verged toward black, a dry cough, sinking spells, pressing pain in the head, swelling of jugular veins, and "an agitation or a throbbing in the jugular veins." Toward the end stage of the disease, Sandifort observed swelling of the feet and face. Therapy was concerned with venesection, mild laxatives, and leeches which, at the beginning, seemed to have some effect, but later were to no avail. He made special mention that this child was a "clever boy." Sandifort very carefully searched the literature and quoted Vieussen, Morgagni, Meckel, and others (7).

At autopsy, he found that the foramen ovale was widely patent. He wrote:

> How great was the surprise of the onlookers, how great equally was my
> own surprise, when we saw the point of the finger to stretch into the
> aorta, which is not at all accustomed to maintain communications with
> the right ventricle, in conformity with otherwise constant laws of na-
> ture! Thus, the arterial aorta was springing from both ventricles, and
> had to receive all the blood from both.

He found the pulmonary artery to be very small, almost rigid, and blocked by a certain granular substance. Sandifort came to the conclusion that he was dealing with a truly congenital malformation. Scientist and historian that he was, he quoted Stensen. He mentioned that Stensen also had been able to push a probe upward next to the septum directly into the aorta from the right ventricle (7).

Not much changed in the field of congenital heart disease until the middle of the nineteenth century. In 1858 Thomas B. Peacock published a book on malformations of the heart. The book is based on lectures delivered to medical students in 1854 at the St. Thomas's Hospital in London (8). Peacock carefully describes anatomical studies on congenital heart disease by Burns, Corvisart (Napoleon's physician), Berthis, Laennec, Boilland, and Hope. The book contains beautiful illustrations of various congenital malformations such as ventricular septal defects and pulmonary stenosis, with and without foramen ovale. He discusses transposition of the aorta and pulmonary artery described by Baillie in 1797. Peacock's biography was briefly featured in the *London Medical and Provincial Directory* (1858) (9), which was advertised as "the only cheap medical journal, instructive in its matter, independent in its policy, and honest in its purpose." (Few journals nowadays can make *this* claim.) Peacock received his medical degree in Edinburgh in 1852, became a Fellow of the Royal College of Physicians, assistant physician at St. Thomas's Hospital, physician to the City of

London, and medical superintendent and pathologist at the Royal Infirmary in Edinburgh (9).

In 1921 A. Spitzer published a book on congenital heart disease that was very different from that of Peacock (10). He was particularly interested in the origin of the malformations, assuming that many congenital malformations were due to arrested development of the heart and could be explained by an arrested state through which the evolutionary process of the species was carried out. The evolution of the species, therefore, appears to him to be reflected in the formation of the individual, and malformations are explained on an evolutionary basis. To make this theory clear, he repeatedly tried to explain the cor triatriatum by comparing it with the reptile heart. He mentions that in the reptile, the aorta originates from the right ventricle, since in the reptile, when there is enough oxygen available, blood can be shunted directly into the body. According to Spitzer, the force and capacity of the right ventricle is "temporarily placed in service of the larger circulation, when there is no particular need for the pulmonary circulation. The dextraposed aorta converts the right chamber into an auxiliary pump of the larger circulation" (10).

Wilhelm Ebstein (1836–1912) was the discoverer of a malformation that bears his name (11). He was professor of medicine and director of the medical clinic at Goettingen, and he studied at the universities of Breslau and Berlin. This was Berlin's greatest period in the medical sciences, with Von Graefe, Traube, DuBois-Reymond, Langenbeck, Romberg, Schoenlein, and Virchow. In 1898 Ebstein published an article in which he grouped obesity, gout, and diabetes mellitus as inheritable cellular metabolic diseases. On the basis of this, he was called "the forgotten founder of biochemical genetics" (12). One of Ebstein's often cited observations, which lead to the eponym Pel-Ebstein's fever, was his description, in 1887, of the periodic fever of lymphoma (13). Today, the major source of Ebstein's fame is his work on congenital heart disease carried out early in his career and largely ignored until after his death. In 1864 he performed an autopsy on a patient in whom he described three cardiac anomalies: severe malformation of the tricuspid valve, absence of the pulmonary valve, and a patent foramen ovale (14). A. Arnstein published his case in 1927, fifteen years after Ebstein's death, and named it "Ebsteinsche Krankheit" (Ebstein's disease) (15).

A Canadian physician, Maude Abbott, forms the connection to today's diagnosis of congenital heart disease (Fig. 4.2). Abbott graduated in arts from McGill University in Montreal in 1890, with the third class of women. She was elected president of her class and was the valedictorian. She wrote sometime later that she was "in love with McGill" (16). This passionate affection was clearly not reciprocated. The medical school, in spite of pressures from faculty, public agitation, and headlines in the press, refused to consider her because she

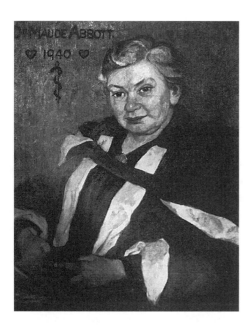

Figure 4.2. Maude Abbott. *(Courtesy of the New York Academy of Medicine)*

was a woman. The professor of surgery said he would resign if women were allowed to take the medical course. And this was only one hundred years ago.

Since the doors of her beloved McGill Medical School were shut tightly at that time (and did not open to women until 1918), Abbott accepted an offer from the University of Bishops College in Montreal. She graduated from this small school in 1894 as the only woman in her class. After graduation from medical school, she undertook the required pilgrimage to the European centers of learning—from London to Vienna. Abbott returned to Montreal after spending three years in Europe and opened an office for the practice of medicine in 1897. She apparently was not comfortable with the requirements of private practice and dealing with patients, so she obtained an appointment as an assistant curator of the medical museum the next year. This is how she became acquainted with the Osler Collection, described the Holmes heart, and devoted all of her life to the study of congenital heart disease.

It was customary, until the middle of the twentieth century, to collect pathologic specimens in museums. William Osler, when at McGill University in Montreal, had started such a collection. Abbott met Osler in Baltimore in 1898, and he mentioned to her his collection at McGill, which was later referred to as the Osler Collection (17). He saw the teaching possibilities of such a museum, calling the collection "pictures of life and death together." Abbott wrote, "And thus he gently dropped a seed that dominated all my future work. This is but an illustration of how his influence worked in many lives." When she returned to Montreal, she gave herself entirely to the work at this museum. "The work was very demanding," she wrote, "and it seemed at first a dreary and unpromising drudgery; but as Dr. Osler had prophesied, it blossomed into wonderful things. I shall never forget him as I saw him walking down the old museum toward me, with his great, dark, burning eyes fixed fully upon me" (17).

Abbott's interest in congenital heart disease began at that time. She traces her original interest in congenital heart disease to her work in this museum. Probably Osler's help in identifying some of the specimens focused her attention on the subject, but what made her devote herself to it completely was having been asked by Osler to write the section on congenital heart disease in his *System of Medicine* of 1907 (17). She asked Osler how to approach writing this chapter and his answer was: "Statistically." Thus, she analyzed all the initial cases in large charts arranged according to the special features and symptoms. Finally, she had a large quantity of facts and figures from which she could draw conclusions, with illustrations of many of the types of conditions drawn from the museum specimens. She completed this atlas in 1907. Osler was delighted. He wrote her, "This is by far and away the best thing ever written on the subject in English— possibly in any language." And he added, "I have but one regret, that Rokitansky and Peacock are not alive to see it." Thus, Osler gave direction and intensity to her work.

In Osler's book, *The Principles and Practice of Medicine*, published in 1892, eleven years prior to Abbott's publication, he commenced his chapter on congenital heart disease as follows: "These (congenital affections of the heart) have only limited clinical interest, as in a large proportion of the cases the anomaly is not compatible with life, and in others nothing can be done to remedy the defect or even to relieve the symptoms" (18). Within the next eleven years, thanks largely to Abbott, the knowledge of congenital heart disease increased. The advances of cardiac surgery and pediatric cardiology would have been impossible without her contribution.

In the 1940s congenital heart disease grew from a field of limited clinical interest into one of considerable practical importance. This progress was to a large extent the result of the development of cardiac surgery and of new diagnostic tools. Robert E. Gross in Boston, Clarence Craaford in Stockholm, and Alfred Blalock in Baltimore were the pioneers.

August 26, 1938, may be identified as the date when surgery to correct congenital heart disease was born. Gross, at thirty-three, chief resident of Surgery at the Children's Hospital in Boston, successfully ligated the patent ductus arteriosus of a seven-year-old girl. There had been previous attempts to obliterate the ductus arteriosus; a patient of John Strieder, at Boston University, survived the operation, but succumbed to postoperative infection. Gross, having worked for years in the pathology laboratory and the dog lab of the Children's Hospital and of the Peter Bent Brigham, was intellectually prepared for the undertaking. He was skillful with his hands, knew where he was going, and was lucky. His colleagues, to put it mildly, were not totally supportive of his vision. It was surely no coincidence that the daring tour de force was attempted during the month when his chief, William E. Ladd, was away on vacation. Legend has it that after the little girl seemed to have come through surgery without complications, Gross and his group of young people went to celebrate the success by attending one of the Longwood tennis matches, where they met Ladd. The chief asked Gross after the tennis game, according to the story, "Anything new, Bob?" The chief resident said, "Nothing much," or some such thing. In fact, cardiac surgery had been born.

The medical cardiologists, as expected, were no more courageous than the surgical community. At the time, Green and Emerson ran the congenital heart clinic at the Children's Hospital every Thursday afternoon. Neither of their names appeared on Gross's original publication (19). Instead, the co-author was John Hubbard, who ran the rheumatic fever clinic. How the head of the rheumatic fever clinic had access to a patient with patent ductus arteriosus remains a mystery, but it certainly happened and is another example of Gross's firm determination, skill, and good luck.

Gross was born in Baltimore, Maryland. After graduating from high school, he went to Carleton College in Minnesota. As an undergraduate, he received a scholarship to the University of Wisconsin for postgraduate studies in chemistry. During summer vacation, however, he read Harvey Cushing's biography of Sir William Osler (the Osler influence once again), and decided to go to medical school. He chose, and was admitted to the Harvard Medical School, where Cushing was professor of surgery. (Note the difference between the career opportunities for men and women, such as Maude Abbott and Helen Taussig.)

Having graduated from Harvard in 1931, Gross had training in pathology under S. Burt Wolbach, surgery under Elliot Cutler at Peter Bent Brigham, and Ladd at the Children's Hospital. These three people had major influences on his career. Eventually he became the second Ladd Professor of Children's Surgery at the Harvard Medical School. Clearly, surgery was to be his career, but he carried a strong conviction to the very end that thorough training in pathology and the experimental laboratory were indispensable parts of academic surgical training.

Gross's surgical career had two distinct and separate but overlapping chapters. The first was that of pediatric surgery; the text *Abdominal Surgery of Infancy and Childhood*, by Ladd and Gross, bears witness to his seminal contributions to the field (20). Gross was the first to repair diaphragmatic hernia in a newborn, to resect lobar emphysema, and to perform the first successful pneumonectomy in an infant. He contributed significantly to the diagnosis and treatment of Wilms' tumors. He learned to manage atresias of the GI tract and choledochal cysts

(21). Not only did Gross contribute significantly to the techniques in pediatric surgery, and really established the discipline, but, in addition, most of the heads of pediatric surgical departments in the United States today are either children or grandchildren of the Gross training program.

The second chapter, which overlapped the first, was the start of cardiac surgery. There is no question that Gross opened the field with his ligation of the patent ductus arteriosus in 1938. There is some argument about the first treatment of coarctation of the aorta. The first report of successful surgical treatment appeared in 1945, and was authored by Craaford (22). Gross always maintained, although seldom articulated, that Craaford visited his laboratory, learned his end-to-end anastomosis technique there, and beat him to the first report. With Edward Neuhauser, head of Radiology at Children's Hospital, Gross worked out the diagnosis and treatment of vascular rings. He designed an ingenious approach to atrial septal defect surgery through suturing of a rubber sleeve to the anterior wall of the right atrium, allowing the blood to rise in the sleeve through the atriotomy, to the level of right atrial pressure (usually low in secundum atrial defects). He then sewed blindly, but highly successfully, through the blood with a needle attached to a long hemostat. The procedure worked in hundreds of cases, and other surgeons continued to use it even after he abandoned the technique, using the pump oxygenator.

Gross was an ingenious, meticulous, and inventive person. He and Savage, from the machine shop at the Children's Hospital (who formerly worked in the Springfield armory on machine guns before he retired to come to Children's) constructed their own pump oxygenator. He would not use "store-bought stuff." He was clearly a do-it-yourself, independent person. He wanted to make everything simple. There was (and maybe still is) a sign in the Children's Hospital operating room saying, "If an operation is difficult, you are not doing it properly." He did not tolerate "messy" things. He never took to the hypothermia technique of Henry Swan. To put an anesthetized child in a tub of ice water offended his sense of aesthetics. At catheterization conferences, he barely would listen to the complex physiologic data presented and hardly looked at the angiograms. He wanted to know what the final diagnosis was, and mainly, how old the child was and how much he or she weighed—just the facts. Indicative of his dual careers, Gross was surgeon in chief at the Children's Hospital from 1947 to 1967 and he acted as cardiovascular surgeon in chief from 1967 to 1972.

Alfred Blalock was the second in this constellation of cardiac surgeons. By the time Blalock came to Hopkins from Vanderbilt University, he was superbly prepared for the surgical work which was to challenge him. He had already excelled in research on shock (the role of the depletion in plasma volume), which was surely his greatest contribution, and later on the role of the thymus in myasthenia gravis (23, 24).

Longmire in an authoritative book on Alfred Blalock concisely stated the relative role of Blalock and Taussig in the initiation of the shunt operation (25).

Taussig's role on the tetralogy event has been the subject of some controversy and has been enlarged or diminished, in part, depending upon whether the narrator is a surgeon or a cardiologist. The view that I obtained from working with Alfred Blalock, and from hearing his comments, was, of course, that he had originally performed the subclavian pulmonary anastomosis while working in the experimental laboratory at Vanderbilt during a period when he was interested in the general subject of hypertension. His object at that time was to create pulmonary hypertension, and he was somewhat disappointed in the procedure when, due to the low resistance in the pulmonary circulation, such an anastomosis did not immediately produce an increased tension in the pulmonary artery. Obviously his experimental animals were not followed long enough, or he would have seen some element of hypertension develop. In any event, he had developed the technique of the anastomosis. . . . When the first three operations were reported in the *Journal of the American Medical Association*, and in the general conversation in the operating room with early visitors, and others, I recall that Blalock adopted his usual gracious—some would say—overly-generous attitude toward his associates and colleagues, including Helen Taussig, occasionally giving them somewhat lavish credit and praise for their roles in various undertakings. . . . Initially, it was only because of Blalock's custom of giving generous recognition to his associates that Helen Taussig began to receive a share of the acclaim. As time wore on, however some thought that Taussig's somewhat contentious nature and her tendency to assume a greater degree of credit for the success of the procedure than was justified began to undermine this mutually productive relationship; indeed a quite subtle distrust slowly evolved into a thinly suppressed hostility. Blalock, I know, became quite annoyed by some of her statements, reactions, and claims. Fortunately, I believe that there was never any public or open disruption of the Blalock–Taussig team.

Harry Muller, Stephen H. Watts Professor of Surgery Emeritus at the University of Virginia, has recounted, in a letter to me (RJB), the point to which this controversy degenerated during his tenure as chief resident on the cardiac team (1948–1949):

"At this time [Blalock] was having a great deal of difficulty with Dr. Helen Taussig because she would not recommend patients for operation even though to most of us the patient seemed to merit an operative procedure. . . ." Thomas Turner, dean of the Johns Hopkins School of Medicine during the latter part of the Blalock era, wrote to Longmire recently: "I knew Al Blalock from his house officer days on; upon his return to Hopkins my admiration for him continued to grow and our

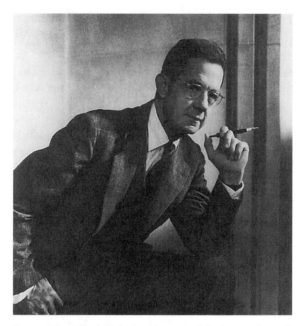

Figure 4.3. Alfred Blalock. *(Courtesy of the New York Academy of Medicine)*

friendship deepened. I view with dismay the tendency to underestimate the seminal role he played in developing the so-called Blue Baby operation and related surgery" (25).

It is certain, however, that Helen Taussig's idea that an increase in pulmonary blood flow would be beneficial was not correct. It was not the diminution in pulmonary blood flow, but the right to left shunt, or the decrease in effective pulmonary blood flow, which was responsible for the cyanosis and clinical symptoms of these patients. Nonetheless, the idea led Blalock to the correct surgical treatment (26; Fig. 4.3). Blalock had already carried out experimental anastomoses between the subclavian and the pulmonary arteries many years before at Vanderbilt together with Sanford E. Levi to see whether he could produce pulmonary hypertension by increasing pulmonary blood flow (27). But an operation is a surgical and not a medical or pediatric procedure. The best ideas often run afoul in the experimental laboratory, or worse, the operating room. Thus, the early surgical treatment of some types of cyanotic congenital heart disease should be credited to Blalock (28). It was certainly fortunate for the future of cardiac surgery that these divergent and completely different personalities happened to be there at the same time and in the same place.

The worldwide acceptance of the designation of the Blalock–Taussig shunt

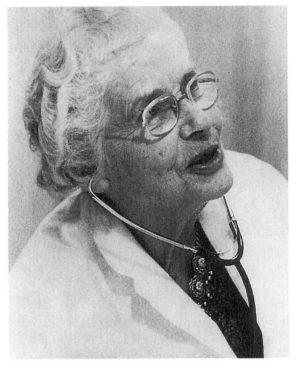

Figure 4.4. Helen Taussig. (*Courtesy of the Johns Hopkins University Library*)

(B-T shunt as it is colloquially referred to) speaks for itself. Suffice to say that the shunt operation (systematic artery to pulmonary artery) was a landmark achievement. For the first time, miserable, blue, squatting little children became pink, and could run, play, and join the human race. With all the enormous progress in the surgery of congenital heart disease since 1944, one could still argue that more actual suffering was alleviated by this palliative procedure than with any other subsequent corrective operation.

Taussig was born in 1898 (Fig. 4.4). Her father was the Henry Lee Professor of Economics at Harvard. Taussig went to Radcliffe for the first two years of her college education; she transferred to the University of California at Berkeley and graduated from that institution. She wanted to study medicine, but the president of Harvard, a frequent visitor to the house, advised her that as a woman in 1922 she had no chance of being admitted; she should try the Harvard School of Public Health. The dean of that institution told her that she could audit classes but would not obtain a degree. This was Harvard's first rebuke to Taussig.

Taussig then applied to the Johns Hopkins School of Medicine, where she was admitted. (Nearly fifty years before, a wise and wealthy lady had pledged a half million dollars to Hopkins under the condition that the school would admit women on the same basis as men.) After graduating from medical school, Taussig decided to become a cardiologist. (In those days, and even twenty-five years later, this meant a cardiologist for adults.) She was steered toward pediatrics, an appropriate career track for females in those days. Edward A. Park, chairman and head of the Harriet Lane Home for Invalid Children, a major influence in American pediatrics, took Taussig under his wing and encouraged her to establish a cardiac clinic that would concentrate on rheumatic as well as congenital heart conditions. This clinic at Harriet Lane became her base of operations for the next fifty years. With the virtual disappearance of rheumatic fever in the United States and the growing field of surgery of congenital heart disease, the clinic population shifted largely toward congenital malformations. Taussig hovered over her large patient population; she knew the children and their families intimately and as time went on the cardiology fellows also became her children. This was her family, a tightly knit group of young patients and young doctors from all over the United States and overseas with a marvelous esprit de corps.

Taussig's tools in understanding cardiac malformation were based first on pathology. She personally dissected hundreds of specimens and was a close friend and disciple of Abbott. She thoroughly understood the anatomy of congenital cardiac malformations. Among clinical tools, the fluoroscope might have been her favorite. Her hearing was seriously impaired from an early age, thus auscultation was not her forte. Under the fluoroscope, however, she could see the anatomy very clearly and could correlate it with her profound knowledge of pathology. Significant also was her understanding of each individual child as a total person, physical and emotional. Taussig was at first antagonistic toward cardiac catheterization. It is not clear whether her antagonism was due to aversion to performing additional invasive tests on children, or due to her lack of understanding of physiological concepts. Seeing many cyanotic children, she gradually defined the clinical, radiologic, and electrocardiographic profile for tetralogy of Fallot, the most common subgroup of blue babies. She noticed that among this group, those who had continuous murmurs were significantly less blue than the others. From this observation came the original idea of attempting to create an artificial ductus to increase pulmonary flow in children with tetralogy of Fallot.

Taussig's idea led to her second rebuke from the Harvard Medical School. One of Taussig's most striking characteristics was her straight, uncluttered, even unsophisticated thinking. In many ways she was similar to Gross in this regard. She knew that Gross had successfully interrupted a patent ductus arteriosus in 1938 and had done this new operation many times since then. If a surgeon could ligate and divide the ductus, why couldn't he create an artificial one? Taussig actually traveled to Boston in the early 1940s to propose the shunt operation for blue babies to Gross. He listened but was not interested. He was at the crest of his career and ductus surgery was highly successful and safe. Coarctation treatment was on the horizon. Taussig returned to Baltimore, where Blalock had been appointed professor and head of Surgery. Baltimore became the Mecca for blue babies. When the Harvard Medical School, years later, gave Taussig an honorary degree, she recited both earlier Harvard rebuffs (29).

Blalock and Taussig were indeed completely different personalities (30). Probably because of her deafness, Taussig guarded her territory closely. Blalock appeared on the surface as an urbane Southerner, suave and polite. Actually, he was a determined surgeon and the glove hid an iron fist. In contrast to Taussig, he was thoroughly trained in physiology and experimental surgery. Blalock had the ability to cut through nonessentials and arrive at the core of a problem, an important attribute of greatness. This ability demands a singularity of purpose and simplicity of thought. Minds of greater intellectual capacity who lack this quality sometimes cannot find their way through the maze of false leads to arrive at the goal of discovery. Directness of thought, mistaken by some as simplemindedness, is essential to scientific discovery. Directness of thought combined with tenacity, or doggedness, were characteristic of Blalock. For years, he and his assistant Vivien Thomas worked on animals before attempting surgery for the tetralogy of Fallot (31).

Clearly, fundamental changes have occurred in the care of patients with heart disease in this century. The changes are not only quantitative (establishment of boards and subboards with a dramatic increase in the number of certified cardiologists) and qualitative (the technical advances), but also philosophical. Today the cardiologist must be like the surgeon, a technically involved clinician who is familiar with invasive as well as noninvasive techniques.

A man who best represents the new breed of cardiologists was William J. Rashkind. He took the great step forward from diagnostic to therapeutic catheterization in congenital heart disease. Rashkind, born in New Jersey in 1922, had both his undergraduate and graduate education at the University of Louisville, Kentucky, with an M.D. degree in 1946. After a rotating internship at Michael Reese Hospital in Chicago, he entered the Navy and worked for two years in physiology and hemodynamics at the Naval Medical Institute in Bethesda, Maryland. He pursued his hemodynamic interests for another four years in the Physiology Department at the University of Pennsylvania. Rashkind finally decided that he really wanted to be a doctor and began his training in pediatrics in 1953 at the Children's Hospital in Philadelphia, where he remained for the rest of his life, eventually becoming professor, senior staff member, and head of the catheterization laboratory.

Conceptualization and practical application of balloon atrial septostomy for palliation of transposition of the great arteries was Rashkind's major contribution to the field. The results were presented first at the annual meeting of the American Academy of Pediatrics in Chicago in 1965, and published in the *Journal of the American Medical Association* (JAMA) in 1966 (32). This relatively simple, ingenious maneuver consists of introducing a deflated balloon into the foramen ovale through a catheter inserted into the inferior vena cava through fluoroscopy control. Once the balloon is lodged in the left atrium, it is blown up with contrast material and pulled back forcefully into the right atrium, causing a large tear in the atrial septum, resulting in an increase in arterial oxygen saturation and venting of the high-pressure left atrium. The procedure was simple but needed consummate courage and skill. As Rashkind, with characteristic wit, once said, "The important thing is the big jerk at the end of the catheter." Balloon atrial septostomy significantly improved the clinical course of critically ill babies with transposition of the great arteries. The maneuver was accepted globally and became an eponym. "The Rashkind" was announced with distortion, but was clearly recognizable in all languages.

Important as this brilliant maneuver was in the care of children, perhaps more important was establishment of the principle that the cardiac catheter can also be used for treatment purposes in congenital heart disease. This approach had been used for some time in the treatment of coronary heart disease, but its application in pediatric cardiology should be credited to Rashkind. Following publication of his paper on balloon septostomy (32), he reported on palliative measures for transposition of the great arteries and certain other critical congenital cardiac defects (33).

Rashkind was a spectacular human being. Academically, he was brilliant; he was a consummate gadgeteer and physiologist; clinically, he was a warm, dedicated, compassionate physician and he enjoyed life. He loved good food and good wine; in search of these devotions he traveled widely in the disguise of medical education. He loved and was very knowledgeable in the fine arts, good books, movies, theater, and opera. He said once that one of the major advantages of living and working in Philadelphia was that you could take the train to New York early Saturday afternoon, go to dinner and the theater in the city, pick up the Sunday *New York Times*, read it on the train, and still be at home in bed at a reasonable hour.

The prototype of the modern cardiac pediatric surgeon is Aldo R. Castaneda. Castaneda was born in Genoa, Italy, where his parents landed, in transit from Guatemala to Germany. He spent his childhood and adolescence in Munich; he was deeply affected, fascinated, and repelled by the horrors of the Nazi regime. Castaneda came from a distinguished medical family in Guatemala; both his father and his uncle were professors at the medical school there. It was, thus, a logical move for him to return home from postwar Germany and enroll in the Medical School of the University of Guatemala, obtaining his M.D. degree in 1957.

While a medical student in Guatemala, Castaneda had his initial contact with the Children's Hospital in Boston, Massachusetts. Louis K. Diamond, senior physician at Children's and professor of pediatrics at the Harvard Medical School, visited Guatemala as the guest of the local Pediatric Society to give a few lectures and, of course, to admire the Inca treasures of Tical and the scenic beauties of Lake Atitlan. Young Castaneda acted as an interpreter for Diamond, a brilliant teacher and an expert talent scout, who was much impressed by Castaneda, and was anxious to help him obtain the best possible training in surgery, his chosen career. He arranged for Castaneda to come to Boston and be interviewed by his good friend Robert E. Gross for a job in his surgical training program. Castaneda indeed came to Boston and saw Gross, but nothing came of it. His internship was at the Guatemala General Hospital.

Castaneda entered the surgical training program at the University of Minnesota, from where he obtained a Ph.D. in surgery in 1963 and an M.S. in physiology in 1964. These were heady days in surgery in Minnesota. Owen Wangensteen was chief and Walt Lillehei was deeply involved in developing circulatory support for open heart surgery first through cross-circulation and later through the use of a pump oxygenator, a modification of the Gibbon pump. Castaneda was strongly influenced by these two mentors, as well as by Richard Varco, whose right-hand man he eventually became. Castaneda's surgical brilliance was recognized early, and by 1970 he became full professor of surgery at Minnesota.

It is interesting to contemplate the cosmopolitan background of Castaneda—born in Italy, of Guatemalan parents, raised in Germany, educated to the M.D. level in Guatemala, and trained in surgery in the United States. Castaneda arrived in Boston in September 1972. Gross retired on June 30 of that year. Gross was very pleased by the selection of the committee; he liked the fact that a practical, no-nonsense operating surgeon was chosen as his successor. He appreciated Castaneda's youth and liked the fact that he was interested in the laboratory (having worked on lung autotransplants in primates prior to leaving Minnesota). However, there was no doubt that his prime responsibility was the meticulous care of patients. He espoused close collaboration and mutual support among surgeons and cardiologists, intensivists, anesthesiologists, radiologists, nurses, basic scientists, and pathologists. The result is the Cardiology Department at the Children's Hospital, a highly successful experiment in patient care, medical education, and research.

An important contribution to the understanding of congenital heart disease is the work of Charlotte Ferencz and her co-workers, who published a monumental volume dealing with "a systematic search to achieve complete ascertainment of all live born infants with cardiovascular malformation in whom the diagnosis was confirmed before one year of age" (34). This ascertainment took into account factors such as genetics, heterogeneity, environmental factors, and socioeconomic status. In systematic order the various malformations of the heart and great vessels were subjected to scrutiny. For example, the study revealed that in malformations of the cardiac outflow tract there was exposure of the mother to benzodiazepin as well as a history of diabetes. An examination of the background of ventricular defects revealed as major risk factors for the chromosomal subset an increased risk of advancing maternal age, the use of hair dyes, and paternal cocaine exposure. In coarctation of the aorta a number of findings were of importance, for example, predominance among infants among the white race, a coexistence with noncardiac malformations, maternal epilepsy, and several medical therapies. It is clear that this study is essential; it offers guidelines to the geneticist, the physician, and the patient.

Congenital heart disease is a field of medicine in which the surgeon has shown the way. Without the surgical pioneers, cardiac malformations would have remained interesting abnormalities with no further hope for successful therapy.

References

1. Stensen, N. Embryo monstro affinis Parisiis dissectus 1665. Acta Med. Philos. Hafniensis, 1:200–304, 1673.
2. Warburg, E. Niels Stensen's Beskrivelse af det forste publicerede Tilfaede af "Fallots Tetrade." Nord. Med., 16:3550–3551, 1942.
3. Moller-Cristensen, A.G. The Medical Faculty 1479–1842. Copenhagen, Kobenhavns Universitet, 7:39–43, 1979.
4. Miller, W.S. Niels Stensen. Johns Hopkins Hosp. Bull., 25:44–51, 1914.
5. Willius, F.A. An unusual early description of the so-called tetralogy of Fallot. Cardiac Clinics 124. Proc. Staff Meetings Mayo Clinic, 23:316–320, 1948.
6. Scherz, G. Pioneer der Wissenschaft: Niels Stensen in seinen Schriften. Copenhagen, Munksgaard, 1963.
7. Bennett, L. R. Sandifort's "Observationes." Chapter 1, Concerning a very rare disease of the heart. I. Tetralogy of Fallot or Sandifort? Bull. Hist. Med., 20:539–570, 1946.
8. Peacock, T.B. On Malformations of the Human Heart: With Original Cases and Illustrations. London, Churchill, 2nd ed., 1866.
9. The London and Provincial Medical Directory, 1858.
10. Spitzer, A. Ueber den Bauplan des normalen und missbildeten Herzens. Versuch einer phylogenetischen Theorie. Virchows Arch. Pathol. Anat. Physiol. Klin. Med., 243:81–272, 1923.
11. Mann, R.J., and J.T. Lie. The story of Wilhelm Ebstein (1836–1912) and his almost overlooked description of a congenital heart disease. Mayo Clinic Proc., 54:197–204, 1979.
12. Bartalos, M. Wilhelm Ebstein: a forgotten founder of biochemical genetics. Humangenetik, 1:396, 1965.
13. Ebstein, W. Das chronische Rueckfallfieber, eine neue Infektionskrankheit. Berliner Klin. Wochenschr., 24:565–568, 1887.
14. Ebstein, W. Ueber einen sehr seltenen Fall von Insufficienz der Valvula Tricuspidalis, bedingt durch eine angeborene hochgradige Missbildung derselben. Arch. Anat. Physiol. Wissenschaftl., 33:238–254, 1866.
15. Arnstein, A. Ein seltene Missbildung der Trikuspidalklappe (Ebsteinsche Krankheit). Virchows Arch. Pathol. Anat. Physiol. Klin. Med., 266:247–254, 1927.
16. Dobell, A. Maude Abbott: Portrait of a Pioneer. The Second Clinical Conference on

Congenital Heart Disease: B.L. Tucker, G.G. Lindesmith, and M. Takahashi. Gruber & Stratton, 1982.

17. MacDermot, H.E. Maude Abbott: A Memoir. Toronto, Macmillan, 1941.
18. Osler, W. The Principles and Practice of Medicine. New York, Appleton, 1892.
19. Gross, R.E., and J.P. Hubbard. Surgical ligation of patent ductus arteriosus. Report of first successful case. JAMA, 112:729, 1939.
20. Ladd and Gross. Abdominal Surgery of Infancy and Childhood. Philadelphia, W.B. Saunders Co., 1941.
21. Folkman, M.J. Harvard Medical Alumni Magazine, obituary, 1988.
22. Craaford, C. Congenital coarctation of the aorta and its surgical treatment. J. Thorac. Surg., 14:347, 1945.
23. Ravitch, M.M. Alfred Blalock, 1899–1964. In: The Papers of Alfred Blalock. Baltimore, Johns Hopkins Press, 1966.
24. Ravitch, M.M. Progress in resection of the chest wall for tumor with reminiscences of Dr. Blalock. Johns Hopkins Med. J., 151:43–53, 1982.
25. Longmire, W.P. Jr. Alfred Blalock: His life and times, 1991.
26. Bahnson, H.T. Classics in thoracic surgery: surgical treatment of pulmonary stenosis: a retrospection. Ann. Thorac. Surg., 33:96–98, 1982.
27. Levy, S.E., and A. Blalock. Experimental observations on the effects of connecting by suture the left main pulmonary artery to the systematic circulation. J. Thorac. Surg., 8:525–530, 1939.
28. McNamara, D.G. The Blalock–Taussig operation and subsequent progress in surgical treatment of cardiovascular diseases. JAMA, 251:2139–2141, 1984.
29. Nadas, A. Personal communication.
30. Bing, R.J. Johns Hopkins: the Blalock–Taussig era. Persp. Biol. Med., 32:85–90, 1988.
31. Thomas, V. Pioneering Research in Surgical Shock and Cardiovascular Surgery: Vivien Thomas and His Work with Alfred Blalock. Philadelphia, University of Pennsylvania Press, 1985.
32. Rashkind, W.J. Creation of an atrial septal defect without thoractomy. A pallative approach to complete transposition of the great arteries. JAMA, 196:991, 1966.
33. Rashkind, W.J. Balloon atrioseptostomy: a pallative measure for transposition of the great arteries and certain other critical congenical defects. Advances in Cardiology, 11:2–10, 1974.
34. Ferenz, C., C.A. Loffredo, A. Correavillasenor, and P.D. Wilson (eds). Perspectives in Pediatric Cardiology. Volume 5: Genetic and Environmental Risk Factors of Major Cardiovascular Malformation. The Baltimore-Washington Infant Study: 1981–1989. Armonk, NY, Futura Publishing Co., 1997.

Chapter 5

Transplantation of the Heart

J.C. BALDWIN
S.A. LEMAIRE
R.J. BING

MORE THAN ANY OTHER cardiac operation, successful transplantation of the heart requires a combination of meticulous surgical technique and lifelong multifaceted medical management. Despite early perfection of the technical aspects, cardiac transplantation did not become a clinical success until substantial advances were made in the control of graft rejection.

The pioneer in both the technical and immunologic aspects of heart transplantation was Alexis Carrel (1873–1944) (Fig. 5.1). Carrel was cut from a different cloth than his contemporaries at the Rockefeller Institute (1, 2). He was gregarious and interested in matters other than science, such as politics, religion, and philosophy. He published articles in popular journals and wrote a book dealing with his philosophy concerning man's relationship to his environment and his fellow man. He was a hardworking and dedicated scientist who collaborated with his associates in the laboratory every day. What distinguished him from his colleagues was primarily his desire to extrapolate his research into the general panorama of the world outside the laboratory. He used his scientific observations as springboards into philosophical, cultural, and even parapsychological fields. In this respect, he was akin to the men of the Renaissance, such as Roger Bacon, who could not separate the occult from the proven truth and saw no distinction between truth and speculation.

Carrel's surgical innovations had a profound effect on the development of cardiovascular surgery, organ transplantation, and tissue culturing. His work on the technique of blood vessel anastomoses, which he mastered as a young physician in Lyon, France, became the cornerstone of his research. He once said that

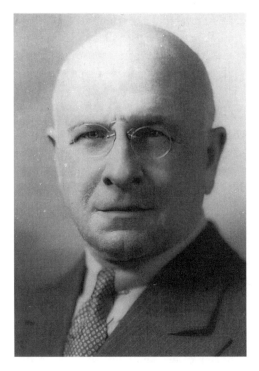

Figure 5.1. Alexis Carrel. (*Courtesy of the New York Academy of Medicine*)

he became interested in "suturing things together" from watching a seamstress who came to his home. By perfecting the triangulation technique for blood vessel anastomoses (which he carried out with unusual dexterity, having practiced the technique in a match box with one hand), he demonstrated that a simple, purely technical accomplishment can lead to extraordinary technical and physiological progress.

Carrel repeatedly carried out experimental bypass operations in which all types of veins were transplanted to all types of arteries in end-to-side and end-to-end configurations (3, 4). Carrel reported that xenografts of blood vessels were possible if the grafts had been previously maintained in cold storage for several days prior to implantation (5). In the *Johns Hopkins Hospital Bulletin*, he noted that when veins were used as arterial transplant conduits, the venous wall would thicken in response to its exposure to the increased blood pressure (6). Carrel anastomosed the peripheral end of the renal artery to the splenic vein (splenorenal shunt) and produced a stenosis of the portal vein near the liver; "venous blood flowed through the renal artery, the kidney, the renal vein and into the vena cava." An accidental finding was that transplantation of one or two large veins of the thyroid gland into the carotid artery produced a "strong arterial hyperemia, which in one animal suffering from myxedema, led to improvement of this state; the animal lost excess fat, hair grew rapidly on the bald spots and it became very lively and pugnacious." Replantation of the kidney with vascular anastomoses was performed several times, including into the abdominal cavity (7, 8). Coronary bypass operations and replantation of limbs were also successfully performed.

Carrel also transplanted skin and, on December 6, 1911, he wrote (5):

> The cadaver of an infant who had died during labor was used for the extirpation of cutaneous and other grafts. Several hours after death, the body of the child was washed with soap and water and with ether. Dermoepidermic grafts and flaps of skin were extirpated in large numbers and washed in Ringer's solution. Bones were also extirpated. With the Wasserman reaction negative, the dermoepidermic grafts and the flaps of skin, preserved in petrolatum and in Ringer's solution, were used at the Rockefeller Hospital for the treatment of three large ulcers and one circular ulcer of the leg in two patients.

Reference to transplantation of the heart was made in several of Carrel's publications prior to 1912. In 1905, in a paper in *American Medicine*, Carrel described the transplantation of the heart of a small dog into the neck of a larger one achieved by anastomosing the cut ends of the jugular vein and the carotid artery to the aorta, the pulmonary artery, the vena cava, and a pulmonary vein (9). About one hour and fifteen minutes after the initial cessation of contractions, the circulation was reestablished through the heart; twenty minutes later, blood was actively circulating through the coronary system. Strong fibrillar contractions were observed initially, followed by contractions of the auricles, and, about an hour after implantation, effective contractions of the ventricles. The transplanted heart beat at the rate of 88 per minute, while the rate of the normal heart was 100 beats per minute.

Carrel's experiments with Lindbergh in the early 1930s regarding methods for cardiopulmonary bypass, originating from Lindbergh's wish to operate on a bloodless heart, were indeed visionary. Their attempts were premature, however, and Carrel and Lindbergh ultimately settled for the development of a technique to maintain the viability of organs outside the body (10).

Carrel was quick to recognize that even the most perfect surgical technique combined with careful avoidance of infection were insufficient to guarantee successful organ transplantation because of graft rejection. His insight into the importance of transplantation immunology was one of Carrel's outstanding contributions. As he wrote in his article, "The Transplantation of Organs,"

> As yet these methods (surgical) cannot be applied to human surgery, for the reason that homoplastic transplantations are almost always unsuc-

cessful from the standpoint of the function of the organs. All our efforts must now be directed toward the biological methods, which will prevent the reaction of the organism against foreign tissue and allow the adapting of homoplastic grafts to their hosts (11).

Carrel discovered, together with James Murphy of the Rockefeller Institute, that while tumor cells grew very rapidly on chick fetuses to which they had been grafted alone or together with chick kidney, liver, or connective tissue, they grew very little or not at all when pieces of spleen or bone marrow were grafted to the fetus. At the same time, he and Murphy discovered that when mouse tumors—which previously had never survived on rats—were grafted onto splenectomized rats, the tumors exhibited active growth for twelve or thirteen days. In the presence of benzol, which diminished the activity of leukocytes and lymphocytes, the mouse tumor survived even longer and resorption did not occur before fifteen days. Furthermore, exposing the rats to radiation led to survival of mouse tumors beyond thirty-five days. Carrel concluded that (1) the ability of the organism to eliminate (reject) foreign tissue was due to organs such as the spleen and bone marrow, and (2) when the activity of these organs was impaired, a foreign tissue could develop rapidly after grafting. Carrel received the Nobel prize for these studies, which constituted early recognition of the role of lymphoid cells in the rejection of transplants (11).

Unfortunately, Carrel's tendency to discuss general politics in public and his admiration of strong personalities offended many of his colleagues. He was a genius of a highly contradictory nature, who justified his prejudices to himself with a high degree of naiveté and honesty. Although Simon Flexner, the director of the Rockefeller Institute, was well aware that Carrel did not fit the pattern of the rest of his faculty, Flexner considered Carrel an asset to the Institute and was patient with him. When Flexner retired, however, Herbert Gasser became director of the Institute and all of this changed. Gasser, a Nobel prize winner himself, was the antithesis of Carrel. A punctilious and proper man, administrator and investigator, he considered Carrel a gadfly and a foreign body at the Rockefeller Institute. Gasser, along with the majority of the faculty, soon made Carrel feel terribly unwelcome.

Carrel returned to his native France, a most ill advised venture, given the Nazi occupation. Being isolated from his friends and his adopted country, he suffered a great deal during his last years (12). Carrel was a multifaceted, scintillating, but eventually tragic genius, whose characteristics were bound to conflict with those of his colleagues, who viewed him as a proponent of scientific and political extravagance.

Carrel's work, however, was the stimulus for subsequent studies on cardiac transplantation. His example was followed by Frank C. Mann (1887–1962), director of the Mayo Foundation Institute of Experimental Medicine from 1914 to 1948. Mann was a world authority on liver physiology and surgery of the kidneys, blood vessels, and gastrointestinal tract (13). He pioneered experimental surgery by bringing rigid surgical technique to the laboratory. One of Mann's most remarkable achievements was his work on complete removal of the liver, which made it possible to study the function of this organ. Mann published an article on transplantation of the intact mammalian heart performed using the procedure outlined by Carrel (14). He described that the heart usually began to contract immediately after the coronary circulation had been reestablished. He made the statement, as previously formulated by Carrel, that "failure of the homotransplanted heart to survive is not due to the technique of transplantation but to some biological factor which is probably identical to that which prevents survival of other homotransplanted tissues and organs."

In Carrel's experiment, the transplanted heart was in essence an in situ Langendorff preparation; unlike a heart transplanted into the chest, where it would serve as a replacement for the recipient's heart, the heart in the neck did not perform work. Therefore, this preparation was well suited for determining the graft's metabolism and speed of rejection; such valuable information was obtained using the Carrel preparation. Based on this model, Downie, for example, speculated that rejection was the result of a "humoral agency" that was responsible for the destruction of the transplant (15). In 1948 Sinitsyn maintained the coronary circulation of a homografted heart through the action of its own ventricle (16). The model was later used by Reemtsma and his associates to study myocardial oxygen consumption and carbohydrate utilization of the transplanted heart (17). They reported no marked difference in myocardial glucose consumption of the transplant as compared to the in situ working heart of the recipient. However, in the majority of their experiments, they observed myocardial lactate production rather than consumption. Similar results were obtained by Lee and Webb, who also reported that, in the normothermic canine homograft, coronary flow averaged 128 cc per 100 g of left ventricle per minute and myocardial oxygen consumption of 6.4 cc per minute (18).

Chiba, Bing, and their co-workers described in detail the metabolism of the heart transplanted to the neck of a recipient dog by the method of Carrel and Mann (19, 20). They found that the homografted heart generally extracted glucose and released lactate, pyruvate, malic dehydrogenase, and aldolase. In the setting of accelerated rejection, however, the release of pyruvate and lactate was more pronounced and the glucose concentration in coronary venous blood was increased. The elevated respiratory quotient of the transplanted heart may have signified conversion of carbohydrate to fat (20). The absence of graft anoxia was indicated by a positive redox potential across the transplanted heart, suggesting that myocardial ischemia was not a component of rejection. Many histologic

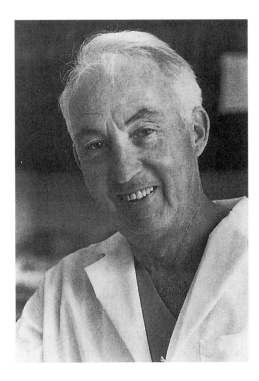

Figure 5.2. Norman E. Shumway.
(*Courtesy of the New York Academy of Medicine*)

findings were similar to those later found in the human cardiac transplants: swelling of the vascular endothelium; polar perivascular cellular infiltration by lymphocytes, plasma cells, macrophages, and histiocytes; Aschoff cells; and Anitschkow-like cells. After eight days, necrosis of the myocardium became prominent. Endothelial hyperplasia, which occurred at fourteen days, may have represented an early stage of the severe coronary artery changes later reported in human transplants.

Several groups laid the technical groundwork leading to the human heart transplant operation. Marcus and co-workers had described techniques for the transplantation of a heart into the chest of a dog in 1953 and speculated on the ultimate use of a transplanted heart as a functioning replacement organ, although they concluded that it "must be considered at present a fantastic dream and does not fall within the scope of present considerations" (21). Neptune and associates were the first to perform orthotopic transplantation of combined heart and lungs in dogs and reported six-hour survival (22). In 1958 Webb and co-workers described a practical method of homologous cardiac transplantation (23). Of twelve technically successful transplants utilizing refrigerated hearts, ten were able to maintain normal blood pressure from thirty minutes to seven and one-half hours.

Norman Shumway (Fig. 5.2) deserves enormous credit for the development of human heart transplantation. Shumway's work with Dick Lower in the late 1950s was facilitated by Stanford Medical School's move from San Francisco to Palo Alto and the reluctance of many of the senior clinical scientists to join those who were willing to make the risky trek. Shumway and Lower borrowed from a wide range of others' experiences and assimilated the accumulating knowledge regarding cardiac transplantation, culminating in the landmark studies that were reported in *Surgical Forum* in 1960 (24). Shumway had a strong interest in myocardial preservation and was a pioneer in the use of cold immersion for induction of hypothermic metabolic inhibition in cardiac tissue. By combining this work with the use of an early cardiopulmonary bypass machine and the midatrial excision and reimplantation technique of Lord Russell Brock, he achieved the first successful orthotopic cardiac transplant in the canine model (24, 25).

Later, Shumway and others in the Stanford transplant laboratory borrowed from the developing fields of kidney transplantation and cytotoxic chemotherapy for malignancy to develop a means of preventing rejection. Without a noninvasive means of reliably diagnosing graft rejection, however, cardiac transplantation would not be truly conscionable because survival of the recipient depends on survival of the graft. The loss of electrocardiographic voltage in transplanted canine hearts, described by Lower and associates, allowed the detection of rejection and thus made clinical cardiac transplantation truly feasible (26). This loss of voltage, which was based on the development of intramyocardial edema, remained a useful and reliable diagnostic method until the introduction of cyclosporin; after that time, intramyocardial edema became a less prominent histological feature of cardiac graft rejection, and hence the electrocardiogram, even with signal averaging, became insufficiently sensitive (27).

The rapid progress made in the late 1950s and early 1960s ushered in the era of clinical cardiac transplantation, which began with the first human transplant in 1964, a xenograft operation performed by James Hardy in Mississippi (28). Hardy and colleagues had carefully explored different operative procedures and ultimately replaced a human heart with the heart of a lower primate (28). Unfortunately, within one hour after removal of the bypass catheter, the primate heart became unable to accommodate the large venous return without intermittent decompression by manual cardiac massage. Although the patient did not survive, Hardy's report in the *Journal of the American Medical Association* stimulated the progression of clinical implementation.

Shumway's 1960 *Surgical Forum* paper, which remains the paradigm for cardiac transplantation techniques to this day, was the basis for the technique used by Christian Barnard when he performed the first allograft operation in December 1967 at the Groote Schuur Hospital in Cape Town (29). The patient survived a mere eighteen days, but the widespread publicity associated with this effort served to further accelerate the clinical implementation of cardiac transplantation. Shumway began his clinical program at Stanford two weeks later and this proved to be the only uninterrupted program in the world from January 1968 to the present.

While the operation itself had been based on the assimilation of a wide range of laboratory experiences, clinical success required an even greater collaboration of cardiac surgeons, cardiologists, infectious disease specialists, clinical immunologists, pulmonary medicine specialists, and nephrologists. Even with the tremendous collaborative effort at Stanford, the early experience was extremely challenging. During the first year, one-year survival was approximately 20 percent (30). This seemingly bleak outcome was actually remarkable when contrasted to the natural history of end-stage cardiac failure: among candidates waiting for operation, the mean survival time was only three months and none survived more than a year. During 1968 one hundred cardiac transplants were attempted at more than sixty centers worldwide with abysmal results. The poor results caused widespread condemnation of cardiac transplantation as a procedure, culminating in the *Life Magazine* cover story entitled "The Tragic Record of Heart Transplants" in the September 17, 1971 issue. The conclusion of the scientific community seemed to be that heart transplantation was an example of medical practice outstripping the associated basic science, resulting in tragically unsuccessful clinical outcomes.

Opposition remained pervasive in the medical and scientific community for several years. Even those who did accept the Stanford program regarded it as an exotic hybrid that could be tolerated but should not be emulated elsewhere. Shumway had to overcome many other types of adversity, including the absence of brain death laws, when he began his program. Newspaper headlines suggested that doctors removing donor hearts from gunshot wound victims were in fact the real murderers. A tremendous political and legislative effort was required to establish brain death criteria for organ procurement.

The Stanford results steadily improved through refinement of surgical technique, meticulous attention to detail in recipient selection and postoperative care, improving antibiotics, and improved immunosuppression with the introduction of rabbit-derived antithymocyte globulin in 1977. Although the results were difficult to ignore, many outstanding academic medical institutions refused to embark on cardiac transplantation, often with great fanfare, attracting the attention of the federal government and others. Despite ongoing public and scientific skepticism, Shumway and his Stanford colleagues doggedly persisted, and, by the end of the 1970s, 80 percent of the transplant recipients were surviving to one year with 87 percent rehabilitation—results superior to those following any other cardiac operation at that time.

Carrel had already clearly demonstrated that the problem in cardiac transplantation was not surgical techniques, but rejection of the graft. Although a chronicle of the development of transplant immunology is beyond the scope of this chapter, certain aspects deserve mention.

The graft versus host reaction was discovered by James B. Murphy, whom we encountered previously in his work with Carrel at the Rockefeller Institute. To grow neoplastic cells in an embryo, he carefully cut out a rectangular opening in the shell of fowl eggs, inoculated the exposed chorioallantoic membrane with the neoplasm, and reincubated the eggs. When the eggs were opened, he found that the chick embryo displayed characteristic changes, including nodules in the membranes and enlargement of the spleen. To Murphy's great surprise, similar changes also occurred in embryos injected with normal spleen cells or spleen fragments, indicating that the changes had nothing to do with the neoplastic nature of the inoculum.

In 1956 the graft versus host reaction was rediscovered by Peter Brian Medawar, the director of the National Institute for Medical Research in London who received the Nobel prize in physiology and medicine in 1960. Medawar was born in Rio de Janeiro, studied at Oxford under Sir Howard W. Florey, and became professor of zoology in the University College, University of London (31). One of his greatest accomplishments was his work regarding the mechanism of rejection (cellular versus humoral), the host versus graft and graft versus host reactions, and the importance of sensitized lymphoid cells. In order to induce tolerance in mice of one strain to tissues from another strain, Brent and Medawar injected donor spleen cells into the veins of newborn mice and later grafted the adult with the skin from the same donor (32). They observed that tolerance could be induced in a high proportion of injected mice in some strain combinations, but that the injected animals in other combinations stopped growing as if suffering from a mysterious runt disease. This disease was interpreted as being the consequence of an immunologic attack by grafted cells on the immunologically immature recipient. As Medawar wrote,

> In the orthodox homograft reaction a relatively small graft is transplanted into a relatively large animal, whereupon it excites and eventually succumbs to an immunological response. In the graft versus host reaction the cells suspected of being responsible for that reaction are removed from one animal and injected into another, so that they can attack the animal into which they are put, the host now playing the part of the graft in the conventional reaction. The host animal is either rendered incapable of counter-attacking the injected cells by irradiation, or is naturally incapable of doing so by being too young (33).

In his Nobel lecture, Medawar paid tribute to the remarkable work of Ray Owen (Fig. 5.3), who discovered that most twin cattle are born with, and may retain throughout life, a stable mixture (not necessarily 50-50) of each other's

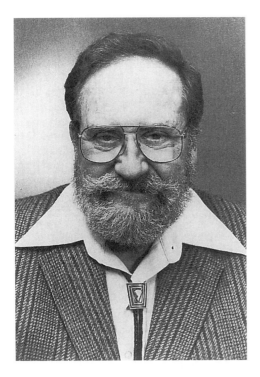

Figure 5.3. Ray Owen. *(With permission)*

red blood cells (34); it followed then, that the twin cattle must have exchanged erythrocyte precursors, and not merely red blood cells, in their mutual transfusion before birth. This was the first example of chimerism. It was also shown that most dizygotic cattle twins exhibited specific mutual tolerance; the twins would accept skin grafts from each other, but skin transplanted from third parties was rejected in the expected fashion. Owen's phenomenon was duplicated in chickens by Hasek, who made deliberate synchorial parabioses between chick embryos in the shell (35). After hatching and separation, the parabions accepted each other's skin grafts and remained incapable of making antibodies against each other's red blood cells.

Several years before the advent of cyclosporin, Brent and Medawar drew attention to the importance of immunosuppressive agents, which they categorized as nitrogen mustards, deoxyribonucleic acid (DNA) base analogues, folic-acid antagonists, and antibiotics that degraded DNA (32).

Cyclosporin was discovered serendipitously in 1970 at the Sandoz Laboratory in Basel, Switzerland (36, 37). As the result of a fundamental search of soil samples from Norway and Wisconsin, the products of two fungi were discovered to have antimycotic activity. Subsequent fermentation of *Trichoderma polysporum* and *Cylindrocarpon lucidum* produced a compound that ultimately had surprisingly disappointing antibiotic ability. If the workers at Sandoz had used a different cell strain, however, cyclosporin A would not have been discovered. Although the drug was a failure as an antimicrobial, it was an unsuspected success in a completely different field. In January 1972, Borel observed important immunosuppressive reactions that were not related to cyclosporin's general toxicity. Staehelin writes,

> The results obtained in December and January 1971 and 1972 in the screening program already disclosed the three most important features of the biological effects of this preparation which was later found to consist mainly of cyclosporin A: effective immunosuppression with a well tolerated dose, no general inhibition of cell proliferation and impairment of kidney function at high doses. Elucidation of the chemical structure soon followed and a purer preparation of cyclosporin A was found to reduce the immune response in a number of tests: hemaglutinin production, formation of antibody-producing cells, rejections of skin grafts and grafts versus host disease. The drug exerts its main effect on T lymphocytes by interfering with the activity of Interleukin-2. The first public report on the biological effects of cyclosporin A was an oral presentation at the meeting of the Union of Swiss Societies Experimental Biology in 1976. Later, Borel reported his findings before the British Society for Immunology. In 1978, Calne of Cambridge, England undertook the first clinical trials in renal transplantation (37).

The pathway of cyclosporin discovery, so writes Staehelin, demonstrates that

> pharmaceutical research quite often proceeds in a path with many windings; and they illustrate how many people, groups of people, strokes of luck, serendipity, preceding events, etc. contribute to research endeavors of this kind and that they are those factors which make the difference between the usual, frequent failures and the rare success (37).

Cyclosporin therapy for cardiac transplant patients was introduced in December 1980 at Stanford (38). Although the incidences of rejection and infection were not reduced, these two major complications were both ameliorated by the new agent. Rejection episodes tended to be less catastrophic, and, for the first time, outpatient treatment of rejection was introduced. While infection was not less frequent, patients tended to respond more reliably to appropriate antimicrobial therapy. The improved results associated with cyclosporin gave many institutions an opportunity to rethink their prior reluctance in accepting cardiac transplantation, and therefore a multitude of programs sprang up across the nation; by the mid-1980s, more than two thousand cardiac transplants were being performed in more than one hundred centers in the United States each year. In addition, active programs began in Europe, including at the Papworth Hospital in Cambridge, the Harefield Hospital in London, and LaPitié in Paris. In 1981 the International Society for Heart Transplantation was founded, with Norman Shumway as its honorary president. Cardiac transplantation is currently established worldwide as an effective mode of therapy for patients with end-stage heart failure.

Transplantation of the entire heat-lung bloc was developed to provide a means of treating patients with heart failure and pulmonary hypertension. The Stanford group had considered an elevation in pulmonary vascular resistance exceeding 6 to 8 Wood units and unresponsive to vasodilator infusions to be a strict contraindication to orthotopic cardiac transplantation; the normal donor right ventricle was unable to sustain the circulation against high pulmonary pressures. Because fixed pulmonary hypertension was a common problem, the Stanford group was keenly interested in pursuing the work of Neptune, Webb, Castaneda, and others in replacement of the entire heart-lung bloc. Monkeys who underwent the operation, with careful preservation of the phrenic nerves, were weaned from the ventilator and resumed normal ventilation. Following the introduction of cyclosporin, successful intermediate term survival in monkeys was demonstrated in the lab by Shumway, Reitz, and others (39). This achievement led to clinical implementation; the first successful combined heart-lung transplant operation in man was performed at Stanford in March 1981 (40). Despite the technically demanding operation and the formidable scientific and clinical challenges regarding lung preservation, heart-lung transplantation has emerged as a highly successful mode of therapy for patients with end-stage pulmonary and pulmonary vascular disease (41, 42).

The future of cardiac transplantation will involve wider application of the operation, particularly in congenital heart disease cases. Newer immunosuppressive agents will further reduce postoperative rejection while minimizing treatment toxicity. While expansion of the donor pool will partially address the shortage of available organs, the ultimate solution to this problem will require further refinement of mechanical heart replacement devices and the introduction of xenograft transplantation. Past experience would indicate that biological replacement is likely to remain preferable to mechanical devices in terms of quality of life. Successful xenograft transplantation may eventually be achieved through the creation of transgenic lines of animals in which histocompatibility antigen expression is diminished or absent. As previously recognized by Carrel and demonstrated by Shumway, future progress in cardiac transplantation will continue to require a combination of technical innovations and fundamental scientific advances.

References

1. Edwards, W.S., and P.D. Edwards. Alexis Carrel, Visionary Surgeon. Springfield, IL, Charles C. Thomas, 1974.

2. Malinin, T.I. Surgery and Life: The Extraordinary Career of Alexis Carrel. New York and London, Harcourt, Brace, Jovanovich, 1979.
3. Carrel, A., and C.C. Guthrie. Results of the biterminal transplantation of veins. Am. J. Med. Sci., 132:415–422, 1906.
4. Carrel, A. Results of the transplantation of blood vessels, organs and limbs. JAMA, 51:1662–1667, 1906.
5. Carrel, A. The preservation of tissues and its applications in surgery. JAMA, 59:523–527, 1912.
6. Carrel, A. The surgery of blood vessels, etc. Johns Hopkins Hosp. Bull., 190:18–26, 1907.
7. Carrel, A., and C.C. Guthrie. Successful transplantation of both kidneys from a dog into a bitch with removal of both normal kidneys from the latter. Science, 23:394–395, 1906.
8. Carrel, A., and C.C. Guthrie. Complete amputation of the thigh with replantation. Am. J. Med. Sci., 131:297–301, 1906.
9. Carrel, A. and C.C. Guthrie. The transplantation of veins and organs. JAMA, 10:1100–1102, 1905.
10. Bing, R.J. Lindbergh and the biological sciences: a personal reminiscence. Texas Heart Inst. J., 14:231–237, 1987.
11. Carrel, A. The Transplantations of Organs. 1915.
12. Chambers, R.W., and J.T. Durkin. Papers of Alexis Carrel centennial conference, Georgetown University. Washington, Georgetown University, 1973.
13. Institute's Dr. Mann dies at 75. Mayovox, 13:2, 1962.
14. Mann, F.C., J.T. Priestly, J. Markowitz, and W.M. Yater. Transplantation of the intact mammalian heart. Arch. Surg., 26:219–224, 1933.
15. Downie, H.G. Homotransplantation of the dog heart. Arch. Surg., 66:624–636, 1953.
16. Sinitsyn, H. Transplantation as a new method. In: Experimental Biology and Medicine, Moscow, 1948, as quoted by Sayegh, S.F., and O.J. Creech. Transplantation of the homologous canine heart. J. Thor. Surg., 34:692–703, 1957.
17. Reemtsma, K., J.P. Delgado, and O. Creech. Transplantation of the homologous canine heart: serial studies of myocardial blood flow, oxygen consumption, and carbohydrate metabolism. Surgery, 47:292–300, 1960.
18. Lee, S.S., and W.R. Webb. Metabolism of the isolated normothermic and rewarmed heart. Surg. Forum, 9:284–291, 1958.
19. Bing, R.J., C. Chiba, A. Chrysohou, P.L. Wolf, and S. Gudbjarnason. Transplantation of the heart. Circulation, 25:273–275, 1962.
20. Chiba, C., P.L. Wolf, S. Gudbjarnason, et al. Studies on the transplanted heart: its metabolism and histology. J. Exp. Med., 115:853–866, 1962.
21. Marcus, E., S.N. Wong, and A.A. Luisada. Homologous heart grafts. Arch. Surg., 66:179–191, 1953.
22. Neptune, W.B., B.A. Cookson, C.P. Bailey, R. Appler, and F. Rajkowski. Complete homologous heart transplantation. Arch. Surg., 66:174–178, 1953.
23. Webb, W.R., H.S. Howard, and W.M. Neely. Practical methods of homologous cardiac transplantation. J. Thor. Surg., 37:361–366, 1959.
24. Lower, R.R., and N.E. Shumway. Studies on orthotopic homotransplantation of the canine heart. Surg. Forum, 11:18–19, 1960.
25. Cass, M.H., and R. Brock. Heart excision and replacement. Guys Hosp. Rep., 108:285, 1959.
26. Lower, R.R., E. Dong Jr., and F.S. Glazener. Electrocardiograms of dogs with heart homografts. Circulation, 33:455–460, 1966.
27. Keren, A., A.M. Gillis, R.A. Freedman, et al. Heart transplantation rejection monitored by signal-averaged electrocardiography in patients receiving cyclosporin. Circulation, 70:I-124–I-129, 1984.

28. Hardy, J.D., C.M. Chavez, F.D. Kurrus, et al. Heart transplantation in man. JAMA, 188:1132–1140, 1964.

29. Barnard, C.N. The operation: a human cardiac transplant: an interim report of a successful operation performed at Groote Schuur Hospital, Cape Town. S. Afr. Med. J., 41:1271–1274, 1967.

30. Baldwin, J.C., E.B. Stinson, P.E. Oyer, V. Starnes, and N. Shumway. Cardiac transplantation and followup care. In: The Heart, Hurst, J.W. (ed.). New York, McGraw-Hill, 7th ed, 1990, pp. 2248–2254.

31. Medawar, P.B. Do advances in medicine lead to genetic deterioration? Mayo Clinic. Proceed., 40:23–33, 1965.

32. Brent, L., and P.B. Medawar. Cellular immunity and the homograft reaction. Brit. Med. Bull., 23:55–60, 1967.

33. Gibson, T., and P.B. Medawar. Homografts, Chapters 1–15. In: Modern Trends in Plastic Surgery, vol. 2, Butterworth, Washington, DC, 1966.

34. Medawar, P.B. Immunologic tolerance, the phenomenon of tolerance provides a testing ground for theories of the immune response. Science, 133:303–306, 1961.

35. Hasek, M. Vegetative hybridization of animals by joining their blood circulations during embryonic development. Cs. Biol., 2:265–277, 1953.

36. Heimbecker, R.O. Transplantation: the cyclosporin revolution. Can. J. Cardiol., 1:354–357, 1985.

37. Staehelin, H. (Cyclosporin) Historical background. Prog. Allergy, 38:19–27, 1985.

38. Oyer, P.E., E.B. Stinson, S.W. Jamieson, et al. One year experience with cyclosporin A in clinical heart transplantation. Heart Trans., 1:285–289, 1982.

39. Reitz, B.A., N.A. Burton, S.W. Jamieson, J.L. Pennock, E.B. Stinson, and N.E. Shumway. Heart and lung transplantation. J. Thor. Cardiovasc. Surg., 80:360–372, 1980.

40. Reitz, B.A., J.L. Wallwork, S.A. Hunt, et al. Heart-lung transplantation. N. Engl. J. Med., 306:557–564, 1982.

41. Franco, K.L., and J.C. Baldwin. Heart-lung transplantation for cystic fibrosis: an overview. J. Appl. Cardiol., 4:571–580, 1989.

42. Baldwin, J.C., W.H. Frist, T.D. Starkey, et al. Distant graft procurement for combined heart and lung transplantation using pulmonary artery flush and simple topical hypothermia for graft preservation. Ann. Thorac. Surg., 43:670–673, 1987.

Chapter 6   Atherosclerosis

R.J. BING

ATHEROSCLEROSIS MANIFESTS ITSELF in a variety of cardiovascular abnormalities, such as cerebral vascular accidents, myocardial infarction, and peripheral vascular disease. We know that the disease has been present since ancient times, as it has been discovered in Egyptian mummies dating from 1580 B.C. to A.D. 525. During embalming, the whole of the viscera and most of the muscles of the body were removed, while the body cavity and the holes, left in the limbs after removal of the muscles, were filled with mud, sand, or rags. The sole of the foot was packed with sawdust mixed with some resinous material. The aorta, fortunately owing to its deep location, often escaped the embalmer's knife. In 1911 M.A. Ruffer isolated the mummy's aorta by placing the parts to be examined in a solution containing carbonate of soda and formalin, and soaking it for twenty-four to forty-eight hours; the skin could then be taken off and the arteries could be dissected out (1). Atheromas were found in almost all of the arteries examined. As Ruffer stated, "The lesions were of the same nature as we see at the present day, namely calcification following an atheroma." He said that he "could not exclude the theory that a high meat diet was the cause of the severe atherosclerosis in the mummies, as the mummies examined were mostly those of priests and priestesses who, owing to their high position, undoubtedly lived well" (1).

Arteriosclerosis (atherosclerosis) was first described by the anatomists; the early reports were concerned with "bone in the heart," a condition that already had been described by Aristotle in certain animals (2). It is likely that this calcification of the heart was synonymous with calcified aortic valves, a fact already recognized by Morgagni (2). While Antonio Benevieni did not define atherosclerosis, he reported that on fifteen necropsies "wounds of the arterial system" were among them (possibly atheromata) (2). It is, however, known that Vesalius was familiar with aortic aneurysms (2). At that time, no distinction was made between aneurysm due to syphilis or that due to arteriosclerosis. The Dutch anatomist Volcher Coiter, while in Bologna, heard from "men worthy of credit" that they had seen the great artery (aorta) universally bony in a body dissected by Fallopius at Padua. By the year 1600, it was likely that all educated physicians had become aware of the condition of ossification of arteries, particularly the aorta. William Harvey, forever the physiologist, had emphasized the difficulty of transmission of the pulse in these arteries (2).

A fascinating description of early atherosclerosis was provided by Johann Conrad Brunner, who witnessed the necropsy of his father-in-law, Johann Jacob Wepfer (1620–95). Wepfer was the discoverer of the relationship between cerebral hemorrhage and stroke. Brunner described the aorta, which contained bone-like plaques throughout, especially in the upper abdominal aorta; "touching this structure hurt the fingers from the roughness of the bones" (2). In 1740 Johann Frederich Crell published his findings, in which hardening of the coronary arteries was described (2). He took a great step forward by writing that the ossifications were in fact not bony, but of tophaceous nature and were derived from atheromatous matter. In 1755 Haller, of Bern, discussed the indurations of the aorta, placing particular emphasis on the atheromatous element existing in senile changes of this artery (2). Morgagni, in 1761, noticed the increased size of the heart in some cases with extensive hardening of the arteries; he was the first who took notice of the changes in the smaller arteries. Antonio Scarpa, who was Morgagni's pupil, while teaching in Modena and Pavia, Italy, was particularly interested in the relationship of the atheromatous ulcer to the aneurysm and rupture of the vessel. He referred to the report of Nichols on the necropsy of George III of England, in whom at postmortem, a fissure in the internal coat of the artery was discovered into which blood had diffused to form an ecchymosis. In 1801 Bichat stated that the initial lesions of arteriosclerosis were in the intima; he reached this conclusion by careful dissection (2).

We owe the term "arteriosclerosis" to Jean Frederick Martin Lobstein, the incumbent of the chair of pathological anatomy at the University in Strasbourg (3; Fig. 6.1). In his textbook we find the term "arteriosclerosis" ("nom composé d'artere et de sclerose"). He published a chemical analysis of the calcified arterial plaques. In 1839 the Viennese pathologist C. Rokitanski spoke of "excessive deposition in the inner membrane of the vessel," and believed that abnormalities in blood lay at the bottom of these conditions (4). But the idea of imbibition of the aortic wall by material in blood was proposed in a more complete form by the great German pathologist R. Virchow, who postulated a deposition (imbibition) of material from the blood stream into the arterial intima (5). The alterations following blood imbibition were not purely passively degenerative, because he noticed proliferation of the connective tissue together with an increase in the

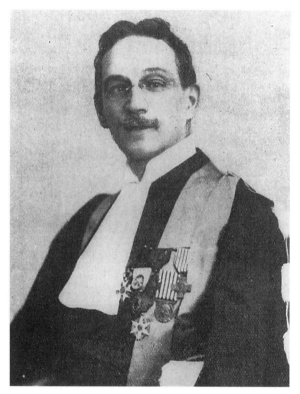

Figure 6.1. Jean Frederick Lobstein. (*Courtesy of the New York Academy of Medicine*)

associated ground substance. An amazing look into the future! The participation of blood pressure in imbibition was later suggested by Virchow's pupils.

The second phase in atherosclerosis research was concerned with the etiology of this condition. This quest continues unabated to the present and undoubtedly will continue into the future.

At the onset, it was necessary to develop an animal model to study the mechanism and etiology of atherosclerosis. This development is credited to A. Ignatowski, N.W. Stuckey, Sergius Saltykow, and N.N. Anitschkow. Ignatowski, from Odessa, who worked in the laboratory of diagnostic clinical science in St. Petersburg, had the good sense, favored by serendipity, to use the rabbit in his experiments (6). In 1907 he presented a lecture before the Military Medical Academy in St. Petersburg entitled "To the Question of the Influence of Animal Nutrition on the Organism of the Rabbit." An article on the influence of animal nutrition on the young rabbit appeared in the transaction of the Clinical Military Hospital in St. Petersburg in May 1907 (7). In these lectures and articles, Ignatowski

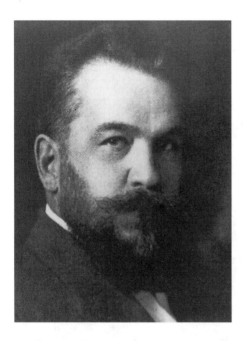

Figure 6.2. Sergius Saltykow. *(Courtesy of the New York Academy of Medicine)*

demonstrated that a high "protein" diet produces atherosclerosis in the aorta of rabbits. However, the "protein" was in reality a mixture of milk and egg yolk. Among other pathological findings, he discovered atheromata of the aorta. Thus, he should be given credit for developing the rabbit model, which is still used in the study of atherosclerosis. At the time, laboratory-bred rats were unavailable— fortunately, because rats fed cholesterol do not show these changes. Stuckey, also in St. Petersburg, was quick to follow and in 1910 discovered similar changes resulting from administration of egg yolk and "brain extracts" (8). In the paper, "On the Changes of Rabbit Aorta after Feeding Different Fatty Material," he reported that the administration of egg yolk was responsible for the aortic changes (9). Stuckey reported identical results with the feeding of brain substances. After four months, he noticed atherosclerotic changes in the aorta.

In 1908 Saltykow, prosector at the Kanton Hospital in San Gallen, Switzerland, experimented with the effect of staphylococcal injection on experimentally produced atherosclerosis in rabbits, reporting that he had observed typical yellow-spotted thickening of the mitral valve (10, 11; Fig. 6.2). Saltykow also administered cholesterol-rich food to these animals. The changes observed probably were the result of the diet rather than the staphylococcal injection, although the presence of bacterial endocarditis was a remote possibility. In several articles, Saltykow summarized his findings, which consisted of meticulous description of the histological changes in the aorta (10–12). Of interest here is that he mentioned

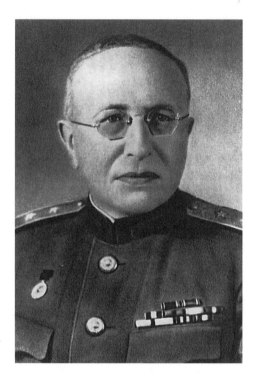

Figure 6.3. Portrait of N.N. Anitsch-
kow as a general in the Red Army.
(*Courtesy of the New York Academy of
Medicine*)

the work of Alexis Carrel and Guthrie, then in Chicago, who transplanted the
terminal aorta to the venous network of an organ with diminished vascular capacity. After a few months they discovered medial hypertrophy followed by sclerosis and calcification of the intima and adventitia. This is an example of the
application of Carrel's surgical technique, which he used so successfully in the
investigation of physiological phenomena.

The central figure in these early Russian studies was Anitschkow (Fig. 6.3).
Anitschkow's life straddled both imperial Russia and the early revolutionary period. His papers from 1913 are listed as from the Pathologic Anatomical Institute
of the Imperial Medical Military Academy at St. Petersburg, while his later publications are from Leningrad, USSR (now again St. Petersburg). Some of his
articles originated from Ludwig Aschoff's Institute in Freiburg, Germany. He
mentioned the role of cholesterol in the production of experimental atherosclerosis in the rabbit (13, 15–22). Anitschkow concluded that the deposit was
cholesterol, since the double refringence of the crystals, according to Aschoff,
"consists in the living organism primarily of fatty acid esters or cholesterol." He
mentioned further the work of A. Windaus, the chemist, who found lipids in the
aortic wall in human atherosclerosis (14). He concluded that "previous and present authors can come to a complete agreement because it is now completely

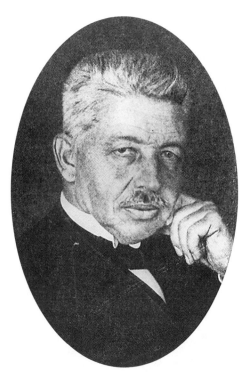

Figure 6.4. Ludwig Aschoff. (*Courtesy of the New York Academy of Medicine*)

clear why such nutritional elements, as for example, egg yolk or brain substance produce changes in the organism." Cholesterol has since then achieved a central position in experimental, clinical, and pharmacological studies on atherosclerosis.

Anitschkow was a prolific writer; most of his publications were more than thirty pages long (13, 15–20). The role of cholesterol in atherosclerosis remains however, the most important of his discoveries. Anitschkow proposed another farsighted concept: participation of smooth muscle fibers in the formation of atherosclerotic processes. "Sometimes one sees layer upon layer of smooth muscle fibers close to the most superficial layers of the intima." The role of smooth muscle proliferation in atherosclerosis has become an important field of research (20). Anitschkow also produced atherosclerotic changes in mitral and aortic valves. This breakthrough could not have been made without the work of the pathologist Aschoff, whose studies in pathologic anatomy pointed to the role of cholesterol, and of Windaus, who demonstrated the presence of cholesterol in human tissue (14; Fig. 6.4). Windaus, in a paper written at the suggestion of Aschoff, concluded that in atheromatous aortas the content of cholesterol is significantly increased. This increase is partially due to the presence of free cholesterol (14). In 1907 Aschoff discussed his finding that cholesterol had been taken up "by the fatty globules, which then became anisotropic" (23). One of

Anitschkow's students, W.D. Zinserling, showed in 1932 that spontaneous atherosclerotic changes could also be present in the aorta of dogs (24). He admitted that, in the rabbit, spontaneous arterial lesions resembling human atherosclerosis are not observed, just as these animals do not exhibit pronounced thickening of the intima in advanced age. In 1924 Zinserling published an extensive article on the presence of fatty changes occurring in the arteries of children (24). He considered fat deposits (fatty streaks) as precursors of atherosclerosis in the adult. He described the typical distribution in children and their increase with age; he found that they originate in the hypertrophic intima, and that they consist of cholesterol. Zinserling mentioned that three factors are, in general, important for their origin: cholesterolemia, mechanical influences, and the condition of the arterial wall. Thus, Zinserling clearly foresaw the most important problems of atherosclerotic research during the next sixty years. He believed that, with time, the lipid mixture which had infiltrated the intima decomposes but that together with the decomposition and resorption of lipid material, reactive tissue originates, which is formed in close proximity to the initial infiltration process.

In this historical review, one must recall the work of Rudolph Schoenheimer (25), whose research stands at the beginning of the modern era of cholesterol metabolism. His work led to the exploration and definition of the pathways leading to cholesterol formation by Konrad Bloch (26) and F. Lynen (27), and the discovery of the low-density lipoprotein receptors by J.L. Goldstein and M.S. Brown (28).

Schoenheimer was born in 1898 in Berlin (Fig. 6.5). His first studies on cholesterol metabolism were published when he was a young physician at a Berlin hospital. In order to obtain additional training in his chosen field, biochemistry, he worked for three years with Karl Thomas in Leipzig, where he developed a new method for peptide analysis. In 1926 Schoenheimer moved to Freiburg, where he began his studies with Aschoff that were to be of fundamental importance in the area of cholesterol metabolism. In 1930 he joined the University of Chicago, strangely enough in the Department of Surgery, where he became a Douglas Smith Fellow. In 1931 he returned to Germany and became the director of the division for physiological chemistry. In 1933 he left Germany and joined the Department of Biochemistry of the College of Physicians and Surgeons at Columbia University, New York, which was under the direction of Hans Clarke (29).

Schoenheimer published his paper on the synthesis and destruction of cholesterol in 1933. The work was done in Aschoff's department in Freiburg, Germany. By the time the paper appeared, Schoenheimer had joined Columbia University. Schoenheimer described studies on the influence of foodstuffs on the synthesis and decomposition of cholesterol in mice. The paper preceded Schoenheimer's studies on the use of isotopes and elucidation of biochemical pathways.

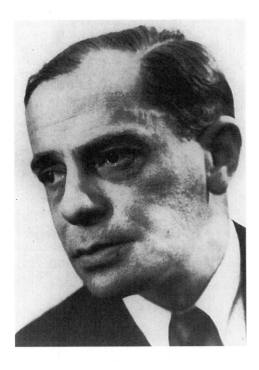

Figure 6.5. Rudolph Schoenheimer at Columbia University College of Physicians and Surgeons, New York. (*Courtesy of the New York Academy of Medicine*)

Schoenheimer was able to follow quantitatively the synthesis and destruction of cholesterol. He confirmed previous work indicating cholesterol can be synthesized in the body. He also showed that in the field of total metabolism, synthesis can play an exceptionally important role. On a diet of bread or bread and fat, mice synthesize as much cholesterol in one month as they had in their bodies at the beginning of the experiment. The administration of large amounts of fat was without significant effect. Schoenheimer furthermore confirmed the data of others according to which cholesterol could also be decomposed.

One of the advances in atherosclerotic research, which was to become the basis of clinical treatment, was the elucidation of cholesterol synthesis by Bloch (26) and Lynen (27). Bloch, who played a major role, was born in Silesia, Germany (Fig. 6.6). He trained with Wieland and Hans Fischer in Munich. After the advent of the National Socialists, he worked in Davos, Switzerland, where he studied the cholesterol content of tubercule bacilli. Like Schoenheimer, he later joined Clarke's department at the College of Physicians and Surgeons, Columbia University. After some period at the University of Chicago, he joined the Department of Chemistry at Harvard. This work, for which he was awarded the Nobel prize together with Lynen, culminated in the elucidation of cholesterol synthesis. Bloch fed acetate, isotopically labeled in its carbon atoms, to rats and found that the cholesterol which synthesized contained the isotopic label (26).

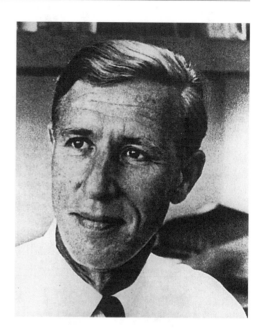

Figure 6.6. Konrad Bloch. (*With permission*)

All 20-7 carbon atoms of cholesterol were derived from acetyl CoA. Of particular importance was the finding that 3-hydroxyl-3-methylglutaryl CoA, an intermediate compound in cholesterol synthesis, can be reduced to mevalonate and that the enzyme catalyzing this step, 3-hydroxyl-3-methylglutaryl CoA reductase, is the control site in cholesterol synthesis which progresses via squalene and lanosterol to cholesterol. This fundamental discovery, made by Folkers et al. in the Merck Laboratories, together with the finding of Brown and Goldstein (28) on receptor-mediated uptake of low density lipoproteins, is the basis for the astonishing progress made in treatment of atherosclerosis by means of HMG-CoA reductase inhibitors.

The discovery demonstrates again the value of fundamental research in the treatment of disease. Bloch, at the end of his article "Summing Up," expresses the feelings of scientists in a manner that might well reflect that of scientists who have enjoyed a lifelong dedication to research:

Whatever the motives, whether curiosity or ambition—usually a combination of both—only near the end does one fully appreciate the rewards and privileges that go with a career in science. So much the better if the results should prove to have some degree of permanence. Science is indeed a glorious enterprise and it has been for me, I admit, glorious entertainment (26).

Why did Konrad Bloch, like so many others such as Rittenberg, Schoenheimer, and Chargaff, flock to Columbia University in New York to the Depart-

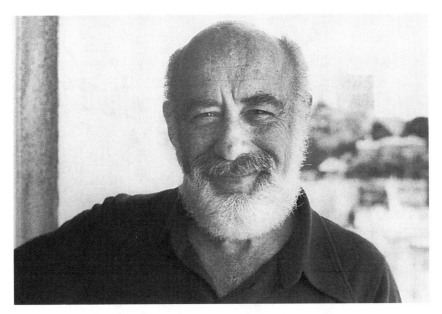

Figure 6.7. John William Gofman. *(With permission)*

ment of Biochemistry of Hans Clarke? The reason was a nurturing environment, particularly because of a departmental chairman whose interest was the promotion of excellent science and scientists. Hans Clarke was a cultured individual who tolerated divergent personalities and understood different cultural backgrounds.

An important discovery in the field of atherosclerosis that shifted the emphasis from cholesterol to lipoproteins was made by John W. Gofman and his co-workers in 1955, working at the Donner Laboratories at the University of California at Berkeley (30; Fig. 6.7). Gofman proceeded to undertake a physiochemical investigation of the giant molecules of serum composed of cholesterol, phospholipids, fatty acids, and protein as building blocks. The basic premise was that it is entirely possible that a defect might exist in certain of these giant molecules, which could be responsible for the development of atherosclerosis, whereas the mere analytical levels of any of these building blocks in serum might be of little or no significance. This work was made possible by the development of the analytical ultracentrifuge. Their studies revealed a considerable diversity of components existing in the low-density group, which they termed B_1-lipoproteins (now beta lipoproteins). By analyzing the ultracentrifugal flotation diagrams of lipids and lipoproteins of humans and rabbits, they concluded that the mechanism of cholesterol transport in the serum of rabbits and humans was in giant lipid and lipoprotein molecules of low density. Defining them as "low or lower density molecules," they showed that these molecules were present in

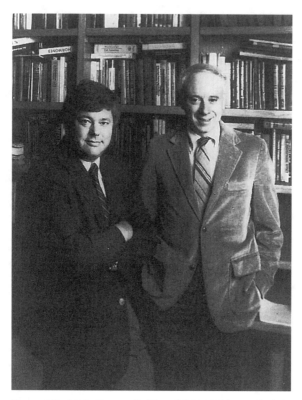

Figure 6.8. M.S. Brown (left) and J.L. Goldstein (right).
(*With permission*)

increased amounts in the cholesterol-induced atherosclerosis in the rabbit, as well as in patients with proved myocardial infarction. They furthermore illustrated that cholesterol intake by the human, as well as by the rabbit, influences the blood level of low-density lipoproteins. This discovery opened the way for the classification of hyperlipoproteinemia of individuals with dominant and recessive types and eventually led to the discovery of abnormal receptors for low-density lipoproteins.

The latest chapter in the study of atherosclerosis deals with the fusion of genetics, biochemistry, and molecular genetics. The central themes are concerned with cholesterol synthesis and transport in blood, cholesterol homeostasis within the cell, and analysis of the origin and progression of vascular lesions of atherosclerosis with special reference to proliferation of smooth muscle cells.

A large number of publications on the low-density lipoprotein (LDL) receptor have appeared from the laboratories of Brown and Goldstein (Fig. 6.8). Their most fundamental contribution concerns the origin of LDL receptors in cell membranes and the mechanism of cellular uptake and transportation of LDL in the cell. Goldstein trained in biochemistry and medical genetics at the National Institute of Health and at the University of Washington in Seattle, and Brown trained at the National Institutes of Health before joining the University of Texas in Dallas.

In 1972, because of their interest in genetics, Goldstein and Brown developed an interest in familial hypercholesterolemia (28). In the two forms of the disease, the heterozygous and homozygous, the blood cholesterol is markedly elevated. Patients with the heterozygous form carry a single copy of a mutant LDL receptor gene, and they may suffer from coronary artery disease at thirty to forty years of age. The homozygotes inherit two mutant genes of the LDL receptor location. These latter individuals may develop heart attacks as children. LDL is internalized into cells after binding to the LDL receptor. Following endocytosis the LDL is delivered to lyosomes, where cholesteryl esters of the LDL are hydrolized to cholesterol and fatty acids. The cholesterol may be used in the biosynthesis of plasma membranes, bile acids, and hormones. The most interesting finding concerns receptor-mediated endocytosis of LDL and the rapidity of internalization in coated pits of the cell membrane. The astonishing fact about these receptors is that they shuttle back and forth: LDL is dissociated from the receptors within intracellular endosomes, and receptors shuttle back to the cell surface to bind another lipoprotein. Each LDL receptor makes a round trip every ten minutes in a continuous fashion whether or not it is associated with LDL.

The impact and ramifications are broad for the therapy of atherosclerosis, for the structure of LDL, and for genetics and molecular biology in general. The action of cholesterol-lowering drugs represents an example of feedback mechanisms involving cholesterol synthesis and LDL receptor activity. HMG-CoA reductase inhibitors inhibit cholesterol synthesis in the liver; this inhibition triggers regulatory mechanisms that result in reduction of the plasma LDL-cholesterol level. Inhibition of cholesterol synthesis in the liver by inhibitors of HMG-CoA reductase elicits a dual compensatory response: hepatocytes synthesize increased amounts of both HMG-CoA reductase and LDL receptors. The increase in HMG-CoA reductase is probably sufficient to neutralize the inhibitor effects of compactin or mevinolin. As a result of the increase in hepatic LDL receptors there is increased clearance of LDL out of the plasma and into the liver and a subsequent decline in plasma LDL levels. Goldstein's earliest papers in this field were published in 1972. His first joint article with Brown appeared in 1973. A new chapter was opened in atherosclerotic research. It represents another victory of basic research, which began with a structure of cholesterol, progressed to its synthesis, and finally to its metabolic fate at the cellular level.

Receptor-related and low-density lipoprotein uptake and disposition are but only one facet of present research work on the pathogenesis of atherosclerosis.

Research also continues on the morphology of the disease. Confirmation of studies of Anitschkow on the morphology of atherosclerosis are being pursued using electron microscopy. Research studies have led to clarification of the fatty streak, the earliest lesion of atherosclerosis, and to the advanced fibromuscular lesions. The role of macrophages and of smooth muscle cells in plaque formation has been studied by means of monoclonal antibodies. The sequence of changes occurring in the development of atherosclerotic lesions has been followed by Russell Ross and his co-workers in monkeys during diet-induced atherosclerosis (31). The role of leukocytes and monocytes, which become macrophages, has been elucidated. Endothelial cells play a major role in the development of atherosclerotic lesions. After exposure to elevated plasma low-density lipoproteins, endothelial cells may become altered (in some as yet undefined way), which thus affects their normal function. In addition, LDL may enter the subendothelial space and become oxidized and stimulate endothelial cells to release various cytokines. The net result is the entry of blood monocytes and LDL into the subendothelial space. Mitogens, derived from adhered platelets, may subsequently result in smooth muscle cell proliferation. There is therefore a close connection among monocytes, macrophage accumulation, endothelial damage, platelet adherence, and smooth muscle proliferation. Endothelial cells also produce vasoactive agents, growth factors, and growth inhibitors. Platelet-derived growth factor (PDGF) was first described by Ross (32). PDGF is not only a mitogen but also a chemoattractant, thus promoting movement of smooth muscle cells from the media to the intima.

Few subjects in medical research are more challenging than atherosclerosis, which involves biochemistry, genetics, morphology, and molecular genetics. It is therefore not surprising that so many different approaches have been used that have been fruitful and rewarding. We now see the spin-off of these fundamental studies in the therapy and prevention of atherosclerosis. From Aristotle's description of "Bone in the Heart," to the experimental production of atherosclerosis in animals by the Russians, and to the discovery of cholesterol synthesis and lipoprotein receptors, the progress has been crescendo, because the basic sciences such as chemistry, physics, and molecular genetics have presented us with the tools. But we should by all means avoid the spirit conveyed by Galen when he wrote, "It is certainly no small advantage that we enjoy living at the present day with the medical arts already brought to such perfection." This concept, expressed by some even now, would surely lead to complacency, scientific stagnation, and the end of progress.

References

1. Ruffer, M.A. On arterial lesions found in Egyptian mummies (1580 B.C.–525 A.D.). J. Path. Bact., 15:453–462, 1911.
2. Long, E.R. Development of our knowledge of arteriosclerosis. In: Arteriosclerosis, Cowdry, E.V. (ed). New York, Macmillan, 1933, pp. 19–25.

3. Lobstein, J.F. Traité d'Anatomie Pathologique. Paris, Levrault, 1829–33.
4. Rokitanski, C. Handbuch der pathologischen Anatomie. Wien, Braumueller und Seidel, 1842–46.
5. Virchow, R. Die Cellularpathologie in ihrer Begruendung auf Physiologische und Pathologische Gewebelehre. Berlin, A. Hirschwald, 1st ed. 1858, 2nd ed. 1859, 3rd ed. 1862, 4th ed. 1871.
6. Ignatowski, A. Influence of animal feeding on the rabbit organism. Trans. Military-Med. Acad. Petersburg, 16:174, 1908.
7. Ignatowski, A. Ueber die Wirkung des tierischen Eiweisses auf die Aorta and die parenchymatoesen Organe der Kaninchen. Virchows Arch. Path. Anat., 198:248–270, 1909.
8. Stuckey, N.W. Ueber die Veraenderungen der Kaninchenaorta unter der Wirkung reichlicher Tierischer Nahrung. Centralbl. Allg. Path. u. Path. Anat., 22:379, 1911.
9. Stuckey, N.W. Ueber die Veraenderungen der Kaninchenaorta bei der Fuetterung mit verschiedenen Fettsorten. Centralbl. Allg. Path. u. Path. Anat., 23:910, 1912.
10. Saltykow, S. Atherosklerose bei Kaninchen nach wiederholten Staphylokokkeninjectionen. Beitr. Path. Anat., 43:147–171, 1908.
11. Saltykow, S. Zur Kenntnis der alimentaeren Krankheiten der Versuchstiere. Virchows Arch. Path. Anat., 213:8–22, 1913.
12. Saltykow, S. Die experimentell erzeugten Arterienveraenderungen in ihrer Beziehung zu Atherosklerose und verwandten Krankheiten des Menschen. Centralbl. Allg. Pathol., 19:321–369, 1908.
13. Anitschkow, N., and S. Chalatow. Ueber experimentelle Cholesterinsteatose und ihre Bedeutung fuer die Entstehung einiger pathologischer Prozesse. Centralbl. Allg. Pathol., 24:1–9, 1913.
14. Windaus, A. Ueber den Gehalt normaler und atheromatoeser Aorten an Cholesterin und Cholesterinestern. Hoppe-Seyler's Zeitschr. Physiol. Chem., 67:174–176, 1910.
15. Anitschkow, N. Ueber die Veraenderungen der Kaninchenaorta bei experimenteller Cholesterinsteatose. Beitr. Path. Anat., 56:379–404, 1913.
16. Anitschkow, N. Ueber die experimentelle Arteriosklerose der Aorta beim Meerschweinchen. Beitr. Path. Anat., 70:265–281, 1922.
17. Anitschkow, N. Ueber die experimentelle Atherosklerose der Herzklappen. Virchows Arch. Path. Anat., 220:233–256, 1915.
18. Anitschkow, N. Ueber die Rueckbildungsvorgaenge bei der experimentellen Arteriosklerose. Verhandl. Deutsch. Path. Gesellsch., 23:473, 1925.
19. Anitschkow, N. Ueber die Atherosklerose der Aorta beim Kaninchen und ueber deren Entstehungsbedingungen. Beitr. Path. Anat., 59:306–348, 1914.
20. Anitschkow, N. Development of our knowledge of arteriosclerosis. Experimental arteriosclerosis in animals. In: Arteriosclerosis, Cowdry, E.V. (ed.). New York, Macmillan, 1933.
21. Anitschkow, N. Das Wesen und die Entstehung der Atherosklerose. Ergebn. Inn. Med. u. Kinderh., 28:1–46, 1925.
22. Anitschkow, N. Zur Histophysiologie der Arterienwand. Klin. Wochschr., 4:2233–2235, 1925.
23. Aschoff, L. Ein Beitrag zur Myelinfrage. Verhandl. Deutsch. Path. Gesellsch., 1906, 166–170.
24. Zinserling, W.D. Untersuchungen ueber Atherosklerose. Virchows Arch. Path. Anat., 255:677–705, 1925.
25. Schoenheimer, R., and R. Breusch. Synthesis and destruction of cholesterol in the organism. J. Biol. Chem., 103:439–448, 1933.
26. Bloch, K. The biological synthesis of cholesterol. Les Prix Nobel, 1964, pp. 179–203.
27. Lynen, F. The pathway from "activated acetic acid" to the terpenes and fatty acids. Les Prix Nobel, 1964, pp. 205–246.

28. Goldstein, J.L., and M.S. Brown. The low-density lipoprotein pathway and its relation to atherosclerosis. Ann. Rev. Biochem., 46:89–93, 1977.
29. Schoenheimer, R. (1898–1942) Ueber den Beginn deu Tracer-Technik bei Stoffwechseluntersuchungen. Inaugural-Dissertation zur Erlangung der Doktorwuerde der Medizinischen Fakultaet der Universitat Zuerich. Juris Druck & Verlag Zurich, 1972, pp. 2–6.
30. Gofman, J.W., F. Lindgren, H. Elliott, W. Mantz, J. Hewitt, B. Strisower, and V. Herring. The role of lipids and lipoproteins in atherosclerosis. Science, 111:166–171, 186, 1950.
31. Ross, R. The pathogenesis of atherosclerosis—an update. New Engl. J. Med., 314: 488, 1986.
32. Ross, R., J. Glomset, B. Kariya, and L. Harker. A platelet-dependent serum factor that stimulates the proliferation of arterial smooth muscle cells in vitro. Proc. Natl. Acad. Sci., 71:1207–1210, 1974.

Chapter 7   Coronary Artery Disease

O. PAUL
R.J. BING

CREDIT FOR THE early work on coronary artery disease should go to clinical observations and judgment. More recently, increased speed of scientific advance has led to a decline in emphasis on purely clinical observations, while at the same time extolling the diagnostic and therapeutic benefits of scientific technology. For a medical student in the late 1920s and early 1930s, training was primarily based on observations and personal experience—the art of medicine—with little hope for successful therapy. Then we paid a price for our ignorance by inability to cure many diseases; today, we pay a price for the emphasis on science and technology, because we are less aware of the patient as a distinct personality, his or her social and economic concerns, and his or her personal response to disease. Reading the early-eighteenth- and nineteenth-century descriptions of coronary artery disease, we see how much can be accomplished by one's eyes, ears, and mind.

Vesalius and Vieussens (1) contributed greatly to the anatomy of the coronary circulation. William Harvey clearly described the second or coronary circulation: "For what should the coronary arteries pulsate in the heart; save to drive blood on by the impulse? And why should there be coronary veins except to acquire blood from the heart?" (2).

The pathologic state of the heart in angina pectoris was recognized by Morgagni (1, 2). In 1761 he published his famous *De Sedibus et Causis Morborum*. Written in the form of letters, *De Sedibus* contains the clinical and pathological description of approximately seven hundred cases. Regarding one of the patients who died of an incarcerated hernia, he wrote: "the left coronary artery appeared to have been changed into a bony canal from its very origin to the extent of

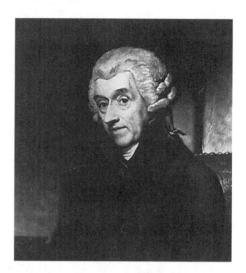

Figure 7.1. William Heberden. *(Courtesy of the New York Academy of Medicine)*

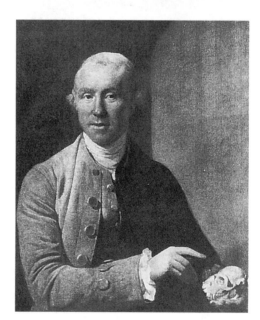

Figure 7.2. John Hunter. *(Courtesy of Special Collections, Health Sciences Library, Columbia University, NY)*

several fingers" (2). Morgagni himself died in his ninetieth year of a ruptured ventricle, presumably infarcted, just seven years before William Heberden's famous lecture on angina pectoris (2).

Heberden was one of the great British physicians who described angina pectoris, without relating it to diseases of the coronary artery (Fig. 7.1). Other clinicians were John Hunter (Fig. 7.2), Edward Jenner (Fig. 7.3), C.H. Parry,

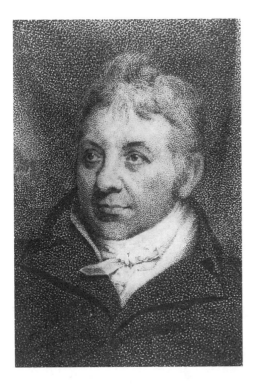

Figure 7.3. Edward Jenner. *(Courtesy of the New York Academy of Medicine)*

J. Fothergill, Marshall Hall, and Allan Burns (1, 2, 3; Fig. 7.4). A vivid description of these great clinicians is contained in James B. Herrick's book, *A Short History of Cardiology*, published in 1942 and in the chapter on the coronary circulation and cardiac metabolism in *Circulation of the Blood: Men and Ideas* (1). These men, except for Burns, were primarily clinical observers rather than experimentalists. The story of Hunter is well known and remains a landmark in medical history. At the age of forty, he began to suffer from recurring attacks of angina pectoris with severe pain in the stomach. He died during an attack that was provoked by a hospital board meeting on October 16, 1793, when "in his usual state of health, he went to St. George's Hospital meeting with some things which irritated his mind and not being perfectly master of his circumstances, he withheld his sentiments in which state of restraint he went into the next room and turned around to Dr. Robertson, one of the physicians of the hospital, gave a deep groan and dropped down dead." On autopsy, performed by Jenner, the discoverer of small pox vaccination, there was intense "ossification of the coronary arteries" (1).

Parry wrote a book entitled *Syncope Anginosa* that was based on cases similar to those of Hunter (1, 2, 3). He, too, correlated the clinical symptoms with autopsy findings. Parry paid more attention to the suddenness of the attack of weakness "due to the loss of strength of the heart muscle" than to the pain.

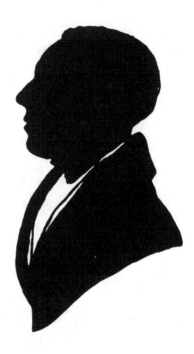

Figure 7.4. The only known picture of Allan Burns, in silhouette. *(Courtesy of Alfred P. Fishman, M.D.)*

It remained for Heberden, who studied many patients with angina pectoris, to draw a clear picture of what he called angina pectoris. Heberden was not concerned with the relationship between chest pain and coronary artery disease (1). Yet his description of angina pectoris became a classic and the disease has sometimes been referred to as Heberden's angina. He described clearly the symptoms: "They who are afflicted with this disease, are seized while they are walking (more especially if it be uphill, and soon after eating), with a painful and most disagreeable sensation in the breast which seems as it would extinguish life if it were to increase or to continue; but the moment they stand still, all this uneasiness vanishes." He mentions many times that the pain may be localized in several places, that males are more likely to be afflicted than females, and that the pain will appear not only when the person is walking, but when she or he is lying down. He ended his chapter by stating, "I know one who set himself a task sawing wood for half an hour every day, and was nearly cured. In one also, the disorder ceased of itself. Bleeding, vomiting, and purging, appear to me improper" (1, 4).

Of all these men, Burns deserves a special place, not only because he related clinical symptoms to pathophysiology, but because he was a most unusual personality in the field of cardiology (1). At fourteen, he began to study medicine and at sixteen he took over the sole direction of the dissecting room from his elder brother. He never obtained a university degree (today he would be without licensure and board certification in internal medicine and cardiology and therefore would be unable to practice!), but he gained experience as a physician and surgeon chiefly by attending and studying the patients of his brother and his friends. Burns accumulated drawings that were subsequently used to prepare his books on the diseases of the heart, on the blood vessels, and on surgical anatomy. He wrote two books during his brief career. The second book, entitled *Observations on the Surgical Anatomy of the Head and Neck*, is illustrated by cases and engravings. Published in 1811, this book had two printings of the second edition, as well as a German and an American edition. Burn's first book entitled, *Observations on Some of the Most Frequent and Important Diseases of the Heart*, was published in 1809 (5). Chapter 7 is of special interest, because here he connects angina pectoris to coronary blood flow.

> The heart like every other part has particular vessels set apart for its nourishment. In health, when we excite the muscular system to more energetic action than usual, we increase the circulation in every part, so that to support this increased action, the heart and every part has its power augmented. If, however, we call into vigorous action a limb, around which we have with a moderate degree of tightness, applied a ligature, we find then that the member can only support its action for a very short time; for now its supply of energy and its expenditure do not balance each other; consequently, it soon, from a deficiency of nervous influence in arterial blood, fails and sinks into a state of quiescence. A heart, the coronary vessels of which are cartilaginous or ossified, is in nearly a similar condition; it can, like the limb, begin with a moderately tight ligature, discharge its function so long as its action is moderate and equal. Increase, however, the action of the whole body and along with the rest that of the heart, and you will soon see exemplified the truth of what has been said; with this difference, that as there is no interruption to the action of the cardiac nerves, the heart will be able to hold out a little longer than the limb.

He continued: "If however, a person with the nutrient arteries of the heart diseased in such a way as to impede the progress of the blood among them, attempts to do the same, he finds that the heart is sooner fatigued than the other parts are, which remain healthy" (1, 5). Thus, Burns clearly saw the connection between a decrease in coronary blood flow and angina pectoris.

When Burns was twenty-three, he accepted an invitation from the Empress Catherine of Russia to go to St. Petersburg as director and surgeon of a hospital. But he soon returned home to again take up lectures on anatomy and surgery. Burns died in 1813, at the age of thirty-one, probably of a ruptured appendix.

The correlation between coronary artery disease and fatty changes of the cardiac muscle was recognized by Sir Richard Quain, who published a book on

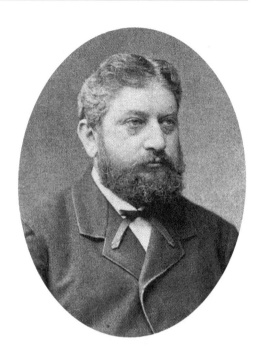

Figure 7.5. Julius F. Cohnheim.
(*Courtesy of Special Collections, Health
Sciences Library, Columbia University,
NY*)

fatty diseases of the heart in 1850 (1, 6). To quote him, "I have seen the coronary arteries extremely ossified going directly to the only part of the heart affected. . . . This connection between fatty softened heart and obstructed arteries suggests an analogy with softening of the brain, in which a like condition of the vessel is known to exist."

M. Hall, who became senior president of the Royal Medical Society of Edinburgh two years after registering as a medical student, expressed the belief that sudden death was often due to arrest of the coronary circulation (1, 7). This suggestion was taken up by another English clinician, J.E. Erichsen, who posed the problem in the following way: "The question, then, is to determine what effect the arrest of the coronary circulation would have on the action of the heart." He therefore ligated coronary vessels of dogs and observed that ventricular action continued for about twenty minutes (1, 8).

Julius Friederich Cohnheim (1839–84) was the initiator of the concept that coronary arteries are end-arteries, in other words, occlusion of one artery would lead to immediate cessation of blood flow to the area of heart muscle supplied by this artery. Cohnheim had commenced the study of medicine in 1856 in Berlin, where he worked under Virchow's guidance in the Pathological Institute (Fig. 7.5). It was there that he resolved to devote his life to science. Following this, he assumed the pathology chair at Kiel. In 1872 Cohnheim removed to Breslau and hence to Leipzig, where he made his mark as one of the early experimental pathologists, and commenced his experiments in dogs on the effect of ligation of a coronary artery. Occlusion of a coronary artery is fatal because blood supply to that part of the heart muscle cannot be furnished from collateral sources (9). Cohnheim cannulated the carotid, femoral, and pulmonary arteries, and fitted cannulas to manometers for the recording of pressures. He and his colleague, A. von Schultheiss-Rechberg, examined the possibility that the consequences of ligating a coronary artery arose from lack of oxygen (9). They did not think this likely, however, since oxygen deprivation of the whole animal had quite different results. Cohnheim even believed in the release of a poison by the heart muscle after occlusion. In the new Sydenham Society *Lectures on General Pathology*, an extensive memoir of Cohnheim was published that gives credit to this unusual and interesting personality (10).

By the end of the nineteenth century, the clinical consequences of coronary occlusion had been clearly defined by two German pathologists, C. Weigert and E. Ziegler. Weigert wrote that "If the occlusion occurs gradually in the absence of collateral circulation producing chronic changes, a slow atrophy and destruction of the muscle fibers without damage to the connecting tissue can be observed—the disappearing muscle fibers are then replaced by connective tissue" (1, 2, 11, 12). Weigert was an extremely productive worker in the field of medicine as well. In 1901 he proposed that myasthenia gravis was related to an abnormality of the thymus (2, 12). He was concise and clear in his description of the pathologic anatomy of myocardial infarction and coronary artery disease. To quote him,

> Atheromatous changes of the coronary arteries are frequently associated with thrombotic or embolic occlusion of their branches. If the occlusion occurs slowly or in such a way that collateral pathways, even though they are insufficient, exist, we will find a slow atrophy degeneration of the muscle fibers without damage to the connective tissue. These injured muscle fibers are then replaced by fibrous connective tissue. The so-called chronic myocarditis is nothing else but such a process. . . . but when there is sudden and complete cutting off of the blood supply to certain parts of the heart, we will find yellowish, dry masses resembling coagulated fibrin. In the surrounding areas there is a reactive infiltration of round and spindle cells (2, 12).

Ziegler also published a concise description of the gross and histologic features of myocardial infarction from onset to healing (1, 2, 13). He wrote: "The appearance of the shortened areas varies according to their age and blood content. Shortly after beginning of the anemia they are firm and manifest themselves only by a dull yellow coloration of the heart muscle." He then described the changes that occur with time and he also described necrosis of muscle cells and what he called "homogenous degeneration." The great step forward was that

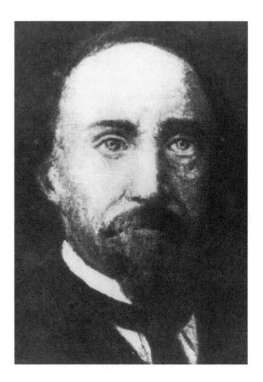

Figure 7.6. Adam Hammer. *(Courtesy of the New York Academy of Medicine)*

he anticipated the work of Herrick when he wrote, "When a certain stage is reached, the reparatory process starts." Thus, he realized that occlusion of the coronary artery may not be fatal, as Cohnheim had proposed, but may lead to chronic changes in the heart muscle that are compatible with life (13).

In a field where great clinicians and personalities abound, Adam Hammer certainly was unique (14; Figure 7.6). He had a checkered career. Born in Germany, he graduated from the University of Heidelberg in 1842, but after participating in the revolution of 1848, Hammer had to flee Germany and sought refuge in America. In St. Louis, Missouri, he first established a practice and later a medical school that survived for only one year. Nine years later, he established another medical school in St. Louis, the Humboldt Institute, where instruction was given in German; this school existed for ten years. In 1877 Hammer returned to Europe and, in 1878 he started a medical practice in Vienna. He died the year after he had presented his detailed report of a patient with coronary thrombosis. Hammer's case report deals with a thirty-four-year-old patient who apparently had rheumatic fever and collapsed. His heart rate was 23 beats per minute. Later, the pulse rate dropped to 8 beats per minute. Hammer reasoned, "In this desperate situation, I wondered if a disturbance of the nourishment of the heart could explain such a condition, and whether this could have been caused by

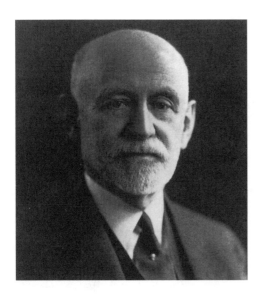

Figure 7.7. James B. Herrick. *(Courtesy of Special Collections, Health Sciences Library, Columbia University, NY)*

a thrombotic occlusion of at least one coronary artery." At autopsy there was a thrombus in the sinus of Valsalva, which extended all the way into the takeoff of the right coronary artery. Incidentally, for some time Hammer was also Felix Mendelssohn's physician (15).

It remained for Herrick to state, in 1912, that a sudden occlusion of the coronary artery might be compatible with life (1, 16). Herrick was a great clinician and innovator and shared with William Osler the ability to present his thoughts and observations in an original and poignant style (1, 17; Fig. 7.7). He knew medical history and presented it with humor and a personal perspective, acquired during his seventy years as a physician (18). Aside from his clear presentation of the clinical symptoms of coronary occlusion, he recognized for the first time the clinical entity, sickle cell anemia. Richard S. Ross has written a delightful essay on Herrick (17). He quotes from Herrick's Billings lecture of 1934: "he would be rash indeed, who would venture to predict what will be the exact stages of medicine or the relation between physician and patient a century from now, yes, even a decade ahead. Toppling thrones, scrapped constitutions, unsettled economic conditions, hostile industrial and social groups, angry nations brandishing loaded weapons, all these things not alone upset the world at present but threaten the stability and tranquility of the future." A truly prophetic statement! Herrick himself made a dramatic attempt to keep abreast of emerging medical science, and Ross reports that, in 1904, when Herrick was forty-three years old and busy with consultation practice, he matriculated at the University of Chicago to take courses in biology and physical and organic chemistry. He subsequently left his practice, went to Germany, and studied with Emil Fischer.

As is the case with many new concepts, it is not surprising that no critical discussion followed Herrick's classical paper on coronary thrombosis presented in 1912 before the Association of American Physicians. Herrick wrote later:

> You know I never understood it. In 1912 when I arose to read my paper at the Association, I was elated, for I knew I had a substantial contribution to present. I read it, and it fell flat as a pancake. No one discussed it except Emanuel Libman, and he discussed every paper read that day. I was sunk in disappointment (17).

In 1918 Herrick again spoke to the Association of American Physicians on coronary thrombosis and this time he included some experimental work done by his colleague, Fred Smith, on occlusion of the coronary artery in dogs (19). He presented electrocardiograms taken on these animals after experimental occlusion and showed the similarity to those obtained from patients. Herrick observed that work done in the laboratory on a dog attracted more attention than that done in the ward on patients. Herrick's broad interest in matters other than medicine is shown by the fact that at the age of seventy he presented a talk on Chaucer at the evening program of the Association of the American Physicians (17). One of the young men in the audience was heard to remark, "Well, I know who Dr. Herrick is, but who in hell is Chaucer?" Herrick took this to indicate that there was a serious lack of cultural background among the physicians of the day and made a strong case for a liberal arts education as a background for medicine (17).

After Herrick, the floodgates opened and today we have seen a major increase in the understanding of coronary artery disease and its effects, including approaches to treatment and prevention. There have been advances in the basic sciences through chemical-pharmological, electrophysiological, and molecular-biological research; there has been the introduction of special catheterization procedures such as selective coronary angiography and coronary angioplasty; new drugs have appeared, including those to alter clotting and assist ventricular function; and there has been the development of surgical techniques to improve the supply of arterial blood to the heart muscle. There have additionally been numerous epidemiological studies to point to predisposing factors leading to coronary artery disease. Yet without the clinical and experimental observations of these pioneers, such advances would not have been possible. In medicine, as in all of science, there is no peak of final accomplishment. If society continues to respect and promote scientific projects, our present advances will seem but the forerunners of greater accomplishments.

Following the work of Herrick, numerous clinical cardiologists made important contributions to the study and treatment of coronary heart disease. In several instances, their contributions were not totally new; others had done somewhat

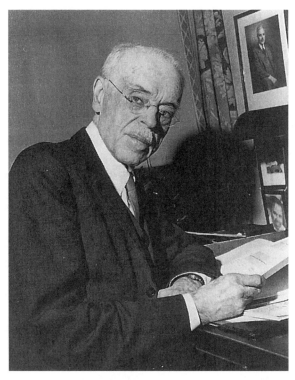

Figure 7.8. Paul D. White. *(Courtesy of the New York Academy of Medicine)*

similar preliminary work but had failed to be as persuasive and effective in their reasoning and presentations.

Paul Dudley White is an example (20; Fig. 7.8). He was raised in the Boston area, attended the Harvard Medical School, and received additional training at the Massachusetts General Hospital. In 1913 he went to London to study under Thomas Lewis (later Sir Thomas Lewis), and then saw service as a medical officer in World War I. White became the head of Cardiology at the Massachusetts General Hospital, where he soon developed a busy clinical service with a heavy load of teaching, research, and patient care. Gifted with boundless energy, a large measure of common sense, broad experience, and a warm and attractive personality, he soon became an international leader. His successful textbook, entitled *Heart Disease*, was first published in 1931, and went into four editions, including translations into Spanish and Italian. White's many research publications included reports about neurocirculatory asthenia in civilians, descriptions with E.D. Churchill of the first resection of the pericardium for chronic constrictive pericarditis to be performed in the English-speaking world (1930), the first report on what came to be called the Wolff-Parkinson-White syndrome (also in 1930), and clinical and electrocardiographic findings in acute cor pulmonale. He served as president of the American Heart Association and of the International Society of Cardiology.

White's role in coronary heart disease was highly influential, not only through the clinical reports published by him and his associates, but especially through his exposition of a prescription for living which he applied with great effectiveness not only to healthy individuals, but also to patients with angina pectoris or who had a history of myocardial infarction. His philosophy had three components: an attitude of optimism, regular physical activity, and avoidance of premature invalidism and retirement from useful living.

As the diagnosis of clinical coronary heart disease became relatively common following the work of Herrick and others, there was a tendency for physicians and the general public to regard persons with such a label as delicate, liable to sudden catastrophe including sudden death, and in need of inordinate protection from the nervous and physical strains of everyday life. Individuals with such diagnoses were often counseled to give up or greatly alter their employment for a routine of rest and quiet living. Surrounding all this was an atmosphere of resignation and pessimism. It was here that White, using his own large experience, but not reflecting any specific physiologic investigations or controlled clinical studies, intervened with great effect.

Beginning as early as 1927, White began to speak and write about the benefits of a routine of regular moderate physical exercise, such as walking and bicycling, for most patients with coronary heart disease; and beginning in 1932, he initiated a campaign to replace pessimism with optimism for such individuals, emphasizing that many persons with coronary heart disease could look forward to years of useful and satisfying living. This more cheerful view was coupled with an admonition to avoid unnecessary invalidism.

White's philosophy was not only presented widely to the medical professions; it was also extensively discussed before lay audiences, as White was a master in lay education. He reached the peak of his influence in this area when he was called in as consultant to President Dwight D. Eisenhower, when the president had a myocardial infarction while in Denver, Colorado, in September 1955. Fascinated by the daily bulletins regarding this very visible illness, the media concentrated on the often quotable pronouncements of White at periodic press conferences. He became the center of attention, particularly when he stated that despite the history of an undoubted recent myocardial infarction, the president might resume playing golf and campaign for a second term. This decision was of course influenced by the uncomplicated course of Eisenhower's illness, his good recovery, and the absence of unfavorable factors such as hypertension, diabetes, or hyperlipidemia. White's optimistic prognosis was borne out, and Eisenhower

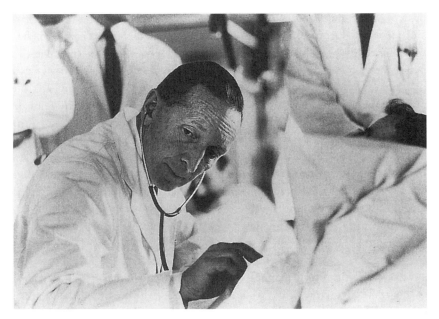

Figure 7.9. Herrman L. Blumgart. (*Courtesy of the New York Academy of Medicine*)

not only lived through his second term, but survived eight more years after he left the White House. This Boston physician's realistic message regarding coronary heart disease was widely disseminated, and without question permitted many patients with angina pectoris or a history of myocardial infarction to look to the future without the grim foreboding so common earlier in the century.

A major correlation of the pathology of coronary artery disease, and its complications, with its clinical manifestations appeared in 1940. This undertaking began with the work of Monroe J. Schlesinger, pathologist at the Bet Israel Hospital in Boston, who described in 1938 an ingenious technique for injecting coronary arteries postmortem with a colored radiopaque lead phosphate in agar mass, followed by cutting open the heart and completely dissecting the coronary tree (21). In this fashion, he was able to accurately locate areas of narrowing and obstruction, as well as visualize anastomoses. Two years later, making good use of this new approach, Schlesinger and Herrman L. Blumgart, who would soon become physician-in-chief at Beth Israel, completed the classic paper, "Studies on the Relation of the Clinical Manifestations of Angina Pectoris, Coronary Thrombosis, and Myocardial Infarction to the Pathologic Findings" (22; Fig. 7.9). Blumgart had received his training at the Harvard Medical School and the Peter Bent Brigham Hospital, followed by a year in London, and then four years at the Thorndike Memorial Laboratory of the Boston City Hospital, a famous incubator of research talent. He was a gracious and charming teacher and physician, in many ways resembling his mentor, Francis W. Peabody. Blumgart and Schlesinger had taken a series of 125 autopsy cases, in which "all subjects were studied who, during life, had had angina pectoris, coronary thrombosis, or congestive failure, or, on postmortem examination, showed coronary occlusion or myocardial infarction or fibrosis." This was a large and detailed undertaking, and the report of the findings occupied ninety-one pages of the *American Heart Journal.*

Blumgart and Schlesinger's conclusions were important and have stood the test of time. The cardiologist and the pathologist together found that normal hearts did not show intercoronary anastomoses of any size, and that larger anastomoses clearly developed in response to the presence of stenotic or occlusive disease. Cases with a history of angina pectoris were usually associated with one or more coronary occlusions; on the contrary, coronary occlusions existed in several cases with no history of angina. Congestive heart failure most often was seen when hearts showed a diffuse fibrosis. Blumgart and Schlesinger also found that the presence of coronary thrombosis and occlusion did not "necessarily produce any characteristic clinical manifestations," and that the clinical syndrome called at that time "coronary occlusion" in reality signified the presence of myocardial infarction. Finally, they emphasized "the extraordinary significance of the collateral circulation in bridging the discrepancy between supply and demand." This significant publication was indeed a high point in the collaboration between clinical cardiologist and pathologist. Its conclusions were supported and extended over the years as technological advances permitted other new approaches.

Very different from the work of Blumgart and Schlesinger was the introduction of an exercise test for patients suspected of having coronary heart disease; such a test was promoted chiefly in its early phase by Arthur M. Master, of Mount Sinai Hospital, New York. Others had also been involved in its development. Master and Oppenheimer had published, in 1929, tables setting out criteria for a test employing repeated ascent and descent of two steps by the patient (23). Each step was nine inches high, and the pulse and blood pressure were to be recorded two minutes after completion of the exercise. This was first described in general terms as "helpful in the diagnosis and the grading of circulatory efficiency and insufficiency," but with further experience, Master wrote in 1935 that the test "is particularly useful in the anginal syndrome" (24).

Six years later, in 1941, Master modified his original protocol by taking a control three-lead electrocardiogram prior to the exercise, and repeating this immediately after completion of the step-climbing. He referred in his first brief report on the revised technique to a fifty-eight-year-old man with a history of chest and arm discomfort, both with and without effort, who had a normal control electrocardiogram, but "immediately after the climb of the required number of steps, the RS-T segment became depressed in the three standard leads, the depression reaching 3 mm. in lead 2" (25). The findings were thus helpful in confirming a diagnosis of underlying coronary artery disease. Actually, others had made similar observations a few years before this. Katz and Landt in 1935 reported on the use of arm exercise with the patient reclining in bed, and produced typical ischemic changes in the electrocardiogram (which included a single chest lead) (26). Also, Missal (27), and independently Puddu (28), in 1938, had comparable experiences, the former employing Master's own two-step test, and the latter a slightly different stair-climbing technique. Because the Master protocol was a standard one, required no large, expensive equipment, could provide valuable information, and was associated with minimal risk, it was widely used during the 1940s and 1950s. It was gradually supplanted by the treadmill and the stationary bicycle with improved monitoring capability. Thus, the application of exercise testing to the study of coronary heart disease, first introduced in 1929, became a much-used—and sometimes overused—feature of office and hospital cardiologic practice and research.

A controversial aspect of the therapy of coronary heart disease and its complications was the use of oral anticoagulants to retard thrombin formation, introduced in the years immediately after the Second World War and widely prescribed for some years thereafter. Spotty use of these anticoagulants, with and without heparin, had been undertaken for a decade beginning in the late 1930s. Irving S. Wright, professor of clinical medicine at Cornell, became a forceful proponent of their use in 1945. Wright, a large, genial, bald-headed physician, led a multihospital cooperative controlled study, with a distinguished group of clinical investigators, which was sponsored by the American Heart Association. This short-term study, employing the drug dicumarol, included 1,031 patients with acute myocardial infarction (29). It was found that after six weeks of drug treatment, the mortality in the treated group was 7 percent lower than in the controls and that thromboembolic events were almost twice as frequent among the controls as among those receiving dicumarol.

The report of this study, published in 1954, was praised and criticized. Certain other investigators obtained similar results; others did not. Expectations of great benefit from the short-term use of such an agent in the management of acute myocardial infarction were not realized. In addition, a small number of patients experienced serious and even fatal hemorrhage. Further, the design and execution of the project were, in retrospect, far from ideal. Despite its shortcomings and the findings of only modest benefit, the 1954 report by Wright and his collaborators was a useful stepping-stone to further investigations.

Wright's study ushered in an era of multi-institutional controlled tests for coronary heart disease, studies that became steadily more sophisticated in design, quality control, and statistical expertise. They focused attention on the role of clotting, not just in the coronary circulation but also in the complications of venous thrombosis and pulmonary and peripheral embolism. General conclusions of these studies were supported in 1977 by Chalmers et al. after they had reviewed thirty years of experience in the treatment of acute myocardial infarction with oral anticoagulants; this was at a time when the enthusiasm for the routine use of these agents had waned (30).

In the decades after 1954 a vast number of other investigations approached the issue of clotting complications in coronary disease, including the use of aspirin and other drugs to alter platelet aggregation, and of several potent thrombolytic substances to attack the clot directly (the observations of DeWood and his collaborators in 1980 pointed once again to the importance of the freshly formed occlusive thrombus in a major coronary artery in the first few minutes and hours of the acute process) (31). In the 1990s as in the 1950s, the complex subject of clotting and its modification was at the forefront of scientific interest.

It was a clinician, Samuel A. Levine, who revolutionized the medical treatment of myocardial infarction by drastically shortening the period of bed rest. He was a feisty, astute, experienced cardiologist, short in stature and widely respected for his diagnostic ability and good sense. Born in Poland and trained at the Harvard Medical School, his professional career was spent in Boston at the Peter Bent Brigham Hospital, where he was deservedly popular as a teacher and practitioner. In 1936 he published a short, readable, and wise text entitled *Clinical Heart Disease*, which went into five editions. He and his associates contributed numerous clinical articles to the medical literature, with one on the "'Armchair' Treatment of Acute Coronary Occlusion," written with Bernard Lown and published in 1952, becoming a classic (32). This was at a time in which strict and prolonged bed rest for several weeks had become enshrined as a prerequisite for recovery from acute infarction.

Levine and Lown stated that "It has been our view that recumbency in bed affords less rest to the heart than the sedentary position in a chair with the feet down." In this brief but influential study, patients with acute myocardial infarction were allowed to be lifted from the bed to the chair for increasing periods, beginning no later than seven days after the onset of the attack, with apparent benefit and without deleterious consequences. The authors wrote: "The prompt improvement shown by some of those desperately ill with congestive heart failure after being placed in a chair was particularly impressive," and "This method of treatment also appeared to have beneficial effects on the psychological state of the patient, and facilitated the rehabilitation process." This was not an impressive publication in terms of later standards. The number of patients in the series was not large, there were no true controls, and the modification of the treatment routine was minor (32). But, the senior position of Levine and the influence of his writings (this was a lead article in the *Journal of the American Medical Association*) were such that this recommendation served to encourage others to open the door to successive steps to liberalize the treatment of acute myocardial infarction. In a few years, earlier use of the bedside chair and ambulation became widely accepted. These changes brought great economic and psychological advantages, facilitating and not compromising the optimal recovery of the patient.

Cardiac arrest had long been known to occur in a variety of situations, including in the presence of underlying heart disease. With the introduction of routine electrocardiograms, documentation of the terminal ventricular arrhythmias and of asystole was frequently made. This "act of God" was usually viewed as irreversible, although several methods of resuscitation had been proposed since 1880, including mouth-to-mouth artificial respiration and attempts to maintain the circulation. In 1947 Beck et al. reported the first successful open chest defibrillation of a human heart by a technique using electric shock developed by Hooker, W.B. Kouwenhoven, and Langworthy (33). This was followed by the important work of Zoll (34) and of Lown (35), making closed chest defibrillation feasible.

No satisfactory method of restoring both ventilation and circulation of patients experiencing cardiac arrest, especially as a consequence of coronary heart disease, was available until the 1961 landmark work of James R. Jude from the Department of Surgery at Johns Hopkins, assisted by Kouwenhoven and by G.G. Knickerbocker (36). These investigators introduced a remarkably simple combination of closed chest cardiac "massage" by compression of the lower sternum toward the thoracic spine sixty to eighty times a minute, coupled with intermittent mouth-to-mouth or mouth-to-nose ventilation. Their original report included 138 cardiac arrests in 118 patients, 24 of whom had acute myocardial infarction, and in many of whom external electrical defibrillation was also attempted. Five of the 24 with infarction were successfully resuscitated, but only 3 survived to leave the hospital. This technique was soon widely adopted and became the established one for treating the earliest phase of cardiac arrest. Hospital personnel including physicians and nurses were trained in the method, as were policemen, firemen, and emergency staff. Many lay individuals attended classes in the technique.

The combination of the ability to sustain life for a precious few minutes using the Jude–Kouwenhoven–Knickerbocker approach, better trained emergency staff and improved equipment in emergency rooms and ambulances, and the capacity for closed chest external cardiac defibrillation as described by Zoll and by Lown, permitted the rescue of a significant number of lives which would otherwise have been lost (see Chapter 14).

Dovetailing nicely with the growing popularity of this active program for treating cardiac arrest was the appearance of the coronary care unit. For decades, patients hospitalized with signs of acute myocardial infarction or unstable angina had been placed on the regular hospital medical wards or in single- or two-bed units. The advantage of doing otherwise was not obvious. With the availability of a more effective approach to the management of cardiac arrest, should it occur, and the ability to monitor the electrocardiogram constantly, there was a reason for change. In June 1962 Wilburne and Fields, from the Cedars of Lebanon and Mount Sinai hospitals in Los Angeles, described before a meeting of the American Medical Association "a central coronary care unit together with 1) a program of physiologic and closed circuit television monitoring, and 2) an organized step-by-step plan of resuscitation in cardiac arrest due to coronary artery disease" (37). Simultaneous with this innovative report Day at the Bethany Hospital, Kansas City, and Meltzer at the Presbyterian University of Pennsylvania Medical Center in Philadelphia published similar studies (38). Such a sequestration of acute coronary cases, together with provision for a specially trained nursing staff and monitoring equipment, was rapidly adopted by most hospitals in the belief that patient lives might thus be saved.

The existence of an acute coronary care unit became overnight not only a useful facility, but also a hospital status symbol, as well as providing business for manufacturers of electronic equipment. Equally important was the delegation of new duties to nurses. Of necessity, nurses became well trained in recognizing cardiac arrest, and often they were the ones to initiate and carry out resuscitative measures. Their level of competence, and their role in applying techniques previously applied only by physicians, increased their professional image and enhanced their importance especially in the area of coronary heart disease. A true cardiac team was usually the result, a happy and unexpected dividend. By the 1990s the period of hospitalization of most acute coronary cases had been drastically shortened from the four- to six-week period common fifty years earlier, to several days, with a great savings in cost and a favorable result in mental and physical recovery.

The history of coronary heart disease in the twentieth century would be incomplete without reference to the recognition of risk factors in coronary heart disease formulated by scientists and epidemiologists. Now accepted without question as important in the genesis of coronary atherosclerotic disease, it was not always so. Earlier in the century, investigators working in the areas of nutrition, blood lipids, cigarette smoking, and other factors, were often regarded as harmless and of no significance. Recognition therefore should be given to a few whose often lonely work has proved fundamental in the risk factor concept. A recent review of the background of cardiovascular disease has pointed to individuals or groups who have been particularly significant in the area of coronary heart disease (39). Information on this subject is also available from the comprehensive textbooks on cardiology by Braunwald (40) and Hurst (41). In the field of diet, the lineage of contributing investigators goes back a hundred years. Ancel Keys of the University of Minnesota was one individual who in the twentieth century has provided especially significant additions to our knowledge, particularly about blood lipids.

In the area of hypertension, Fisher in 1914 was the first to associate an elevated arterial pressure with an excess mortality among life insurance policyholders. Allan in 1934 correctly concluded, from uncontrolled observations, that hypertension was a major factor in the occurrence of angina pectoris and coronary occlusion. Later, several long-term population studies amply confirmed this. The cigarette smoking habit was first linked to coronary heart disease by English, Willius, and Berkson of the Mayo Clinic in 1940, but was particularly well documented by the classic investigation of Hammond and Horn of the American Cancer Society in 1954. These few examples—and many other pertinent reports—have served to provide the basis for the ever-expanding field of the prevention of coronary heart disease (see Chapter 6). The impact of all this and perhaps other factors on the incidence of coronary heart disease as a health problem has been astonishing. Among most developed countries, the death rates from this condition have declined, in particular, in the United States. As noted by Farmer and Gotto: "The coronary artery disease mortality rate [in the United States] fell 54% 1963–1990. In 1950, the annual age-adjusted death rate from myocardial infarction was 226.4 per 100,000; in 1991, it was 108.0. The period of 1982-1992 alone saw a thirty-one percent decline in myocardial infarction death rate" (41).

References

1. Bing, R.J. Coronary circulation and cardiac metabolism. In: Circulation of the Blood: Men and Ideas, Fishman, A.P., and D.W. Richards (eds.). Oxford University Press, 1964, pp. 199–264.
2. Lie, J.T. Recognizing coronary heart disease. Selected historical vignettes from the period of William Harvey (1578–1657) to Adam Hammer (1818–1878). Mayo Clin. Proc., 53:811–817, 1978.
3. Herrick, J.B. A Short History of Cardiology. Springfield, IL, Thomas, 1942.
4. Heberden, W. Commentaries on the History and Cure of Diseases. London, Payne, 1802.
5. Burns, A. Observations on Some of the Most Frequent and Important Diseases of the Heart; An Aneurysm of the Thoracic Aorta; on Preternatural Pulsation in the Epigastric Region; and on the Unusual Origin and Distribution of Some of the Large Arteries of the Human Body. Edinburgh, Bryce, 1809.
6. Quain, R. On fatty acid diseases of the heart. Med. Chir. Trans., 33:121, 1850.
7. Hall, M. On the mutual relations between anatomy, physiology, pathology and therapeutics, and the practice of medicine. The Golstonian Lectures for 1842. London, Bailliere's, 1842.
8. Erichsen, J.E. On the influence of the coronary circulation on the action of the heart. London Med. Gaz., 2:561–564, 1842.
9. Cohnheim, J.F., and A. von Schultheiss-Rechberg. Ueber die Folgen der Kranzarterienverschliessung fuer das Herz. Virchows Arch. Path. Anat., 85:503–537, 1881.
10. McKee, A.B. Lectures on General Pathology. Trans. of Julius Cohnheim, Vorlesungen ueber allgemeine Pathologie. London, New Sydenham Society, 1889–90.
11. Talbott, J.H. A Biographical History of Medicine: Excerpts and Essays on the Men and Their Work. New York, Grune & Stratton, 1970, pp. 837–840.

12. Weigert, C. Ueber die pathologischen Gerinnungsvorgaenge. Virchows Arch. Path. Anat., 79:87–123, 1880.
13. Ziegler, E. Lehrbuch der allgemeinen Pathologie und der pathologischen Anatomie fuer Aertze und Studierende. Jena, Fischer, 1881–1906.
14. Lie, J.T. Centenary of the first correct antemortem diagnosis of coronary thrombosis by Adam Hammer (1818–1878): English translation of the original report. Am. J. Cardiol., 42:849–852, 1978.
15. Neumayr, A. "Musik und Medizin: am Beispiel der deutschen Romantik" Edition Wien, 1989, p. 118.
16. Herrick, J.B. Clinical features of sudden obstruction of the coronary arteries. JAMA, 59:2015–2020, 1912.
17. Ross, R.S. A parlous state of storm and stress. The life and times of James B. Herrick. Circulation, 67:955–959, 1983.
18. Herrick, J.B. The coronary artery in health and disease. Harvey Lectures, 26:129–151, 1931.
19. Herrick, J.B. Concerning thrombosis of the coronary arteries. Trans. Assoc. Am. Physicians, 33:408–418, 1918.
20. Paul, O. Take Heart: The Life and Prescription for Living of Paul Dudley White. Boston, MA, Harvard University Press for the Francis A. Countway Library of Medicine, 1986.
21. Schlesinger, M.J. An injection plus dissection study of coronary artery occlusions and anastomoses. Am. Heart J., 15:528–568, 1938.
22. Blumgart, H.L., M.J. Schlesinger, and D. Davis. Studies on the relation of the clinical manifestations of angina pectoris, coronary thrombosis, and myocardial infarction to the pathologic findings. Am. Heart J., 19:1–91, 1940.
23. Master, A.M., and E.J. Oppenheimer. A simple exercise tolerance test for circulatory efficiency with standard tables for normal individuals. Am. J. Med. Sci., 177:223–243, 1929.
24. Master, A.M. The two-step test of myocardial function. Am. Heart J., 10:495–510, 1935.
25. Master, A.M., and H.L. Jaffe. The electrocardiographic changes after exercise in angina pectoris. J. Mt. Sinai Hospital, 7:629–632, 1941.
26. Katz, L.N., and H. Landt. The effect of standardized exercises on the four-lead electrocardiogram. Am. J. Med. Sci., 189:346–351, 1935.
27. Missal, M.E. Exercise tests and the electrocardiograph in the study of angina pectoris. Ann. Int. Med., 11:2018–2036, 1938.
28. Puddu, V. Alterazioni elettrocardiografiche da sforzo, in sogetti normali e anginosi, con particolare riguardo alla derivazione foracica. Cardiologia, 2:183–192, 1938.
29. Wright, I.S., C.D. Marple, and D.F. Beck. Myocardial Infarction: Its Clinical Manifestations and Treatment with Anticoagulants: A Study of 1031 Cases. New York, Grune & Stratton, 1954.
30. Chalmers, T.C., R.J. Matta, H. Smith Jr., and A.M. Kunzler. Evidence favoring the use of anticoagulants in the hospital phase of acute myocardial infarction. N. Engl. J. Med., 297:1091–1096, 1977.
31. DeWood, M.A., J. Spores, R. Notske, L.T. Mouser, R. Burroughs, M.S. Golden, and H.T. Lang. Prevalence of total coronary occlusion during the early hours of transmural myocardial infarction. N. Engl. J. Med., 303:897–902, 1980.
32. Levine, S.A., and B. Lown. Armchair treatment of acute coronary thrombosis. JAMA, 148:1365–1369, 1952.
33. Beck, C.F., W.H. Pritchard, and H.S. Feil. Ventricular fibrillation of long duration abolished by electric shock. JAMA, 136:985–986, 1947.
34. Zoll, P.M., A.J. Linenthal, W. Bibson, M.H. Paul, and L.R. Norman. Termination of

ventricular fibrillation in man by externally applied electric countershock. N. Engl. J. Med., 254:727–732, 1956.

35. Lown, B., J. Neuman, R. Amarasingham, and B.V. Berkovits. Comparison of alternating current with direct current electroshock across the closed chest. Am. J. Cardiol., 10:223–233, 1962.

36. Jude, J.R., W.B. Kouwenhoven, and G.G. Knickerbocker. Cardiac arrest. Report of application of external cardiac massage on 118 patients. JAMA, 178:1063–1069, 1961.

37. Wilburne, M., and J. Fields. Cardiac resuscitation in coronary heart disease. JAMA, 184:453–457, 1963.

38. Meltzer, L.E., and A.J. Dunning (eds.). Textbook of Coronary Care. Philadelphia, Charles Press, 1972, pp. 5–7.

39. Paul, O. Background of the prevention of cardiovascular disease. Circulation, 79:1361–1368; 80:206–214, 1989.

40. Braunwald, E. Heart Disease: A Textbook of Cardiac Medicine. Braunwald, E. (ed.). Philadelphia, Saunders, 4th ed., 1992.

41. Hurst, J.W. The Heart, Arteries and Veins. New York, McGraw-Hill, 7th ed., 1990.

Chapter 8   Coronary Artery Surgery

J.C. BALDWIN
M.J. REARDON
R.J. BING

Coronary artery disease, the greatest killer in the Western world, has been the focus of attention for cardiologists and surgeons more than any other single affliction. The earliest attempt at the surgical relief of angina pectoris in man is believed to have been undertaken in 1916 by Jonnesco (1). He treated angina by ablation of the upper thoracic sympathetic ganglia. Nonoperative approaches to sympathetic ablation, which included paravertebral alcohol injection, were ultimately abandoned due to the high incidence of complications and the frequency of inducing increased angina (2).

With the knowledge that diminished coronary blood flow was the cause of angina, attempts to increase collateral blood flow or introduce extracardiac sources of blood to affected areas of the heart were undertaken. In 1931 Moritz made the observation that pericardial adhesions appeared to confer a beneficial effect on the course of coronary artery disease. This notion had first been suggested by Thorel in 1903 in a patient with complete obliteration of both coronary arteries and extensive pericardial adhesion (3).

Claude S. Beck (Fig. 8.1) joined the faculty at the Western Reserve University in Cleveland following training in surgery at the Peter Bent Brigham Hospital in Boston. Beck was interested in the problem of cardiac blood flow and made the astute observation that adhesions between the pericardium and the heart bled profusely from both ends when severed (4). This led to discussions with Moritz regarding his study of naturally occurring collaterals to the heart and the early studies of treatment of suppurative pericarditis by instillation of Dakin solution into the pericardium. Beck began a series of brilliant experiments in

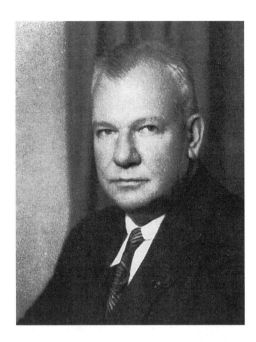

Figure 8.1. Claude S. Beck. *(Courtesy of the New York Academy of Medicine)*

dogs in 1932, which demonstrated the efficacy of recruiting collateral blood flow between coronary arteries and from the adjacent pericardium by mechanical and chemical irritation (4, 5). His paper, published in 1935, began as follows: "It is perversity of nature that the most important muscular structure in the body is the most defenseless" (5).

By 1943 Beck had published his experience with the procedure on thirty patients, reporting partial or complete relief of pain in survivors (6). The technique initially involved the installation of mechanical irritants such as ground beef bone dust. Later, Beck found chemical irritants more efficacious and suggested the use of asbestos. The use of talc and magnesium silicate was popularized by Thompson, who reported favorable results in 70 percent of thirty patients (7). Later, mechanical abrasion of the epicardium was performed using specially designed burrs and even sandpaper (6). Vineberg proposed placement of the Ivalon sponge in the pericardial space to achieve adhesion and improved blood flow (8). Others reported an increase in the vascular supply of the pericardium following ligation of the internal mammary arteries (9).

Although the pericardium became a convenient vehicle for the enhancement of blood supply, because of the development of adhesions it soon became clear that more direct means were required to increase supply of blood to the myocardium. Beck and O'Shaughnessy independently tried various vascular conduits, including the pectoral muscles and the omentum in "cardiopexy" procedures

(10, 11). Lezius, working in Germany in 1939, established that lung adhesions to the heart after pericardiectomy allowed ligation of a coronary artery without adverse effects in animals in 1939 (12). These "pneumopexy" techniques were later popularized by Carter and Vidone (13, 14). Other ideas included the use of pedicle grafts of jejunum by Key and of skin by Moran, as sources of augmented blood supply to the heart (15, 16). Deaths occurred often with these techniques and were thought to be a result of coronary thrombosis brought about by release of thromboplastic materials from the abraded tissues, as well as by direct injury to already diseased coronary intima (17).

Beck's subsequent experimental efforts revolved around the feasibility of increasing myocardial tissue perfusion by "arterialization" of the coronary venous system (18). This concept was an expansion of work done by Gross, who reported his results with coronary sinus occlusion to the Society of Experimental Biology and Medicine in 1935 (19). Fauteux later studied the effect of coronary vein ligation, which was believed to result in an increase in oxygen uptake by an ischemic myocardium (20). Beck, however, focused on the establishment of retrograde perfusion through the coronary sinus via arterial or venous conduits such as the internal mammary artery or venous grafts to the descending aorta (18). This technique was subsequently incorporated clinically by Beck and by others as part of revascularization operations. The bold concept of retrograde perfusion has now been resurrected, with the use of retrograde infusion of cardioplegia solutions through the coronary sinus for intraoperative myocardial protection (21).

Methods for perfusion of the myocardium directly from the cardiac chambers were investigated by several groups. These efforts were based on Wearn's studies on the capillary bed of the heart and those of Beck on venous stasis in the coronary circulation (22, 23). Goldman placed explanted carotid grafts into the myocardium that communicated with the left ventricle (24). The grafts contained a number of small openings that directed theoretically ventricular blood into the sinusoidal network within the myocardium. This procedure reportedly protected against ligation of the anterior descending coronary artery in dogs. Similarly, Massimo and Boffie inserted T-shaped polyethylene tubes of 4 mm in diameter which were embedded in the myocardium of dogs (25).

The direct implantation of the internal mammary artery into ischemic myocardium by Arthur Vineberg of Montreal in 1945 was a continuation of the search for optimal sources of extracardiac blood (26, 27). Although the clinical results were difficult to assess, experimental and clinical data suggested significant increases in myocardial blood flow with this approach (28). Furthermore, recognition that many of these patients had persistently patent mammary arteries and established collateral blood flow when studied many years later sustained interest in the internal mammary artery as a conduit. By 1965 Vineberg had reported on 115 patients with an operative mortality of only 2.9 percent and a graft patency rate of approximately 75 percent. Based on these encouraging findings, seventy-six Vineberg procedures were performed at the Cleveland Clinic by Effler between April 1962 and December 1963 (29). However, the long time period required to achieve maximal revascularization (at least nine months) significantly diminished the appeal of this approach to the urgent problem of myocardial ischemia.

Confidence derived from surgical successes in the treatment of congenital lesions of the heart and in "closed" techniques for relief of mitral stenosis suggested bolder methods in the treatment of coronary disease. Coronary endarterectomy was pursued by Szilagyi and others in animals and in postmortem specimens (30). As a result, a series of endarterectomy procedures were performed on patients and reported by Bailey and by Longmire the following year (1958) (31, 32). As experience accumulated, improvements in survival followed. Modifications, such as the use of the vein patch in 1959 by Senning, were incorporated (33). A high operative mortality, however, resulted in restrained enthusiasm and remained an impetus for the search for safer methods of myocardial revascularization.

The introduction of selective coronary arteriography by Sones in 1959 offered precise localization of lesions preoperatively as well as an assessment of postoperative results (34). The Cleveland Clinic group studied various techniques in the surgical treatment of coronary artery disease, including Vineberg's operation, endarterectomy, and techniques involving direct coronary artery anastomoses (34, 35).

In 1910 Carrel bypassed coronary arteries in the laboratory, using a segment of explanted carotid artery that was interposed between the aorta and the left coronary artery (36). Sustained experimentation with direct coronary artery anastomoses, however, was not undertaken until the early 1950s, when Murray reported interposition arterial grafts following resection of proximal segments of coronary arteries in dogs (37). Experimental work at the University of Minnesota in the late 1950s investigated the feasibility of direct anastomosis to coronary arteries with the internal mammary artery (38, 39). These experiments with internal mammary graft pedicles were expanded by Ormond Julian in Chicago (40). Julian used free arterial grafts interposed between the aorta and the left circumflex coronary artery in dogs on cardiopulmonary bypass. Several other studies were conducted with refinements in the technique (41, 42, 43, 44).

The use of aortocoronary bypass in man was first reported in 1962 by David C. Sabiston at Duke University in a patient following an unsuccessful right coronary endarterectomy (45). Sabiston described a patient in whom a complete occlusion of the right coronary artery was demonstrated by coronary arteriography. Endarterectomy was unsuccessful and a reversed saphenous vein graft was placed. The patient died of a cerebral vascular accident three days later. At autopsy, a thrombus was present at the aortic end of the coronary anastomosis. Two years later, again as a result of difficulties following endarterectomy, Garret performed aortocoronary bypass to the left anterior descending artery (46). This case, however, was not reported until seven years later.

In the popular medical mind, the origin of the current era of coronary surgery was the Cleveland Clinic, and the prodigious efforts of Effler, Favaloro, and Grove, which were truly historic in gaining wide acceptance for this procedure in a relatively short period of time. Their experience began in May 1967, when surgery on an occluded right coronary artery required its excision and replacement with an interposed segment of saphenous vein. The patient recuperated fully and was discharged.

> With timidity, we slowly repeated this experience. First to the right and later to the left coronary artery. In a short period, the interposed grafts gave way to the bypassed grafts from aorta to coronary artery. As results improved and enthusiasm escalated, all combinations of single and multiple grafts were tried and efforts were made to find the simplest and best procedures and then to standardize them. *Letter from Dr. Effler to Dr. Bing.*

In 1967 37 bypass operations were performed at the Cleveland Clinic. By 1968 the number rose to almost 200. In 1969 1,500 patients underwent coronary artery bypass procedures at the Clinic and, in 1976, the number was 3,000. The surgical results by Effler and his colleagues were singular for their low operative mortality and the Clinic became a magnet for surgeons around the world interested in learning these techniques. The success of the operation depended on careful selection of low-risk patients and standardized teamwork, as emphasized by the Cleveland group. This approach involved coordination of surgeons, anesthesiologists, cardiologists, and nursing and other health care personnel committed to caring for these patients in a reliable and consistent fashion.

Although no one individual can be credited for the ultimate success of the bypass procedure, Rene Favaloro stands out as one of the most innovative surgeons of this era. The career of Favaloro, like many of the pioneers, was a circuitous one (Fig. 8.2). After graduation from La Plata University School of Medicine in 1948, and obtaining an M.D. degree in 1949, Favaloro moved to a small village in a farming area of Argentina with approximately 1,100 inhabitants. There he worked as a country doctor with the help of his physician brother, providing medical care for the population until the end of 1961. As Favaloro wrote, "I could no longer watch the revolution in cardiac surgery any longer. I wanted to be part of it" (47). In early 1962 he moved to the United States and started work in the Department of Thoracic and Cardiovascular Surgery at the Cleveland Clinic, under the guidance of Effler. Favaloro also credited Sones, saying "there is no question that without his introduction of coronary arteriography the operation would have not been feasible. Initially there was considerable concern about the

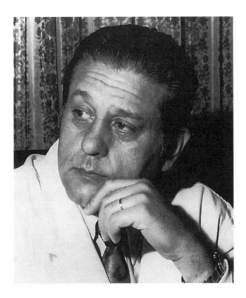

Figure 8.2. Rene G. Favaloro. *(Courtesy of the New York Academy of Medicine)*

prolonged patency of the saphenous vein graft." Favaloro quotes Sones, who would often shake his head, saying to him, "Oh Rene, I wonder what will happen to all of us if those grafts occlude two or three months after the operation." Favaloro mentions that the first operation was performed on one of the relatives of an executive at the Cleveland Clinic who had suffered a myocardial infarct. A single bypass was performed to the anterior descending coronary artery and the patient made an uneventful recovery. Favoloro has recently published an extensive analysis of coronary artery bypass graft surgery (48). Favoloro describes the evolution of the surgical technique, the controversies arising from the procedure, the clinical trials, and the relationship to percutaneous transluminal coronary angioplasty (PTCA).

The medical community was slow to accept the bypass operation as a legitimate surgical procedure. Favaloro remembers a discussion during a meeting of the World Congress of Cardiology in London in 1979, when he and Charles Friedberg, a prominent clinical cardiologist, had serious arguments about this type of surgery (47). Finally, in the discussion, when Friedberg said that it was difficult to accept the very low mortality rate, Favaloro wrote, "My Latin blood flared up and I said emphatically that the work of our team was an honest effort under the leadership of Effler and Sones and that our records at the Cleveland Clinic were at the disposal of anyone who wanted to study them."

Although the mammary arteries were identified early as suitable arterial conduits for coronary bypass, they were employed sparingly in the United States during this time (49). In Leningrad, Vasilii Kolessov, as chairman of the Surgical

Department of the First Medical Institute, performed a series of internal mammary anastomoses to the left coronary circulation. His accomplishments and contributions to coronary surgery were virtually unknown in the Western medical literature at the time (1967) (50, 51). He used direct internal mammary artery to coronary artery anastomoses, describing his procedure in detail and reporting the results on five patients. The main difference between the Cleveland Clinic group and Kolessov was that the latter eschewed coronary angiography "lest it should result in fibrillation of heart ventricle." Kolessov graduated in 1931 from the Second Leningrad Institute. After serving in the war, he returned to Leningrad, where he was awarded the title of professor in 1949. In 1952 he became the chief of the Department of Military Surgery in the Military Medical Department in Leningrad. At the time of his publication, he was the chairman of the Surgical Department of the First Leningrad Medical Institute.

As cardiopulmonary bypass technology improved and familiarity and safety were achieved, longer pump runs and more complete revascularizations were undertaken. Important in this regard was the refinement of the techniques of myocardial protection. Although the concept of cardioplegia was initially advanced by Melrose, it received intensive and widespread attention with the advent of the "bypass revolution." More recently, the work of Buckberg and many others has made possible extended periods of arrest, thereby allowing surgeons of widely varying skills and speed to operate with relative safety (52).

Given the lack of long-term follow-up data, bypass operations were not initially embraced by the general medical community. Acceptance came slowly as the efficacy of the procedure at relieving angina was recognized. Large multicenter trials were instituted to investigate the efficacy of coronary bypass in comparison to standard medical therapy. The first of these studies was the Veterans Administration (VA) Cooperative Study, which began its pilot phase in 1970 (53). Although this study was undertaken during the early days of the coronary artery bypass operation, it clearly demonstrated the benefit of surgery for patients with significant (> 50%) left main coronary artery stenosis. This was followed by the European Cooperative Surgery Study, which demonstrated the superiority of surgery over medical management for symptomatic patients with three-vessel coronary disease or two-vessel disease in which the left anterior descending coronary artery is involved (54). This study also corroborated the findings of the VA study for patients with left main coronary artery disease. The Coronary Artery Surgery Study, which was sponsored by the National Institutes of Health, studied patients who were randomized to medical or surgical therapy between 1975 and 1979 (55). This study attempted to define the role of surgery as initial therapy for patients with significant coronary disease and limited symptoms. It demonstrated a benefit for those patients with coronary artery disease in three vessels and depressed ventricular function (ejection fraction between 0.35 and

0.5). Although these studies have been instrumental in defining the benefits of surgery, differences in study design and data collection have resulted in continued controversy. Nonetheless, proponents of the need for national statistical and longitudinal analysis of the efficacy of new medical interventions can find gratification in the area of coronary surgery. It is perhaps the best studied of the newer technological innovations in medicine.

Newer developments in the surgical treatment of coronary artery disease involve the increased use of multiple arterial grafts for myocardial revascularization (56). The left internal mammary artery to left anterior descending coronary bypass has been unequivocally shown to improve survival and have significantly increased long-term patency when compared to saphenous vein graft to left anterior descending coronary artery bypass (57). This has led to the use of internal mammary arteries, radial arteries, and right gastroepiploic arteries as routine for many surgeons. In addition to the use of novel arterial conduits, the surgical procedure itself has evolved novel "minimally invasive" approaches. The definition of minimally invasive coronary artery bypass is generally divided into two groups: (1) beating heart coronary artery bypass to avoid the negative effects of cardiopulmonary bypass itself; and (2) port access coronary artery bypass with femoral cardiopulmonary bypass to minimize the incisional violation of the body wall integrity. Both have been achieved in recent years but their exact place in the surgical armamentarium for the treatment of coronary artery occlusive disease remains to be determined. Issues still under consideration with these procedures revolve around the technical and judgmental development necessary to allow accuracy and patency of the anastomosis vis-à-vis conventional bypass, issues of complete revascularization, the ability to teach this procedure in a consistent fashion to new cardiac surgeons, and long-term outcomes. During the past few years angioplasty rather than bypass surgery or the use of thrombolytic agents has become the preferred treatment for acute myocardial infarction, provided certain clinical conditions are present. Angioplasty is less invasive and more cost-effective than coronary bypass surgery. However, coronary bypass surgery remains a unique and irreplaceable treatment for many patients.

An additional approach is the use of transmyocardial laser revascularization (TMR) to attempt to treat coronary artery disease via the heart's own microvascular structure. This approach is a modification of the methods described by Goldman and by Massimo and is based on the myocardial sinusoidal network concept developed by Wearn and Beck nearly half a century ago. Although the initial theory of perfusion through the myocardial sinusoid appears to be nonfunctional, newer theories revolve around the concepts of angiogenesis initiated by the laser injury or denervation of the heart from laser injury. TMR continues to have appeal on a theoretical basis as it is not limited to patients with adequate distal coronary arteries and therefore significantly broadens the range of candidates for treatment. Also, since many small channels are made, the failure of any one channel to perform its role would probably be of little consequence, unlike the failure of macroscopic bypass graft, which can have catastrophic consequences. Currently the two main laser types are the CO_2 laser and the holmium-YAG laser. The advantage of the CO_2 laser is that it is a more powerful (150 watt) laser necessitating a shorter pulse duration and causing less tissue necrosis than the holmium-YAG laser (40 watt). However, the holmium-YAG laser has the advantage in that the laser energy can be controlled via a fiberoptic, thoracoscopic, and percutaneous catheter. Early clinical results suggest angina relief is excellent, averaging two classes of anginal improvement (58, 59). Currently studies are seeking more objective criteria with exercise improvement and perfusion scans for ischemia.

The dramatic success of cardiac transplantation for "ischemic cardiomyopathy" has resulted in a trend toward increasing prevalence of ischemic disease as an indication for transplant. At present, the majority of patients awaiting heart transplant have ischemic disease. The clinical success of heart transplantation has led to a 80 percent to 90 percent one-year survival and 50 percent to 60 percent five-year survival in these desperately ill patients. The procedure has been limited by a lack of donor availability—only 10 percent of the patients requiring heart transplantation ultimately receive an organ. Because of this and substantial improvement in mechanical support devices, a new interest in permanent mechanical support has arisen and is currently undergoing evaluation in the rematch trial. Lack of donor availability has also led to a high level of interest in developing chimeric xenograft based on the pig for ultimate human transplantation. Ultimately, replacement of the heart with a biological (allograft or xenograft) or mechanical substitute will establish itself as a fundamentally new approach to ischemic heart disease, one that conceptually transcends this century's remarkable efforts at repair and palliation.

References

1. Jonnesco, T. Traitement chirurgical de l'angine de poitrine par la résection du sympathique cervico-thoracique. Presse. Med. Par., 29:193,1921.
2. White, J.C. Cardiac pain: anatomic pathways and physiologic mechanisms. Circulation, 16:644, 1957.
3. Thorel, C.H. Pathologie der Kreislauforgane. Ergebn. Allg. u Path. Anat., 9:559–1116, 1903.
4. Beck, C.S. The effect of surgical solution of chlorinated soda (Dakin's Solution) in the pericardial cavity. Arch. Surg., 18:1659–1671, 1929.
5. Beck, C.S., and V.L. Tichy. The production of a collateral circulation to the heart. (I. An experimental study.) Am. Heart J., 10:849–873, 1935.
6. Beck, C.S. Principles underlying the operative approach to the treatment of myocardial ischemia. Ann. Surg., 118:788–806, 1943.
7. Thompson, S.A., and M.J. Raisbeck. Cardio-pericardiopexy: the surgical treatment of coronary arterial disease by the establishment of adhesive pericarditis. Ann. Int. Med., 16:495–520, 1942.

8. Vineberg, A.M., T. Deliyannis, and G. Pablo. The Ivalon sponge procedure for my-ocardial revascularization. Surgery, 47:268–289, 1960.
9. Battezzati, M., A. Tagliaferro, and G. DeMarchi. La legatura delle due arterie mam-marie interne nei disturbi di vascolarizzazione del miocardio. Minerva Med., 11:1178–1188, 1955.
10. O'Shaughnessy, L. An experimental method of providing a collateral circulation to the heart. Brit. J. Surg., 23:665–670, 1936.
11. O'Shaughnessy, L. Surgical treatment of cardiac ischemia. Lancet, 1:185–194, 1937.
12. Lezius, A. Die anatomischen und funktionellen Grundlagen der kuenstlichen Blut-versorgung des Herzmukels durch die Lunge bei Coronarterienverschluss. Arch. Klin. Chir., 191:101, 1839.
13. Carter, B.N. Discussion of C.S. Beck. Revascularization of the heart. Ann. Surg. 128:861–864, 1948.
14. Vidone, R.A., J.L. Kline, M. Pitel, and A.A. Liebow. The application of an induced bronchial collateral circulation to the coronary arteries by cardiopneumopexy. Am. J. Path., 32:897–925, 1956.
15. Key, J.A., F.G. Kergin, Y. Martineau, and R.G. Leckey. A method of supplementing the coronary circulation by a jejunal pedicle graft. J. Thorac. Surg., 28:320–330, 1954.
16. Moran, R.E., C.G. Neumann, G. von Wendel, J.W. Lord, P.W. Stone, and J.W. Hin-ton. Revascularization of the heart by tubed pedicle graft of skin and subcutaneous tissue. Plastic Reconstruct. Surg., 10:295–302, 1952.
17. King, E.S.J. Surgery of the Heart. William & Wilkins, 1941, p. 437.
18. Beck, C.S. Revascularization of the heart. Ann. Surg., 128:854–864, 1948.
19. Gross, L., and L. Blum. Effect of coronary artery occlusion on the dog's heart with total coronary sinus ligation. Proc. Soc. Exp. Biol. Med., 32:1578–1580, 1935.
20. Fauteux, M. Experimental study of the surgical treatment of coronary disease. Surg. Gyn. Obstet., 71:151–155, 1940.
21. Beck, C.S., E. Stanton, W. Batiuchok, and E. Leiter. Revascularization of the heart by graft of a systemic artery into coronary sinus. JAMA, 137:436–442, 1948.
22. Wearn, J.R. The extent of the capillary bed of the heart. J. Exper. Med., 47:273–291, 1947.
23. Beck, C.S., and A.E. Mako. Venous stasis in the coronary circulation. Am. Heart J., 21:767–779, 1941.
24. Goldman, A., S.M. Greenstone, F.S. Preuss, S.H. Strauss, and E.S. Chang. Experi-mental methods for producing a collateral circulation to the heart directly from the left ventricle. J. Thorac. Surg., 31:364–374, 1956.
25. Massimo, C., and L. Boffie. Myocardial revascularization by a new method of carrying blood directly from the left ventricular cavity into the coronary circulation. J. Tho-rac. Surg., 34:257–264, 1957.
26. Vineberg, A.M., and G. Miller. Internal mammary coronary anastomosis in the sur-gical treatment of coronary artery insufficiency. Can. Med. Assoc. J., 64:204–210, 1951.
27. Vineberg, A.M. Development of an anastomosis between the coronary vessels and a transplanted internal mammary artery. Can. Med. Assoc. J., 55:117–119, 1946.
28. Effler, D.B., L.K. Groves, F.M. Sones Jr., and E.K. Shirey. Increased myocardial perfu-sion by internal mammary implant: Vineberg's operation. Ann. Surg., 158:526–536, 1963.
29. Effler, D.B., F.M. Sones Jr., L.K. Groves, and E. Suarez. Myocardial revascularization by Vineberg's internal mammary artery implant. Evaluation of postoperative results. J. Thor. Cardiovasc. Surg., 50:527–533, 1965.
30. Szilagyi, D.E., R.T. McDonald, and L.C. France. The applicability of angioplastic procedures in coronary atherosclerosis: an estimate through postmortem injection studies. Ann. Surg., 148:447–461, 1958.

31. Bailey, C.P., A. May, and W.M. Lemmon. Survival after coronary endarterectomy in man. JAMA, 164:641–646, 1957.

32. Longmire, W.P., Jr., J.A. Cannon, and A.A. Kattus. Direct-vision coronary endarterectomy for angina pectoris. N. Engl. J. Med., 259:993–999, 1958.

33. Senning, A. Strip grafting in coronary arteries: report of a case. J. Thorac. Cardiovasc. Surg., 41:542–549, 1961.

34. Effler, D.R., L.K. Groves, F.M. Fones, et al. Endarterectomy in the treatment of coronary artery disease. J. Thorac. Cardiovasc. Surg., 47:98–108, 1964.

35. Effler, D.R., F.M. Sones Jr., R. Favalora, and L.K. Groves. Coronary endarterotomy with patch-graft reconstruction: clinical experience with 34 cases. Ann. Surg., 162:590–601, 1965.

36. Carrel, A. On the experimental surgery of the thoracic aorta and the heart. Ann. Surg., 52:83–95, 1910.

37. Murray, G., R. Porcheron, J. Hilario, and W. Roschlau. Anastomosis of a systemic artery to the coronary. Can. Med. Assoc. J., 71:594–597, 1954.

38. Absolon, K.B., J.B. Aust, R.L. Varco, and C.W. Lillehei. Surgical treatment of occlusive coronary artery disease by endarterectomy or anastomotic replacement. Surg. Gyn. Obstet., 103:180–185, 1956.

39. Thal, A., J.F. Perry, F.A. Miller, and O.H. Wangensteen. Direct suture anastomosis of the coronary arteries in the dog. Surgery, 40:1023–1029, 1956.

40. Julian, O.C., M. Lopez-Belio, D. Moorehead, and A. Lima. Direct surgical procedures on the coronary arteries: experimental studies. J. Thorac. Surg., 34:654–660, 1957.

41. Botham, R.J., and W.P. Young. An experimental study of experimental systemic coronary anastomosis. Surg. Gyn. Obstet., 108:361–365, 1959.

42. Baker, N.H., and J.H. Grindlay. Technique of experimental systemic coronary anastomosis. Proc. Staff. Meet. Mayo Clinic, 34:397–501, 1959.

43. Miller, E.W., W.F. Kolff, and L.K. Groves. Experimental coronary artery surgery in dogs employing a pump-oxygenator. Surgery, 45:1005–1012, 1959.

44. Moore, T.C., and A. Riberi. Maintenance of coronary circulation during systemic-to-coronary artery anastomosis. Surgery, 43:245–253, 1958.

45. Sabiston, D.C., Jr., and A. Blalock. Physiologic and anatomic determinants of coronary blood flow and their relationship to myocardial revascularization. Surgery, 44:406–423, 1958.

46. Garrett, M.E., E.W. Dennis, and M.E. DeBakey. Aortocoronary bypass with saphenous vein graft. Seven-year follow-up. JAMA, 223:792–794, 1973.

47. Favaloro, R.G. Coronary bypass surgery: the first decade. Med. Trib., R4–R12, 1976.

48. Favoloro, R.G. Critical analysis of coronary artery bypass surgery: a 30-year journey. JACC, 31:1B–63B, 1998.

49. Green, G.E., S.H. Stertzer, and E.H. Reppert. Coronary arterial bypass grafts. Ann. Thorac. Surg., 54:443–450, 1968.

50. Kolessov, V. Mammary artery-coronary artery anastomosis as method of treatment for angina pectoris. J. Thorac. Cardiovasc. Surg., 54:535–544, 1967.

51. Olearchyk, A.S. Vasilii I. Kolessov: a pioneer of coronary revascularization by internal mammary-coronary artery grafting. J. Thorac. Cardiovasc. Surg., 96:13–18, 1988.

52. Buckberg, G.D., G.N. Olinger, D.G. Mulder, and J.V. Maloney Jr. Depressed postoperative cardiac performance. Prevention by adequate myocardial protection during cardiopulmonary bypass. J. Thorac. Cardiovasc. Surg., 70:974–988, 1975.

53. Murphy, M.L., H.N. Hultgren, K. Detre, et al. Treatment of chronic stable angina. A preliminary report of survival data of the randomized Veterans Administration Cooperative Study. N. Engl. J. Med., 297:621–627, 1977.

54. European Coronary Surgery Study Group: Long-term results of prospective randomized study of coronary artery bypass in stable angina pectoris. Lancet, 2:1173–1180, 1982.

55. CASS Principal Investigators and their Associates. Coronary Artery Surgery Study (CASS) a randomized trial of coronary artery bypass surgery. Survival data. Circulation, 68:939–950, 1983.

56. Reardon, M.J., L.D. Conklin, P.R. Reardon, and J.C. Baldwin. Coronary artery bypass conduits: review of current status. J. Cardiovasc. Surg., 38(3):201–209, 1997.

57. Loop, F.D., B.W. Lytle, D.M. Cosgrove, et al. Influence of the internal mammary artery graft on 10-year survival and other cardiac events. N. Engl. J. Med., 314:1–6, 1984.

58. Horvath, K.A., L.H. Cohn, D.A. Cooley, J.R. Crew, O.H. Frazier, B.P. Griffith, K. Kadipasaoglu, A. Lansing, F. Mannting, R. March, M.R. Mirhoseini, and C. Smith. Transmyocardial laser revascularization: results of a multicenter trial with transmyocardial laser revascularization used as sole therapy for end-stage coronary artery disease. J. Thorac. Cardiovasc. Surg., 113(4):645–653, 1997; discussion pp. 653–654.

59. Horvath, K.A., F. Mannting, N. Cummings, S.K. Shernan, and L.H. Cohn. Transmyocardial laser revascularization: operative techniques and clinical results at two years. J. Thorac. Cardiovasc. Surg., 111(5):1047–1053, 1996.

Chapter 9   Isotopes in Cardiology

H. SCHELBERT
R.J. BING

THE USE OF ISOTOPES is one of several important technical contributions of fundamental science to medicine. This contribution has been made by inspired and colorful scientists and physicians whose ideas are projecting cardiology into the next century. One of the early pioneers in this field was George Hevesy (Fig. 9.1). His publications give a rare insight into the development of the use of isotopes in biology and medicine. We are indebted to him for the description of the first use of isotopes in biology and medicine. A native of Hungary, he worked in 1911 with Lord Ernest Rutherford; Hevesy foresaw the possibility of using radioactive radium D as a tracer to study chemical reactions. One of his most important contributions was the discovery of the dynamic state of the body components. Hevesy obtained his Ph.D. in 1908 from the University of Freiburg, Germany, then studied with Rutherford until 1913. He worked at the Vienna Institute of Radium Research and, in 1920, went to the University of Copenhagen on the invitation of Niels Bohr. He then returned to the University of Freiburg as professor of physical chemistry. In 1943 he fled from Copenhagen before the invading Nazis and took refuge in Sweden.

Hevesy's historical papers are informative and entertaining (1–5). He mentioned his cooperation with Rutherford, who asked Hevesy to separate radium D from lead. Rutherford said, "My boy, if you are worth your salt, you try to separate radium D from all that lead." The efforts of Hevesy were unsuccessful. In 1913 Hevesy worked with Paneth at the Vienna Institute of Radium Research; they published the use of labeled lead to determine the solubility of lead chromate and sulphide. Applications of radio sodium in circulatory studies were to follow. The first use of radioactive indicators in plant physiology was carried out by Hevesy in

166

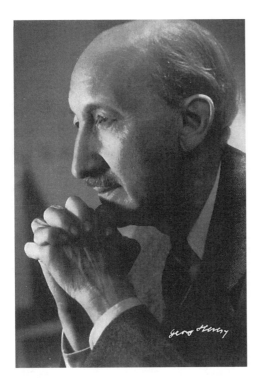

Figure 9.1. George Hevesy. (Courtesy of the New York Academy of Medicine)

1923, using labeled lead in bean seedlings and its release by the plants upon placing them in a culture solution containing nonradioactive lead. Until 1933 only the isotopes of lead, bismuth, thallium, radium, thorium, and actinium had been applied as tracers, none of which played a role in the living organism.

Further advances in this field were not possible until the discovery of heavy water (deuterium) in 1932 by Harold C. Urey, and of artificial radioactivity by Iréne and Frederik Joliot-Curie in 1933 (6–14). Use of radioisotopes in medicine and cardiology was entirely dependent on the discovery of artificial radioactivity. The Joliot-Curies were pioneers in this field (Fig. 9.2). They discovered artificial radioactivity, which made possible preparation of a large number of radioactive isotopes that became of considerable importance in biology and medicine. Iréne Curie became her mother's (Marie Curie) assistant at the Radium Institute in Paris. In 1925 she received her doctorate on her graduate thesis, "Recherches sur les rayons alpha du polonium." In 1934 the Joliot-Curies succeeded in artificially producing radioactive elements, thereby furnishing proof of the possibility of transforming elements (6–14). On Monday, January 15, 1934, Jean Perrin introduced to the session of the French Academy of Science a communication entitled "A New Type of Radioactivity," with the authors Iréne and Frederik Joliot-Curie. The text of the announcement read, "it has been possible, for the

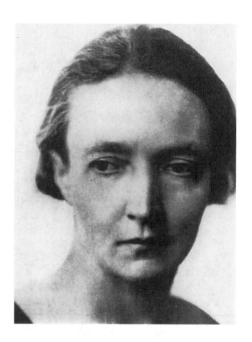

Figure 9.2. Iréne Joliot-Curie. *(Courtesy of the New York Academy of Medicine)*

first time, to create by means of external causes, radioactivity of certain substances which remain stable for a measurable time" (6–14). The authors demonstrated that when an aluminum foil was irradiated on a polonium preparation, the emission of positive-charged electrons did not cease immediately when the active preparation was removed. A new isotope had been produced. They wrote: "the radioelement may be regarded as a known nucleus formed in a particular state of excitation." But they thought it more probable that these new radioactive elements were unknown isotopes that are always unstable (6–14). In 1935 the Joliot-Curies received the Nobel prize in chemistry.

The marriage of Frederik Joliot and Iréne Curie was one of opposites. While Curie was quiet and serene, Joliot was impulsive. By nature reserved, she had difficulty relating to people. She cared little for external appearance and dresses, while he was a handsome, well-groomed man. Curie loved French, English, and German poetry. As Michel Rouze wrote, "Joliot and Iréne had different characters, but they were complementary, for work as well as life. Often valuable associations are not those of individual characters, but of personality features which complement each other" (13).

Joliot and Curie's fundamental discovery was followed by that of Fermi and his colleagues, who produced radioisotopes by neutrons emitted from uranium by a mixture of radon and beryllium in an atomic pile. Identical methods were used for the production of ^{32}P by Hevesy in Copenhagen, an isotope that was soon used for biological studies (1–5). As Hevesy wrote, "It was soon made clear that isotopic methods were the only possibility of studying the organism as a whole under practically equilibrium conditions."

Fermi's method of using uranium-produced radioactive isotopes made possible extended application of radioactive tracers in biology. The first radioiodine was produced by Fermi in Italy in 1934. Study of the activity of the thyroid gland and the synthesis of thyroid hormones began soon afterward. In 1940 John Lawrence and Joseph Hamilton utilized ^{131}I in the treatment of hyperthyroidism and treatment of cancer of the thyroid.

The construction of the cyclotron by Lawrence in Berkeley was an outstanding event in the history of biological application of radioactive tracers (16, 17). The cyclotron found immediate use in medicine. The use of ^{131}I commenced soon and the discovery of radiosodium followed. In 1935 ^{32}P was introduced on both sides of the Atlantic. Lawrence, in 1936, conceived of the idea of *selectively* irradiating leukemic cells. This idea was the beginning of what was called metabolic radiotherapy. In 1939 cyclotron-produced radiophosphorus was used in clinical studies of leukemia; extensive use of these isotopes in other biological fields followed. Lawrence's paper on the production of high-speed light ions without the use of high voltages appeared in April 1932 (17). He described the apparatus for generation of 1,220,000 volt protons. It is noteworthy that this work was partially supported by the industry, including the Federal Telegraph Company and the Chemical Foundation. Soon afterward cyclotron-produced iodine was used in the study of radioiodine uptake by the thyroid. Other isotopes of sodium, potassium, calcium, and strontium soon became available.

The early part of this century was a great period for physics; it was the time of Otto Hahn and Lise Meitner, who discovered nuclear fission, and of Hess, who discovered cosmic rays. The early twentieth century was also the time of the introduction of the quantum theory of the atomic structure by Niels Bohr (1913), Rutherford's fundamental observation on the structure of the atom, introduction of the first counter for radioactivity by Hans W. Geiger at Kiel, and Einstein's theory of relativity.

The pioneering work of Hevesy was soon followed by the studies of Rudolph Schoenheimer and David Rittenberg at the College of Physicians and Surgeons, Columbia University (18; see Fig. 6.5). After his work on cholesterol metabolism in the Department of Pathology in Freiburg, Germany, under Ludwig Aschoff, Schoenheimer carried out his studies in the United States on the use of isotopes in investigating metabolism with Rittenberg. It was Urey who gave them the isotope needed: heavy hydrogen (deuterium). The epochal discovery of Urey appeared in a letter to *Physical Reviews* (15, 19). An argument immediately ensued regarding what to call this new isotope. Names such as bar-hydrogen and diplogen were proposed by Rutherford, but the name "deuterium" was maintained.

Using deuterium as an isotopic tracer, Schoenheimer and Rittenberg (the latter had worked in Urey's laboratory) developed methods of synthesizing isotopically labeled compounds. For example, linseed oil hydrogenated with deuterium was used to study the isotope's fate in experimental animals. They showed that labeled fatty acids were deposited in fat even during starvation (18).

Later, when ^{15}N was concentrated in Urey's laboratory in the form of heavy ammonia, Schoenheimer and Rittenberg turned to the problem of protein metabolism (18). Administering compounds labeled with ^{15}N or double-labeled with deuterium and ^{15}N, they confirmed Hevesy's observation that body constituents are in a highly dynamic state. This led to the concept of a "metabolic pool," with body tissues continually entering and leaving this pool.

Rudolf Schoenheimer, who introduced the application of radioisotopes to the study of metabolic functions, was born in May 1898 and died by suicide in September 1941. The son of a physician who practiced in Berlin, he studied medicine at the University of Berlin, receiving his M.D. degree in 1922. After a year in the Department of Pathology, he recognized his deficiency in biochemistry and studied biochemistry at the University of Leipzig under a Rockefeller Foundation Fellowship for three years. Schoenheimer's productive career commenced at the University of Freiburg with the great pathologist Aschoff, with a short interlude at the University of Chicago; he soon became head of the Department of Pathological Chemistry at the University of Freiburg. In 1933 he moved to New York to the College of Physicians, Columbia University. Schoenheimer was an ingenious and scintillating personality. In a moving obituary, Hans T. Clarke, his friend and chief, wrote:

> Schoenheimer died by suicide at the height of his productive career, September 11, 1941 (20). Few men had more reason for desiring to live; his work gave him intense satisfaction, and its increasing importance was widely recognized. . . . One of Schoenheimer's most striking characteristics was his ability to correlate pertinent facts from highly diversified branches of knowledge and bring them to bear upon problems under immediate consideration.

The application of radioisotopes to cardiology began with G. Liljestrand from Stockholm who, in 1939, determined the normal blood volume in the ventricles of the human heart (21). In 1940 Hevesy used radioactive phosphorus to determine circulation time (2). The method was relatively simple. Blood was withdrawn from the patient and mixed with radioactive phosphorus. The mixture was reinjected intravenously, while an intraarterial needle permitted the collection of fractionated specimens of arterial blood for measurement of radioactivity. Nylin, who worked in Stockholm in close proximity to Hevesy, used isotopes for the determination of residual blood in the cardiac ventricles and also measured circulation time (22, 23). In a paper published in 1945, he referred to the advantage of radioisotopes over the prevalent measurement of circulation time with decholin, a test that relied on the patient's subjective judgment (23).

In 1947 H. Blumgart, at the Harvard Medical School, accomplished accurate measurements of the "velocity of blood flow" (circulation time) using intravenous radium and detection time of arrival at another point of the circulation (24; see Chapter 7). He cited work at the Memorial Hospital in New York dealing with the possible therapeutic effect of radium C in patients with advanced generalized carcinomatosis. In this study, repeated intravenous injections of up to 75 millicuries of radium were administered without any ill effects. Blumgart's detection device was complicated, but he was able to measure normal circulation time (approximately eighteen seconds) from arm to contralateral arm. Much higher values were obtained in myocardial failure. Blumgart was an outstanding physician and investigator, one of a great group of Harvard cardiologists that included Paul D. White (see Chapter 7).

Similar to Blumgart, M. Prinzmetal used a Geiger counter positioned over the heart to record "radiocardiograms" (25). He summarized his efforts by stating that radiocardiography offered a simple and safe method for the determination of the "pumping qualities of the heart." He also studied patients with congenital heart disease (patent ductus arteriosus) before and after surgical correction. Discussing Prinzmetal's paper presented at the Section on Experimental Medicine and Therapeutics at the 97th Annual Session of the American Medical Association, Chicago, in 1948, Nylin voiced astonishment that "it was feasible to study the filling and emptying of both cavities separately." Prinzmetal affirmed that he had consulted several experts in the field of atomic energy in California and elsewhere on the danger of radioactive material; "their opinion was unanimous that the amount of radioactivity used is completely safe by all methods of estimation" (25).

Tracing of isotopes through coronary arteries was described in 1952 by P. von Waser and W. Hunzinger, from Basel, who observed that the descendant slope of the left ventricular component of the radiocardiogram contained a significant amount of radioactivity due to the passage of radioisotopes through coronary vessels (26). In 1955 G. Sevelius attempted to estimate myocardial blood flow with iodinated human serum albumin ^{131}I following the example of Huff and co-workers (27). He employed a "heart channel and a carotid channel." Each channel consisted of a scintillation detector, a rate meter, and a recorder. In this procedure, it was difficult to recognize the coronary flow contribution in the precordial radiogram.

A great step forward for cardiology was achieved by Hal Oscar Anger, who developed the gamma ray camera for in vivo studies in 1952 (28, 29). Anger was born May 24, 1920, in Denver, Colorado, and received his elementary and high school education in southern California. During the war (1942), he devised a special unit for use in radar. This was later referred to as the "Anger Circuit." After graduation, he served on the staff of the Radio Research Laboratory at Harvard University. His cooperation with the Donner Laboratory at the University of California at Berkeley began in 1946, when he became associated with John Lawrence.

"No single person has been as successful as Hal Anger in interrelating physics with nuclear medicine through sound engineering principles and practice," according to William G. Myers (28). Anger first used ^{131}I to visualize thyroid metastases in bone of living patients. In his first device, a 3 mm pinhole in a lead shield was located 20 cm from a photographic plate, placed in contact with a sodium iodine intensifying screen. A useful image was obtained from a 1R exposure to the plate when the ^{131}I density was about 1 mCi per cc thyroid tissue. This instrument pointed the way for development of his more sensitive scintillation camera five years later. In 1958 Anger constructed his scintillation camera, equipped with a sodium iodide crystal only 4 inches in diameter which was viewed by 7 phototubes. In 1963 he completed construction of a larger scintillation camera employing an 11-inch crystal. This camera and its subsequent models are essential for use in scanning of the heart to the present day. The Anger camera was later used to measure regional myocardial blood flow (28, 29).

Early work on myocardial scanning was performed by H.N. Wagner (30), W.D. Love and G.E. Burch (31), E.A. Carr (32), and R.J. Bing (33). Carr, in 1962, used [84]Rb to scan the precordium prior to and after the death of animals (32). Accidental counts resulting from the use of single emission interfered with the accuracy of these determinations.

After these beginnings, the use of isotopes in cardiology increased exponentially. The determination of cardiac wall motions and of cardiac ejection fraction at rest and during exercise have become important clinical tests in patient evaluation.

The Use of Positron Emitters

In 1937 Carl D. Anderson published his Nobel lecture entitled "The Production and Property of Positrons" (34; Fig. 9.3). These new particles in physics were positive-charged electrons (positrons). Anderson had received the Nobel prize for his work in 1936. It is interesting that when his Nobel lecture was published in the *Bulletin of the California Institute of Technology*, Anderson was still an assistant professor of physics. Anderson reported that information of fundamental importance to the general problem of atomic structure had resulted from systematic studies of the cosmic radiation carried out in the Wilson cloud chamber. Energies of atomic particles of 5 billion electron-volts were discovered. It was shown that particles of positive charge occurred about as abundantly as did those

VOLUME 46   NUMBER 2

Bulletin of the
CALIFORNIA INSTITUTE
of TECHNOLOGY

THE PRODUCTION *and* PROPERTIES
of POSITRONS

Nobel Lecture presented before the Swedish Royal Academy
of Science at Stockholm, December 12, 1936.

by CARL D. ANDERSON, Ph.D.
Assistant Professor of Physics,
California Institute of Technology

PASADENA, CALIFORNIA
JUNE, 1937

Figure 9.3. Title page of the Nobel prize winning article by Carl D. Anderson, California Institute of Technology. *(With permission)*

of negative charge, and in many cases several positive and negative particles were found to be projected simultaneously from a single center (34). Anderson had interpreted the particles of negative charge as electrons, but those of positive charge were first tentatively identified as protons—at that time the only known particle of unit was a positive charge. It soon became evident, however, that the positive particles differed in specific ionization only inappreciably from the negative ones. At first, to avoid this assumption, which appeared at the time very radical, Anderson wrote that the positive particles did have electronic mass and appeared to be positively charged, but were in reality negatively charged electrons which, through scattering, had suffered a reversal of direction and were projected upward away from the earth (34). But this explanation soon appeared to be inadequate.

It became clear that the results could be interpreted only in terms of particles of a positive charge and a mass of the same order of magnitude as that normally possessed by the free negative electron. The only possible conclusion seemed to be that these were positively charged electrons. These results were published in September 1932, announcing the existence of free positive electrons (35). The mass and charge of the positive electrons did not differ by more than 20 percent and 10 percent, respectively, from the mass and charge of the negative electron. Soon, production of positrons by agents other than cosmic rays was shown, when it was observed that positrons were produced by the radiation generated in the impact of alpha particles upon beryllium. The Joliot-Curies measured the yield of positrons as a function of the thickness and material of the absorber by a lead block and paraphine and concluded that the positrons arose more likely as a result of gamma rays than of neutrons. Positrons also were soon observed among the disintegration products of certain radioactive substances.

In 1964 ^{84}Rb, which emits positrons 19 percent of the time, was used for determination of coronary blood flow in man (36, 37). Positrons (free positive electrons) travel 1.5 mm in the tissue and disintegrate by striking an electron, ejecting two gamma photons at an energy level of 0.51 mev, 180° apart or back to back. The coincidence method has the following advantages over the single proton emission method: since the counting system registers only coincidence events, background counting rates arising from natural radioactivity, cosmic radioactivity, and the presence of background counting rates are essentially zero. The coincidence counting method gives approximately five times the counting rates of single photon emission for a given field of view. Although coincidence counting is, like simple proton counting, subject to tissue absorption of gamma rays (a phenomenon termed attenuation), the relative time of light of the two gamma protons indicates the relative position of the atom emitting the positron particle. Because of the elimination of single gamma photons, the coincidence method provides a means for distinguishing radioactivity of the heart muscle from that of the surrounding tissue, thereby simplifying collimation, and together with the coincidence counting systems, eliminating interference with accidental counts. This principle offers a higher resolution than simple proton techniques in positron emission tomography (PET).

During early attempts, a continuous infusion of ^{84}Rb for determination of coronary blood flow was used (38). A coefficient had to be obtained that made possible definitions of clearances in ml/min. Furthermore, the first derivative of the myocardial clearance of ^{84}Rb had to be obtained in order to calculate uptake of ^{84}Rb at zero time. This was accomplished by extrapolation of the myocardial clearance to zero. At that time, the activity in coronary venous blood was assumed to be zero and the extraction ratio to be unity. Later, coronary blood flow was measured after a bolus injection of ^{84}Rb, as performed by L. Donato (39) and by S.B. Knoebel (40). According to L.A. Sapirstein, the uptake of rubidium by the heart muscle can be calculated since cardiac uptake equals the fraction of coronary flow supplying the myocardium (41). This method has the advantage that the coronary sinus need not be intubated. Other methods rely on the use of clearances of radioactive materials such as krypton or xenon (42, 43). Superiority of the coincidence method over the use of single gamma photons determination was demonstrated on models (44).

These pioneering experiments with the positron emitter ^{84}Rb sparked future developments in techniques of imaging and in physiological studies. The work became a precursor for the determination of myocardial imaging with thallium-201 and technitium 99 sestamibi using single-photon emission computed tomography (SPECT). Using these isotopes, perfusion defects in the myocardium can be outlined and the amount of myocardium at risk can be estimated. The most important advance originating from the early work on ^{84}Rb was the development of positron emission tomography (PET), discussed later in this chapter.

As a positron-emitting nuclide, ^{84}Rb found itself in good company. Cyclotron bombardment of stable atoms with deuterons or protons produced positron-emitting isotopes of elements like ^{15}O, ^{11}C, and ^{13}N. These elements were major constituents of living matter. Incorporated into biological molecules, their positron-emitting nuclides carried considerable promise for tracing biological processes in vivo. For example, Kamen and co-workers (45) recognized the importance of the ^{11}C label for studies of the carbon dioxide utilization by plants and, in 1941, Cramer and Kistiakowsky (46) conducted metabolic studies with lactate labeled with ^{11}C in the 1, 2, and 3 positions. Several years later, Buchanan and Hastings (47) applied the same radionuclide to studies of intermediary metabolism. In 1946 Tobias and co-workers (48) studied the metabolism of carbon monoxide in humans with ^{11}C. The positron-emitting ^{13}N also found uses in biological studies of nitrogen metabolism in plants (49, 50).

In the mid-1940s interest in these radioisotopes began to fade. Possible reasons were their short physical half-life and associated logistical complexities. Another reason, according to Ter-Pogossian (51), was the availability of more stable isotopes like ^{14}C or ^{3}H, which offered more flexibility in the research laboratory. Both isotopes played important roles in delineating aspects of human substrate metabolism. They also proved useful for mapping the spatial distribution of functional processes in organs, as autoradiography could quantify their regional tissue activity concentrations. It was at that time that Louis Sokoloff, trained in psychiatry and working at the University of Pennsylvania, devised a novel approach to the exploration of regional cerebral metabolism (52, 53). Employing ^{14}C labeled deoxyglucose, he mapped the spatial distribution of regional rates of cerebral glucose utilization and their changes in response to physiologic stimuli in awake rats and cats. Sokoloff's approach took advantage of the specific properties of deoxyglucose. The agent traces the initial uptake and the hexokinase-mediated phosphorylation of glucose to glucose-6-phosphate as a key metabolic step in the glycolytic flux of the brain. Unlike its parent substrate, the labeled glucose analog was a poor substrate for glycolysis, the fructose-pentose shunt, and dephosphorylation. Because the phosphorylated analog is rather impermeable to the cell membrane, it becomes virtually trapped in the brain in proportion to rates of regional cerebral glucose metabolism. The tissue kinetics of this tracer compound were described by a three-compartmental model, which formed the basis for estimating regional metabolic rates. From the arterial tracer input function, the arterial plasma glucose concentrations, and the cerebral ^{14}C activity concentrations determined postmortem by quantitative autoradiography, it yielded metabolic rates of glucose in μmol per minute per gram tissue. In fact, Sokoloff's method possessed the ingredients of the later evolving positron emission tomography except, of course, that measurements of regional tracer activity concentrations relied on quantitative autoradiography. Obviously, the approach was unsuitable for studies in humans. Given the impact more stable radioisotopes had made on biomedical research, Siri in 1949 painted a rather bleak picture of the future of the short-lived positron-emitting radionuclides (54). He noted that "the unstable species of the longest half-life is oxygen-15 (126 sec); this has not been employed for tracer work and does not offer much promise."

Ter-Pogossian was the man who revived interest in short-lived positron-emitting radionuclides for biomedical research in the mid-1950s. Ter-Pogossian (51) saw the earlier perceived weakness of these short-lived radioisotopes as a major advantage. They permitted serial measurements of biological processes. He recognized the fact that they constituted a major part of living matter. Their insertion into biomolecules caused no adverse effects on their very properties. They could be synthesized in high specific activities. Therefore, they exerted no mass effect and did not perturb the very process to be studied. Early work in Ter-Pogossian's laboratory at Washington University in St. Louis included autoradiographic approaches to the study of tumor oxygenation with [15]O. Later work expanded into other areas such as studies of cerebral oxygen metabolism. These pioneering studies gave new impetus to investigations with other positron-emitting nuclides at several institutions that commissioned cyclotrons dedicated to biomedical research. Foremost among these institutions were Hammersmith Hospital in London, the Sloan-Kettering Institute in New York City, the University of Chicago, the University of California at Berkeley, and later at Los Angeles with Schelbert and Phelps.

It must be remembered that this early pioneering work relied on external radiation detectors for monitoring the uptake and clearance of positron-emitting nuclides in whole organs or large organ parts. What these studies lacked were imaging devices for localizing or even mapping the distribution of functional processes evaluated by these radiotracers. Early attempts in Ter-Pogossian's laboratory to determine the spatial distribution of these functional processes prompted the development of the "lead chicken."

The "lead chicken" device resembled a lead helmet spiked with twenty-six detector probes for collecting activity from different regions of the brain. Yet it proved to be less than satisfactory. The lead collimators lowered the count efficiency and required injection of the tracer directly into the carotid artery. At the same time, Hal Anger demonstrated that two-dimensional images of the distribution of tracers in organs could in fact be obtained. Taking advantage of the simultaneous emission of two 511 keV photons in diametrically opposite directions as a property unique to positron decay, he designed a coincidence circuitry for a double-headed gamma scintillation camera. In 1968 Yano and Anger at the University of California at Berkeley presented the first images of the heart and kidney in animals, recorded with the ultra-short-lived [82]Rb (55). Long-standing interests in Gordon Bronell's laboratory at the Massachusetts General Hospital at the time resulted in the first dedicated positron camera (56). It consisted of two large detector banks of sodium-iodide detectors coupled to seventy-two photomultiplier tubes. Coincidence circuits connected each detector in one bank with twenty-five detectors in the opposite bank and provided a total of 2,549 lines of coincidence response. Both Brownell's and Anger's devices yielded planar images of the distribution of positron-emitting nuclides in organs. They fell short of providing information on their spatial or three-dimensional distribution.

David E. Kuhl, at that time at the University of Pennsylvania, had been keenly interested in the development of techniques that would depict the distribution of radionuclide in the form of transverse images. He demonstrated the utility of back projection techniques that produced transverse section images of the distribution of single photon-emitting radionuclides (57, 58). Properties specific to positron decay offered distinct advantages for producing truly tomographic images. As early as 1962 Rankowitz built a device for coincidence collimation (59). It consisted of a ring of *discreet* radiation detectors. Ironically, Rankowitz's system was ahead of its time, as mathematical algorithms for image reconstruction had not yet been developed.

Hounsfield described in 1973 the x-ray computed tomography (60). This event proved pivotal for subsequent advances in the field of tomographic imaging of positron-emitting nuclides. The general principles for reconstructing tomographic images from angular projection of an object were formulated. Michael E. Phelps, an assistant professor with a doctoral degree in nuclear chemistry, together with his Fellow, Edward J. Hoffman, dissembled in Ter-Pogossian's laboratory the "lead chicken" in order to salvage the twenty-six detector probes. They positioned sets of four detector probes in a hexagonal array. Phelps and Hoffman rotated by hand the source of positron-emitting nuclides placed in the center of this array for proper linear and angular sampling while different computers at different locations, at the medical school, in a biomedical laboratory several blocks away, and a large IBM computer at the university campus, collected and mathematically reconstructed the data. Jerome Cox, Donald Snyder, and Sung-Cheng Huang designed the reconstruction algorithms. The first true tomographic image was obtained in 1973. They dubbed the new imaging device PETT II (for positron emission transaxial tomography). The system contained only twelve coincidence lines and offered an intrinsic spatial resolution of only 25 mm in one single image slice. The initial success led to the development of the first tomograph for human studies, called PETT III, and produced the first images on ^{13}N ammonia uptake in the human brain (61, 62) and formed the basis for the first commercially built positron emission tomographer (63). The initial, single-slice imaging approach formed the basis for the soon following multislice positron emission tomography which today acquires simultaneously as many as fifteen to thirty slices with over a million response lines and an intrinsic in-plane resolution of 3 mm to 5 mm. Ironically, Phelps and Hoffman in 1975 moved to the University of Pennsylvania, where Sokoloff had conceived the deoxyglucose method for mapping the spatial distribution of metabolic rates of glucose in rat brain and where in David E. Kuhl's laboratory transverse images of the spatial distribution of deoxyglucose in brain labeled with ^{18}F had been acquired (64, 65). The following years demonstrated the possibility of measuring accurately rather than only depicting the regional ^{18}F deoxyglucose concentrations with positron emission tomography. This imaging device thus could substitute for quantitative autoradiography. This ability permitted in vivo measurements of regional tracer tissue concentrations and resulted in the application of Sokoloff's approach to the measurements of regional metabolic rates of glucose in human brain (66).

With these accomplishments, positron emission tomography began to evolve as an analytical tool for probing biochemical processes in humans. This development would not have been possible without an increasing number of positron-emitting isotopes. Investigators in centers of major activities under Al Wolf at Brookhaven National Laboratory and under Michael Welch at the Mallinckrodt Institute at Washington University have designed and developed synthesis methods for more than two hundred such compounds labeled with positron-emitting radionuclides. Processes that can now be evaluated and measured in the human heart include blood flow, biochemical reaction rates, fluxes of glucose, fatty acid, and oxygen, as well as studies of receptors in the human heart.

As Claude Bernard has stated, "No category of sciences exists to which one could give the name of applied sciences. There are science and application of science, linked together as fruit of the tree that bore it" (67).

References

1. Hevesy, G.A. Scientific career. In: Adventures in Radioisotope Research. New York, Pergamon, 1962.
2. Hevesy, G. Some applications of isotopic indicators. In: Adventures in Radioisotope Research. New York, Pergamon, 1962. (Originally published in Les Prix Nobel 1940–1944, p. 95.)
3. Hevesy, G. Historical progress of the isotopic methodology and its influences on the biological sciences. In: Adventures in Radioisotope Research. New York, Pergamon, pp. 997–1038. (Originally published in Minerva Nucleare, 1:182, 1957. Lecture delivered in 1956 at the International Meeting of Nuclear Medicine in Turin.)
4. Hevesy, G. The application of radioactive indicators in biochemistry. In: Adventures in Radioisotope Research. New York, Pergamon, 1962, pp. 961–996. (Originally published in Chem. Soc. J., p. 1618, 1951. Faraday Lecture, delivered before the Chemical Society in Edinburgh on March 29, 1950.)
5. Hevesy, G. McGraw-Hill Modern Men of Science, J.E. Greene (ed). New York, McGraw-Hill, 1966, pp. 222–224.
6. Joliot-Curie, F., and I. Joliot-Curie. Oeuvres scientifiques complètes. Paris, Presses Universitaires de France, 1961.
7. Amaldi, E., P. Briquard, L. Goldstein, et al. La radioactivité artificielle à 50 ans, 1934–1984. Paris, Centre Nationale de la Recherche Scientifique, 1984.
8. Joliot, F., and I. Curie. Artificial production of a new kind of radio-element. Nature, 133:201–202, 1934.
9. Nobel Prize Winners Charts, Indexes, Sketches, compiled by Flora Kaplan. Chicago, Nobel Publishing, 1941, pp. 37, 38, 58.
10. Cotton, E. Les Curies et la radioactivité. From the series: Savants du Monde Entier. Paris, Editions Seghers, 1963, pp. 74–79.
11. Biquard, P. Frederic Joliot Curie; Choix de Textes, Bibliographie, Portraits, Facsimiles. From the series: Savants du Monde Entier. Paris, Editions Seghers, 1961, pp. 26–31.
12. Chaskolskata, M. Frédéric Joliot-Curie. Essais et Documents (Editions de Moscou), pp. 26–31.
13. Rouze, M. Frédéric Joliot-Curie. Editeurs Francais, Reunis, 1950.
14. La radioactivité artificielle et les sciences de la vie. Synelog L'Edition Artisteque, Paris (1), 228:26, 40.
15. Urey, H.C. Names for the hydrogen isotopes. Science, 78:602–603, 1933.
16. Lawrence, E.O., and M.S. Livingston. The production of high speed protons without the use of high voltages. Phys. Rev., 38:834, 1931.
17. Lawrence, E.O., and M.S. Livingston. The production of high speed light ions without the use of high voltages. Phys. Rev., 40:19–35, 1932.

18. Schoenheimer, R., and D. Rittenberg. The study of intermediary metabolism of animals with the aid of isotopes. Phys. Rev., 20:218–248, 1940.

19. Urey, H.C. Relative abundance of H1 and H2 in natural hydrogen. Phys. Rev., 40:464–465, 1932.

20. Clarke, H.T. Rudolf Schoenheimer, 1898–1941. Science, 94:553–554, 1941.

21. Liljestrand, G., E. Lysholm, G. Nylin, and C.G. Zachrisson. The normal heart volume in man. Am. Heart J., 17:406–415, 1939.

22. Nylin, G., and M. Malm. Ueber die Konzentration von mit radioactivem Phosphor markierten Erythrocyten im Arterienblut nach der intravenoesen Injektion solcher Blutkoerperchen. Cardiologia, 7:153–162, 1943.

23. Nylin, G. The dilution curve of activity in arterial blood after intravenous injection of labeled corpuscles. Am. Heart J., 30:1–11, 1945.

24. Blumgart, H., and O.C. Yens. Studies on the velocity of blood flow. J. Clin. Invest., 4:1–13, 1927.

25. Prinzmetal, M., E. Corday, R.J. Spritzler, and W. Flieg. Radiocardiography and its clinical applications. JAMA, 139:617–622, 1949.

26. Waser, P. von, and W. Hunzinger. Radiocirculographische Untersuchung des Coronarkreislaufes mit Na24Cl. Cardiologia, 22:65–100, 1953.

27. Sevelius, G., and P.C. Johnson. Myocardial blood flow determined by surface counting and ratio formula. J. Lab. Clin. Med., 54:669–679, 1959.

28. Myers, W.G. Nuclear Medicine Pioneer Citation—1974, Hal Oscar Anger, D.Sc. (Hon.). J. Nucl. Med., 15:471–473, 1974.

29. Anger, H.O. Scintillation camera. Rev. Sci. Instr., 29:27–33, 1958.

30. Wagner, H.N., J.G. McAfee, and J.M. Mozley Medical radioisotope scanning. JAMA, 174:162–165, 1960.

31. Love, W.D., and G.E. Burch. A study in dogs of methods suitable for estimating the rate of myocardial uptake of RB86 in man, and the effect of L-norepinephrine and pitressin on RB86 uptake. J. Clin. Invest., 36:468–478, 1957.

32. Carr, E.A., W.H. Beierwaltes, A.V. Wegst, and J.D. Bartlett. Myocardial scanning with rubidium-86. J. Nucl. Med., 3:76–82, 1962.

33. Bing, R.J. Scanning of heart. N.Y. State J. Med., 67:1406–1410, 1967.

34. Anderson, C.D. The production and properties of positrons. Nobel lecture, Bull. Calif. Inst. Tech., 46:3, 1937.

35. Anderson, C.D. The apparent existence of easily deflectable positives. Science, 76: 238–239, 1932.

36. Bing, R.J., C. Cowan, D. Bottcher, G. Corsini, and C.G. Daniels. A new method of measuring coronary blood flow in man. JAMA, 205:277–280, 1968.

37. Cohen, A., E.J. Zaleski, H. Baleiron, T.B. Stock, C. Chiba, and R.J. Bing. Measurement of coronary blood flow using rubidium84 and the coincidence counting method: a critical analysis. Am. J. Cardiol., 19:556–562, 1967.

38. Bing, R.J., A. Bennish, G. Blumchen, A. Cohen, J.P. Gallagher, and E.J. Zaleski. The determination of coronary flow equivalent with coincidence counting technique. Circulation, 29:833–846, 1964.

39. Donato, L., G. Bartolomei, and R. Giordani. Evaluation of myocardial blood perfusion in man with radioactive potassium or rubidium and precordial counting. Circulation, 29:195–203, 1964.

40. Knoebel, S.B., P.L. McHenry, L. Stein, and A. Sonel. Myocardial blood flow in man as measured by a coincidence counting system and a single bolus of 84RbCl. Circulation, 36:187–196, 1967.

41. Sapirstein, L.A. Fractionation of the cardiac output of rats with isotopic potassium. Circ. Res., 4:689–692, 1956.

42. Ross, R.S., K. Ueda, P.L. Lichtlen, and J.R. Rees. Measurement of myocardial blood

flow in animals and man by selective injection of radioactive inert gas into the coronary arteries. Circ. Res., 15:28–41, 1964.

43. Holman, B.L., D.F. Adams, D. Jewitt, P. Eldh, J. Idoine, P.F. Cohn, R. Gorlin, and S.J. Adelstein. Measuring regional myocardial blood flow with 133Xe and the Anger camera. Radiology, 112:99–107, 1974.

44. Ikeda, S., H. Duken, H. Tillmanns, and R.J. Bing. Coincidence counting and noncoincidence counting: a comparative study. J. Nucl. Med., 16:658–661, 1975.

45. Kamen, M.D. Isotropic Tracers in Biology: An Introduction to Tracer Methodology. New York, Academic Press, 3rd ed., 1957.

46. Cramer, R.D., and G.B. Kistiatowsky. The synthesis of radioactive lactic acid. J. Biol. Chem., 137:549, 1941.

47. Buchanan, J.M., and A.B. Hastings. The use of isotopically marked carbon in the study of intermediary metabolism. Physiol. Rev., 26:120–155, 1946.

48. Tobias, C.A., J.H. Lawrence, F.J.W. Roughton, W.S. Root, and M.I. Gregersen. The elimination of carbon monoxide from the human body with reference to the possible conversion of CO to CO_2. Am. J. Physiol., 145:253–263, 1945.

49. Ruben, S., W.Z. Hassid, and M.D. Kamen. Radioactive carbon in the study of photosynthesis. J. Am. Chem. Soc., 61:661, 1939.

50. Ruben, S., M.D. Kamen, and W.Z. Hassid. Photosynthesis with radioactive carbon II chemical properties of the intermediates. J. Am. Chem. Soc., 62:3443–3449, 1940.

51. Ter-Pogossian, M.M. Positron emission tomography instrumentation. In: Positron Emission Tomography. New York, Alan R. Liss, 1985, pp. 43–61.

52. Kennedy, C., M. DesRosiers, M. Reivich, F. Sharp, J.W. Jehle, and L. Sokoloff. Mapping of functional neural pathways by autoradiographic survey of local metabolic rate with [^{14}C] deoxyglucose. Science, 187:850–853, 1975.

53. Sokoloff, L., M. Reivich, C. Kennedy, M. DesRosiers, H. Patlak, K.D. Pettigrew, O. Sakurada, and M. Shinohara. The [^{14}C] deoxyglucose method for the measurement of local cerebral glucose utilization: Theory, procedure and normal values in the conscious and anesthetized albino rat. J. Neurochem., 28:897–916, 1977.

54. Siri, W.E. Isotropic Tracers and Nuclear Radiations. New York, McGraw-Hill, 1949.

55. Yano, Y., and H.O. Anger. Visualization of heart and kidneys in animals with ultrashort-lived 82Rb and the positron scintillation camera. J. Nucl. Med., 9:412–415, 1968.

56. Brownell, G.L., C.A. Burnham, B. Hoop, and H. Kazemi. Positron scintigraphy with short-lived cyclotron-produced radiopharmaceuticals and a multicrystal positron camera. In: Proc. Symp. Med. Radioisotope Scintigraphy, Copenhagen, 1972, Vienna, IAEA, 1973, p. 313.

57. Kuhl, D.E., and R.Q. Edwards. Image separation radioisotope scanning. Radiology, 80:653–661, 1963.

58. Kuhl, D.E., and R.Q. Edwards. The Mark III scanner: a compact device for multiple view and section scanning of the brain. Radiology, 96:563–570, 1970.

59. Rankowitz, S., J.S. Robertson, and W.A. Higginbotham, et al. Positron scanner for locating brain tumors. IRE Int. Conv. Rec. Pt., 9:49–56, 1962.

60. Hounsfield, G.N. Computerized transverse axial scanning (tomography): Part I. Description of system. Br. J. Radiol., 46:1016–1022, 1973.

61. Phelps, M.E., E.J. Hoffman, N.A. Mullan, and M.M. Ter-Pogossian. Application of annihilation coincidence detection to transaxial reconstruction tomography. J. Nucl. Med., 16:210–224, 1975.

62. Phelps, M.E., E.J. Hoffman, N.A. Mullani, C.S. Higgins, and M.M. Ter-Pogossian. Design considerations for a positron emission transaxial tomograph (PETT III). IEEE Nucl. Sci. NS, 23:516–522, 1976.

63. Phelps, M.E., E.J. Hoffman, S.C. Huang, and D.E. Kuhl. ECAT: a new computerized

tomographic imaging system for positron emitting radiopharmaceuticals. J. Nucl. Med., 19:635–647, 1978.

64. Ido, T., C-N. Wan, J.S. Casella, J.S. Fowler, A. Wolf, M. Reivich, and D.E. Kuhl. Labeled 2-deoxy-D-glucose analogs: 18-F labeled 2-deoxy-2-fluro-D-glucose, 2-deoxy-2-fluoro-D-mannose and ^{14}C-2 deoxy-2-fluoro-D-glucose. J. Lable Compds. Radio-pharm., 14:175–183, 1978.

65. Reivich, M., D. Kuhl, A. Wolf, J. Greenberg, M.E. Phelps, T. Ido, V. Casella, E. Hoffman, A. Alavi, and L. Sokoloff. The (^{18}F) fluorodeoxyglucose method for the measurement of local cerebral glucose utilization in man. Circ. Res., 44:127–137, 1979.

66. Phelps, M.E., S.C. Huang, E.J. Hoffman, C. Selin, L. Sokoloff, and D.E. Kuhl. Tomographic measurement of local cerebral glucose metabolic rate in humans with (F-18) 2-fluoro-2-deoxy-D-glucose: validation of method. Ann. Neurol., 6:371–388, 1979.

67. Bernard, C. An Introduction to the Study of Experimental Medicine. Tr. by H.C. Green, New York, Macmillan, 1927.

Chapter 10

Myocardial Failure

A.M. KATZ
W. ABELMANN
G. HASENFUSS
R.J. BING

Early History, Biochemistry, Receptors, and Contractile Proteins

HEART FAILURE IS a pathologic state characterized by the inability of the heart to maintain a cardiac output sufficient to meet the metabolic requirements of the organ systems of the body at rest and during ordinary activity, at normal levels of ventricular filling pressures. A decline in ejection fraction (ratio of stroke volume to end-diastolic volume) is a more sensitive marker of cardiac performance than cardiac output. Heart failure is considered compensated when an adequate cardiac output can be maintained by virtue of the activation of compensatory mechanisms, albeit at elevated ventricular filling pressures. When accompanied by pulmonary or systemic congestion, or when physical activity is restricted by symptoms of pulmonary hypertension or fatigue secondary to inadequate systemic blood flow, heart failure may be considered decompensated.

In recent years, increasing attention has been given to alterations in diastolic function of the ventricles. Impaired diastolic function may result in elevated ventricular filling pressures associated with congestion in the presence of normal systolic function. The first portions of this chapter deal primarily with heart failure secondary to impaired systolic function, that is, impairment of the pump function of the heart.

Although many manifestations of congestive heart failure were recognized early in the history of medicine, the modern concept of congestive heart failure had to await the understanding of the heart as a pump responsible for the circulation of the blood. Only with the recognition of the heart as a muscle could weakness or other impairments of this muscle be associated with failure of the pump and interference with the circulation of the blood.

The attribution of the manifestations of heart failure to this organ was made more difficult by the fact that, unlike disease or failure of other organs, these manifestations generally presented themselves elsewhere in the body, such as dyspnea implicating the lungs, ascites and edema implicating the liver, and oliguria attributed to the failure of the kidneys. Yet even well before William Harvey's description of the circulation, the study of the pulse and its variation in disease led many authorities to relate such changes to afflictions of the heart.

In the scholarly and comprehensive historical monograph, *The Concept of Heart Failure from Avicenna to Albertini* (1), Saul Jarcho analyzed the evolution of the understanding of the symptoms and signs of heart failure from the eleventh to the eighteenth centuries, from the description of dyspnea, orthopnea, ascites, and edema, to the nascent recognition of clinicopathologic correlates, and finally to attribution of these manifestations to disease of the heart and/or circulation. Thus, Avicenna, also known as Ibn Sina (980–1037), in his extensive *Canon of Medicine*, clearly describes dyspnea and orthopnea, as well as pulmonary edema producing foam at the mouth and carrying a grave prognosis, but does not relate these manifestations to the heart (2).

In the chapter on dyspnea and dropsy of the lung in his text on the treatment of internal diseases published in 1619, Ludovivicus Mercatus, a physician and teacher in Valladolid, Spain, was perhaps the first to list as one of the causes of dyspnea the suppression of urine, which he thought collected in the lung (3).

In 1618 Carolus Piso, professor of medicine at the University of Pont-á-Mousson, provided the most descriptive case history of an octogenarian nobleman with paroxysmal nocturnal dyspnea (4).

> After he had first fallen asleep as usual, a suffocation would suddenly excite the old man and interrupt his sleep, so that against his will he was obliged to get out of bed and rush at once to the windows of his bedroom in order to breathe fresh air through dilated nostrils. The old man could be seen, with inflamed face, drawing breath deeply, and with his shoulders trembling. He could not remain quietly in one place and especially he could not stand the fireplace but exposed himself even in a severe winter. Gradually and insensibly as the day advanced he would be relieved of his oppression, especially in the afternoon, but during the next sleep the affection returned and troubled the excellent old man again. . . . I concluded finally that the fluid which was occupying his bronchi and the lung itself, or which more probably was stagnating in the middle of his chest, was of the kind that at the time of sleep through return of the vital spirit flowing back into the precordia received a certain new fervor, so that while bubbling in this way it could not be kept

within its own space as formerly and it would necessarily compress the lungs and block their free motion. However, when this fervor gradually became spontaneously quiescent and the spirit flowed again out of the precordia into the body generally, as is the case in persons who are awake, then the lungs could more freely regain their space and the patient could breathe without such great oppression. Further, the fluid could be aqueous or serous, as I had seen formerly and repeatedly in dissected cadavers. Therefore, the totality of my reasoning led at length to this conclusion: I decided in my own mind that the difficulty of breathing which troubled the patient night after night and remitted somewhat in the daytime was to be attributed to dropsy of the chest.

Yet, in neither the writings of Mercatus nor in those of Piso is there any attribution of the symptoms to disease of the heart. It should also be noted that Harvey's description of the circulation of the blood in his famous monograph *De Motu Cordis* (published in 1628) (5) did not contain any description of the effects of disease.

It remained for Marcello Malpighi to lay the foundation of cardiovascular pathophysiology. This great scientist took advantage of the unusual opportunities northern Italy offered in the seventeenth century: he was a student of the famous anatomist Carlo Fracasati in Bologna, and as a professor in Pisa, his colleagues included the mathematician Giovanni Borelli and the physicist Galileo. It is not surprising then, that Malpighi's work shows evidence of a quantitative bent, and that in his view of disorders of the circulation he may be considered the first hemodynamicist. Aside from two letters published in 1661 (6), in which he first described the pulmonary capillary circulation as well as the erythrocyte, Malpighi's contributions to cardiology are contained in sixty-four consultations, not published until 1747. In his second consultation (7), which deals with the illness of the king of Poland, who suffered from an irregular pulse, Malpighi postulated an altered entry of blood into the heart: "As a result the respiration and pulse are changed, for when blood in the lungs has been delayed, their weight is increased. This causes dyspnea."

In the third consultation, referring to the queen of Poland, also suffering from intermission of the pulse, Malpighi states,

> when the passage of blood through the lungs is clogged by disease of the vessels, when the necessary amount of fluid is denied to the left auricle, the heart contracts but the impulse indeed is not transmitted through the arteries. Therefore, when the freedom of the pathways is impeded by convulsion of nerves or by a static coagulated object, or the diameter of the vessels has become altered, the pulse is varied and does not occur in the periphery of the body even though the heart does not desist from its motion, and indeed it may then be moved more often.

One must recall here that before the twentieth century the vast majority of heart disease was rheumatic heart disease, generally associated with atrial fibrillation.

The fourth consultation addresses a cardinal suffering from dropsy, which Malpighi explains by stating that "the veins were not resorbing the fluids pushed forth by the arteries, stagnation necessarily followed." In the thirty-first consultation, orthopnea is explained as follows: "the movement of the blood is slowed, the mass of the lungs becomes heavier."

Jarcho (1) credits Giorgio Baglivi with the first clinical description of pulmonary edema (8). Describing "suffocative catarrh" Baglivi states: "In this catarrh the patient has a cold, pain in the chest, and difficulty in breathing; also interrupted speech, anxiety, cough, stertor, a widely spaced slow pulse, foam at the mouth, and the like." He also states that "An instant remedy for this disease during the paroxysm is repeated bloodletting."

With Raymond Vieussens (1636–1715) we see the beginning of delineation of heart disease by the method of clinicopathologic correlation. At the St. Eloy Hospital in Montpellier, Vieussens was active clinically but stood out for performing autopsies personally or at least witnessing autopsies on many of the patients he had examined previously. Thus, he was able to describe both pericardial effusion and constrictive pericarditis, and he recognized that the latter "deprives (the heart) of part of its strength and of the liberty that it naturally must have in order to contract and expand" (9). In cardiology, Vieussens is best known for his description of mitral stenosis. An apothecary suffered from dyspnea, orthopnea, and peripheral edema. His pulse was small. At autopsy,

> the lung was extraordinarily bulky and soft, because its entire tissue was drenched in watery lymphatic juices. The posterior part of the lobes on the left appeared inflamed. After having surveyed the condition of the lung, I pulled the heart, together with the common trunks of its blood vessels, out of the thoracic cavity in order to examine all its parts. Its size was so extraordinary as to approach that of an ox heart. The coronary veins and their branches were very greatly dilated. The cavity of the right ventricle and of the right auricle had become excessively large.

Vieussens noted that the columnae carneae of the right ventricle were thickened and that "the common openings of this ventricle have been so greatly dilated that they became perceptible, and the membrane which covered them had become so greatly stretched that it allowed free passage to the blood that came out through them." He also described enlargement of the left auricle, and stated that "the entrance of the left ventricle appeared to be extremely small and that it had an oblong oval shape. In looking for the cause of such a surprising fact I discovered that the triglossine (mitral) valves of this ventricle were truly bony." Vieussens further observed that "some of the bundles of the fleshy ducts which formed the sides of the depression in this ventricle had lost much of their natural thickness because they did not receive as much blood as they were used to receiving before the triglossine valves had turned to bony matter." Hence, he concluded that

> the blood could not pass freely and as abundantly as it should into the cavity of this ventricle. As soon as the circulation became impeded by this, it began to expand to an extraordinary extent the trunk of the pulmonary vein, because the blood remained there too long and accumulated there in too large an amount. The blood had no sooner begun to stay too long in the trunk of this vein than it delayed the course of the blood in all the blood vessels of the lung, so that the branches of the pulmonary artery and vein, spread by all the tissue of this organ, were always too full of blood and hence so dilated.

Here then, we have a fairly complete description of congestive heart failure, including tricuspid insufficiency, secondary to mitral stenosis.

A thirty-five-year-old pauper with epilepsy was found to have a rapid and strong pulse that made resting on the left side most uncomfortable: "it seemed as if he was being beaten on the ribs with a hammer." At autopsy, the left ventricle was markedly dilated and "its semilunar valves were greatly stretched and cut off at the end. All the cut edges in them, which had a certain resemblance to the teeth of a saw, were truly stoney." Vieussens concluded that "since the valves were slashed, their ends could never approach closely enough to leave no opening between them. This is why every time the aorta contracted it sent back into the left ventricle a part of the blood that it had just received." This, then, represents an early description of aortic regurgitation, with remarkable hemodynamic insight. Jarcho concludes that Vieussens should be credited with the first complete explanation of backward heart failure (1).

Vieussens thus described and understood congestive heart failure secondary to structural (anatomical) morbid processes of the heart and pericardium, with remarkable insight into the pathophysiology but no clear recognition of the heart as a muscle.

The Danish anatomist Niels Stensen (Nicolas Steno) (1638–86) is credited with the first description of the heart as a muscle: "I am able to prove that there exists nothing in the heart that is not found also in a muscle" (10) (see Chapter 4). Later recognition of the muscular nature of the heart was to be found in the work of Richard Lower in England in 1669 (11) and in Jean-Baptiste Senac's monumental textbook on cardiology published in 1749 (12). It was, however, the Swiss physician, naturalist, and poet Albrecht von Haller, in 1736, who formulated the myogenic theory of heart action (13) and was most influential in its eventual acceptance.

It was Ippolito Francesco Albertini who in 1748 stated unequivocally "in actual fact the heart is a complex muscle" (14). He recognized that in disease this muscle might be weakened. Thus, he wrote,

> observations of patients and their autopsies have shown me that pericardial dropsy arising spontaneously and alone is differentiated at least partly from other lesions in sick persons. Usually it is associated with comparatively soft pulses, rather frequent and small, when the structure of the heart has begun to soften here and there in its fibers, a sluggish or merely watery fluid accumulating in the pericardium.

And again,

> I have found that edema, which at the start of an illness appears in the external parts of the body together with difficulty of breathing, also occurs in the internal organs and especially in the lungs. At such times much heavier and more difficult respiration is produced by a moderate amount of fluid collected in the interstices of the lungs than is produced by a much greater quantity poured out in the cavity of the chest.

Laennec (15) recognized what we now call cor pulmonale:

> All diseases which give rise to severe and long-continued dyspnoea produce, almost necessarily, hypertrophia or dilation of the heart, through the constant efforts the organ is called on to perform, in order to propel the blood into the lungs against the resistance opposed to it by the cause of dyspnoea. It is in this manner that phthisis pulmonalis, empyema, chronic peripneumony, and emphysema of the lung act in producing disease of the heart; and that those kinds of exercise which require great exertion, and thereby impede respiration, come to be the most common remote causes of these complaints.

The seventeenth and eighteenth centuries were the era of postmortem examination and correlation of the findings with clinical observations. The advances and insights of the nineteenth and twentieth centuries were to be based to a great extent on the assessment of normal and abnormal function by means of technical devices, permitting measurements, and by the devising and application of the experimental method, first to animals and then to man.

A now generally forgotten chapter in the history of cardiology began toward the end of the eighteenth century, when autopsy studies of heart failure began to focus on the architecture of the failing heart. In 1761 Giovanni Battista Morgagni published a series of letters, entitled "De sedibus et causes morborum," which includes the following description of the hypertrophic response to increased left atrial and pulmonary artery pressures caused by mitral stenosis (16).

> both the auricles, with their adjoining [veins] . . . and the trunk of the pulmonary artery, and the right ventricle, were much distended, and the columnae and fibers of the same ventricle, were become very thick;

which might happen because . . . a greater thickness of the muscles is the consequences of their more frequent and stronger actions. (Letter XVII, Article 13).

Forty years later, Jean Nicholas Corvisart (1755–1821) distinguished between concentric and eccentric hypertrophy, which in his *Essai sur les maladies et les lésions organiques du coeur* he called "active" and "passive" aneurysm (17). Corvisart noted not only that these different architectural patterns were associated with different clinical manifestations, but also that active aneurysm (concentric hypertrophy), where the walls of the ventricle were thickened, was associated with obstruction to emptying (aortic stenosis). Similar observations were made at the University of Edinburgh by John Bell (1763–1820). A few years later, Réné-Joseph-Hyacinthe Bertin (1767–1828) replaced Corvisart's term "aneurysm" with the modern term "hypertrophy." Throughout the nineteenth century, most scholarly textbooks of medicine and cardiology included classifications of the different forms of cardiac hypertrophy that were based on these early observations (see Chapter 15).

The early anatomic pathologists recognized the compensatory nature of cardiac hypertrophy, often equating this response to the enlargement of the muscles of an athlete. By the end of the nineteenth century, hypertrophy was also noted to have deleterious long-term effects. In 1876 Leopold Schroetter wrote: "Hypertrophy may exist for many years, and the individual still continue to have relatively good health, but in the end it certainly leads to a so-called catastrophe through some of its sequels, at all events by fatty degeneration and subsequent dilatation to disturbances of the circulation, which are of themselves full of danger to the patient" (18), and in 1884 Constantin Paul stated: "It has frequently been said that the heart hypertrophies in order to establish a sort of compensation, and this process has been called providential. This view would be correct if the hypertrophy remained stationary; but experience has shown that the excess of work imposed upon the heart finally deteriorates its fibres, which become changed either by fatty degeneration or by the process of irritation of the connective tissue, which develops excessively and finally strangulates the muscular fibres" (19). These views were summarized by William Osler, who in the first (1892) edition of *The Principles and Practice of Medicine*, presents a remarkably modern view of hypertrophy when he notes that while enlargement of the overloaded heart is initially adaptive, with time maladaptive features of this growth response cause the hypertrophied myocardium to deteriorate (20):

The course of any case of cardiac hypertrophy may be divided into three stages:

1. The period of development, which varies with the nature of the primary lesion. For example, in rupture of an aortic valve . . . it may require months before the hypertrophy becomes fully

developed; or indeed, it may never do so and death may follow from an uncompensated dilatation. On the other hand, in sclerotic affections of the valves, with stenosis or incompetency, the hypertrophy develops step by step with the lesion, and may continue to counterbalance the progressive and increasing impairment of the valve.

2. The period of full compensation—the latent stage—during which the heart's vigor meets the requirements of the circulation. This period has an indefinite time and the patient may never be made aware by any symptoms that he has a valvular lesion.

3. The period of broken compensation, which may come on suddenly during very severe exertion. Death may result from acute dilatation; but more commonly takes place slowly and results from degeneration and weakening of the heart muscle.

This anatomical approach to the failing heart, however, was eclipsed in the early twentieth century with the shift to the new hemodynamic approach to heart disease pioneered by Starling in England and Wiggers in the United States.

The Reverend Stephen Hales had measured blood pressure in animals by the direct method already in 1726 (21); the contributions of a long line of physiologists who studied circulation in the nineteenth century made possible the study of the circulation in disease in the twentieth century. Thus, Claude Bernard (22), in 1844, carried out the first cardiac catheterization of both the right and left ventricles in a horse, to compare the temperatures in the two ventricles. The veterinarian Chaveau and the physician Marey in 1861 first measured intracardiac pressures by this approach (23), using a modification of the kymograph and recording manometer devised by the German physiologist Karl Ludwig (24).

Karl Vierordt is credited with the first application of graphic recording methods to the clinical study of the pulse in 1855 (25), and Samuel S.K. von Basch (26), in 1883, with the development of the sphygmomanometer, upon which all subsequent clinical noninvasive measurements of blood pressure were to be based.

Based on graphic records, M. Potain in 1855 (27) postulated the following mechanism for gallop rhythm:

> The gallop sound is diastolic and caused by the rapid development of tension in the ventricular wall under the influence of the entry of blood into the cavity. It is the more pronounced the stiffer the wall, and this decrease of sclerotic thickening of the cardiac wall (hypertrophy due to Bright's disease) or of a change in muscular tone, with the result that the wall, having only its elasticity with which to resist the inflow of blood, will stiffen at the exact moment when the filling occurs (thyphoid fever, right ventricular dilatation of abdominal origin).

In 1870 Adolph Fick, a physicist and physiologist of broad interests, described the basic principles of measurement of cardiac output, although, because of a lack of instrumentation that would have allowed him to measure oxygen uptake and carbon dioxide excretion, he never made such a measurement himself (28). The pioneer work of this physiologist, however, as well as the demonstration by Werner Forssmann in 1929 that a urethral catheter could be introduced into the human right heart with impunity (29), enabled Cournand and Richards, in 1941, to develop cardiac catheterization in man (30), first as a tool for physiologic studies, but then rapidly applied to clinical studies of heart disease and heart failure. In 1956 Forssmann, Cournand, and Richards were awarded the Nobel prize (see Chapter 1).

Early in this century, Mackenzie (31), considered by some the first pure cardiologist in Great Britain (32), in his lectures and treatises stressed the effect of atrial fibrillation on the heart's efficiency:

> There can be little doubt that the orderly action of the auricle in regulating the supply of blood to the ventricle, and in stimulating it in normal manner, results in a more efficient action of the ventricle than the variable and irregular stimulation to contraction. When the ventricle is rapidly and irregularly stimulated to contract, there results a gradual exhaustion of the strength of the ventricle, and evidences of heart failure supervene.

Although it would seem that Mackenzie, especially aided by graphic recordings with the polygraph he developed, recognized what we now call the "atrial kick," he did not seem to recognize the implications with regard to ventricular filling or the obligatory reduction of diastolic time that accompanies rapid tachycardia.

For many years the concept that congestive heart failure was due to backward pressure prevailed. We have seen this expressed in the writings of Vieussens (9) and Laennec (15), cited above, and it was stated perhaps most clearly in a treatise by James Hope in 1832 (33).

In 1913 Mackenzie challenged this theory when he hypothesized the forward-failure concept, which holds that the failing heart's inability to maintain a normal cardiac output is the main cause of congestive heart failure (34). When measurements of cardiac output in patients with congestive heart failure found this to be low (35), the latter theory appeared confirmed. On the other hand, hemodynamic studies soon revealed that cardiac output could be high, notwithstanding the presence of congestive heart failure, in conditions such as thyrotoxicosis, beriberi, and cor pulmonale. This led to the introduction of the terms "low output failure" and "high output failure" by McMichael (36). The concept of forward failure also derived support from the demonstration that in heart failure renal blood flow tends to be diminished, along with decreased excretion of sodium and water (37).

Seminal contributions to our understanding of cardiovascular physiology were made by Ernest Henry Starling and by Otto Frank. Frank studied with Carl Ludwig, and later moved to Munich, where he succeeded Voit as professor of physiology and remained in this position until 1934. Frank was a great scientist and a very demanding teacher. He was thoroughly intolerant of mediocrity, which to his regret, he found prevalent among the young medical students who sat for the first medical examination. His work was carried out on the whole frog heart, perfused with diluted ox blood. By making continuous recordings throughout the cardiac cycle Frank was able to register intracardiac pressure as well as volume and output. As he wrote, "I discovered the following law concerning the dependence of the form of the isometric pressure curve, on the initial tensions. The peaks (maxima) of the isometric pressure curve rise with increasing initial tension (filling). I call this part of the family of curves the first part. Beyond a certain level of filling the pressure peaks decline, the second part of the family of curves." He mentions Fick as co-discoverer of the same law for skeletal muscle. Frank also examined isotonic ventricular contractions, the ventricle ejecting blood into an elastic capsule; he found that the increased speed of pressure built up during early systole increases with increased initial filling and the presence of residual blood at the end of systole increased with increased aortic resistance and increased diastolic filling (38).

Ernest Starling of London's University College (1866–1927) trained in both physiology and medicine. His quantitative studies of ventricular volumes, stroke volumes, filling pressure, and vascular resistance in the isolated perfused dog heart, begun in 1912, established that the output of a ventricle is determined by the amount of blood returned to it, and that an increase in filling results in an increase in filling pressure and stroke volume (39). These studies led to the enunciation of the "Law of the Heart." "The Law of the Heart is therefore the same as that of skeletal muscle, namely that the mechanical energy set free on passage from the resting to the contracted state depends on the area of chemically active surfaces, i.e., on the length of the muscle fibres. This simple formula serves to explain the whole behavior of the isolated mammalian heart" (40).

Starling's work was extended in the studies of Stanley J. Sarnoff and Erik Berglund at the Harvard School of Public Health in the 1950s (41). These investigators, studying the intact circulation in the dog, constructed families of ventricular (Starling) curves and demonstrated that a descending limb of the Starling curve did not occur in the healthy heart, but that an alteration of myocardial contractility—for example, myocardial failure—resulted in a shift of the normal function curve to a depressed function curve. Starling curves were to become a standard approach to the definition of effects of disease states and interventions on myocardial function.

Studying the intact cat heart as well as the isolated cat papillary muscle, Sonnenblick and Downing (42) demonstrated that ventricular performance is determined not only by preload, that is, the cardiac muscle length prior to initiation of contraction or shortening, but also by afterload, that is, the arterial pressure. They concluded that "ventricular performance at a given constant inotropic state is the product of two largely independent variables, the preload (establishing initial muscle length) and the afterload" (42). This work was to form the basis of the later development of afterload reduction as a therapeutic approach to ventricular failure (43).

Further elucidation of the pathogenesis of heart failure had to await improved understanding of the mechanism of intrinsic contractility of the healthy heart. The early history of the evolution of knowledge about the biochemical and biophysical mechanisms of contraction of heart muscle in the present century has been well reviewed by W.F.H.M. Mommaerts (44). Here again, major roles were played by methodologic developments.

Myocardial metabolism has already been considered in Chapter 3 of the present volume. Much of what we know initially about heart muscle was derived not from studies of cardiac muscle, but from studies of skeletal muscle by pioneers such as A.V. Hill (45), who studied muscular contraction physiologically, and Szent-Györgyi (46), who recognized that the two contractile proteins actin and myosin combined to form actinomyosin and who delineated the role of ATP.

The nearly fifty years that have elapsed since the end of World War II have seen an explosion of research addressing the physiology and pathophysiology of the circulatory system, both in man and in experimental animals. These studies have been made possible by the development of new methods and concepts of modern cellular and molecular biology (47) as well as by the availability of a number of natural and experimental animal models of heart disease (48). Congestive heart failure is now recognized as a final more or less common pathway of many different forms of heart disease—congenital, valvular, ischemic, cardiomyopathic, metabolic—comprising abnormal cardiovascular structure, function of the myocardium, peripheral and pulmonary circulation, and the humoral regulation of circulation. Considerable uncertainty exists as to the primary and possible causal changes and the secondary, perhaps compensatory effects. These advances have been summarized in a number of recent publications (49, 50, 51, 52).

Historically, during the past fifty years clinical experience has been supplemented by fundamental studies that applied the tools furnished. This is particularly evident in the case of congestive heart failure. Protein chemistry, biological chemistry, physiology of circulation, fluid dynamics, even molecular genetics have helped furnish a basis for the clinical phenomenon known as congestive heart failure. No definite answer appears to explain the total protean clinical picture, but some leads have emerged. They focus primarily on the contractile proteins and receptors.

Receptors

In 1948 an article that was to revolutionize cardiology and pharmacology appeared in the *American Journal of Physiology*, "A Study of the Adrenotropic Receptors" (53). The author was Raymond P. Ahlquist, from the Department of Pharmacology, University of Georgia School of Medicine (Fig. 10.1). This paper had a curious history. In the first place, the project was undertaken to find a remedy for dysmenorrhea. A uterine muscle relaxant was therefore needed. In the second place, Ahlquist had difficulty in publishing his paper, and once published, it remained unnoticed for several years. He compared the effect of a series of sympathomimetic amines on uterine contraction, blood pressure, heart rate, myocardial contractility, peripheral vasoconstriction and dilatation, intestinal motility, ureteral contractility, and nictitating membranes—at that time all standard tests for pharmacological analysis of catecholamines. Ahlquist found that a series of six sympathomimetic amines had an order of potency—1, 2, 3, 4, 5, 6—on the following functions: vasoconstriction, excitation of the uterus and ureters, contraction of the nictitating membrane, dilatation of the pupil, and inhibition of the gut. In contrast, the same series of amines had an entirely different order of potency on the following function: vasodilation, inhibition of the uterus, and myocardial stimulation. At the time Alhquist's article was written, pharmacology had already made peace in the dispute between "soup versus sparks," or chemical transmission versus transmission by electrical impulses (54). The arguments between Nachmanson in New York and Otto Loewi created much heat. In Loewi's experiments, supposedly inspired by a dream, he demonstrated that stimulation of the vagus nerve of a perfused frog heart produced a substance that slowed the heart rate of a second heart, and the work of the group around Henry H. Dale, such as J. Feldberg, Gaddum, H. Blaschko, and others settled the argument in favor of chemical transmission (55).

From the recognition of the importance of chemical transmission of nervous impulses, it was only a step to the discovery by U. Von Euler of the role of noradrenalin as the chemical transmittor (56). Walter B. Cannon and A. Rosenblueth had postulated the role of two transmitter substances for adrenergic impulses, sympathin E and sympathin I (57). Cannon, in a lecture given at the College of Physicians and Surgeons of Columbia University in 1936, made a good point for the difference between adrenaline and the sympathins. Stimulation of the hepatic sympathetic nerves released something into the blood that affected the

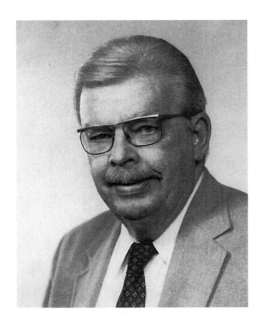

Figure 10.1. Raymond P. Ahlquist. *(Courtesy of the New York Academy of Medicine)*

nictitating membrane differently than adrenalin. Cannon and Rosenblueth therefore concluded that there are two kinds of sympathin, the excitatory (E) and the inhibitory (I). The heart muscle, so they thought, must discharge excitatory sympathin while the coronary circulation discharges inhibitory sympathin. This is a fine example of how uncertainties of different hypothetical transmitter substances, expounded with authority, can be taken as facts. It is not the transmitter that varies, but the receptors that are different. According to Ahlquist, at least two sets of adrenergic responses are present as judged by the comparative potencies of amines (53). His conclusion was that the differences must be due to two types of receptors: alpha receptors and beta receptors. The receptor must be considered to be a part of the effector rather than of the nerve since surgical or pharmacological removal of the nerve does not abolish the effector response to the circulating transmitter. It is the receptor-effector complex rather than the transmitter that ultimately controls the response to stimulation. Ahlquist's concept ran into real difficulties (58, 59, 60). He mentioned that his new concept, arrived at by serendipity, "burst into print in 1948, was ignored for more than five years except when someone referred to the method used or the results obtained, but never to the concept" (58). The reasons for this are obvious: the concept did not fit with the ideas developed since the 1890s on the actions of epinephrine. Ahlquist had difficulties in publishing the paper; it was rejected by the *Journal of Pharmacology and Experimental Therapeutics*, was a loser in the Abel Award Competition, and only could be published in the *American Journal of Physiology* due to

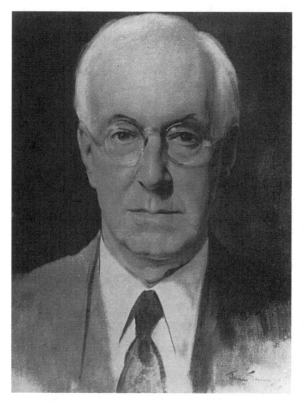

Figure 10.2. Sir Henry H. Dale. *(Courtesy of the New York Academy of Medicine)*

his personal friendship with W.F. Hamilton, the editor. He compared his fate with that of other pioneers of science, for example, to that of Avery who, in 1944, proved that DNA and not protein was the genetic carrier. It was not until 1950 that its correct structure was found, and still later when Watson and Crick showed the double helix. Ahlquist wrote, "Few remember or credit Avery for his concept" (58). In 1977 in the *Post-Graduate Medical Journal*, J.W. Black paid Ahlquist the credit which was his due: "looking back, his paper can be seen to have been hidden in the long shadows cast by two giants—Dale in England and Cannon in the United States" (61; Fig. 10.2).

Looking into the past, we find that the idea of a receptor did not originate with Ahlquist, but earlier with J.N. Langley, professor of physiology in Cambridge, England. His paper in the *Journal of Physiology*, in 1905, is entitled, "On the Reactions of Cells and of Nerve-Endings to Certain Poisons, Chiefly as Regards the Reaction of Striated Muscle to Nicotine and Curari" (62). Reading Langley's paper, which comprises thirty-nine pages, one can only reflect with nostalgia at those happy times when a writer had plenty of space available and when the editors did not object to lengthy introductions, detailed descriptions of the experiments, or a splendid free style of the English language; alas, our scientific language has become ossified in order to be acceptable. Langley reasoned as follows: "Since curari prevents nerve stimulation from having an effect, but does not itself cause muscular contraction, and nicotine, although preventing nerve stimulation from having an effect, does cause muscular contraction, it seems possible that the latter might act on some substance or structure placed more peripherally than that on which the former acts" (62). The professor from Cambridge concluded that

> two poisons, nicotine and curari, act on the same protoplasmic substance or substances. With this proviso, I take it that the action consists in a combination of the alkaloid with the protoplasm. Curari in combining leads to diminished excitability and does not stimulate; nicotine in combining also leads to dimished excitability, but it stimulates in combining.

And then he continues the discussion: "Since this accessory substance is the recipient of stimuli which it transfers to the contractile material, we may speak of it as the receptive substance of the muscle." Langley went further, this being the time of Paul Ehrlich:

> The relation between the receptive and the contractile substance is clearly very close and on the general lines of Ehrlich's immunity theory, it might be supposed that a receptive substance is a side chain molecule of the molecules of contractile substance, but at present there does not seem to me to be any advantage in attempting to refer the phenomena to molecular arrangement. I conclude then that in all cells two constituents at least must be distinguished 1) substances concerned with carrying out the chief functions of the cells, and 2) receptive substances especially liable to change and capable of setting the chief substance in action.

These were the golden years of English physiology. When and where else would it have been possible that, in 1905, in the *Journal of Physiology*, a student in physiology could write a sixty-six-page article on the action of adrenaline that foreshadowed future experiments on chemical transmission of nervous impulses by comparing the action of adrenaline to that of the sympathetic nervous system (63)? That medical student was Thomas Renton Elliott, who four years after he became a student at University College in London, was appointed to the staff, and became the first unit director at London University (Fig. 10.3). A very British wish was expressed to Elliott on the occasion of his retirement: "We hope he will long remain an active player when he goes north to his newly built home among

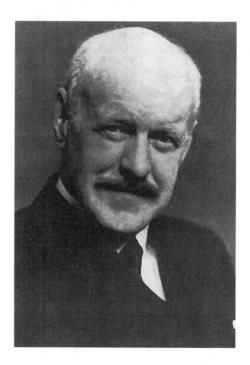

Figure 10.3. Thomas R. Elliott. *(Courtesy of the New York Academy of Medicine)*

the grouse moors of Scotland." The contribution of other great British physiologists and pharmacologists, like Henry Dale and others, are not mentioned here since they contributed only indirectly to the concept of receptors.

Despite the fact that Ahlquist's 1948 paper was ignored for five years, a time came when it was finally noticed, primarily because of the confirmation of his work by C.E. Powell, I.H. Slater, and Black (64, 65). Powell and Slater, working at the Lilly Research Laboratories, published an article in 1957 entitled "Blocking of Inhibitory Adrenergic Receptors by a Dichloro Analog of Isoproterenol" (64). It was found that in the anesthetized dog dichloroisoproterenol did not constrict blood vessels, produce a pressor response, or cause decongestion. Instead, it produced vasodilation, a depressor response, and tachycardia. As Ahlquist explained in *Perspectives in Biology and Medicine*, "This anomalous behaviour was most difficult to explain to medical students" (58). Powell and Slater's discovery in 1958 provided the turning point in the acceptance of the idea of dual receptor mechanism (64). They found that this dichloro analog of isoproterenol selectively blocked some inhibitory effects of epinephrine and isoproterenol. In addition, the pressor actions of isoproterenol and the secondary depressor action of epinephrine were inhibited by the dichloro analog, which of itself had at most caused a transient fall in blood pressure.

The concluding sentence of the paper is worth noting in the line of Ahlquist's work: "It seemed probably that 20522 (the dichloro analog of isoproterenol) was combining with certain adrenergic inhibitory receptor sites and failed to trigger the series of reactions that lead to typical inhibitory effects" (64). In 1964 Black, working with the Imperial Chemical Industries at the Medical Unit of St. Georges Hospital in London, synthetized a new adrenergic beta-receptor antagonist, pronethalol, a specific adrenergic beta-antagonist that was relatively free from sympathomimetic activity on the cardiovascular system (65). He had searched for this compound because of his interest in the treatment of angina pectoris. Unfortunately the compound had some undesirable effects and for this reason Black published his results on a new compound, InderalR, which has been found to satisfy all the criteria of a beta-blocker. Soon this compound was used not only for the treatment of angina pectoris but also for hypertension. Since that time a large series of beta-blockers has been synthetized, some with primarily cardiac receptors (beta 1) and some with primarily smooth muscle receptors (beta 2).

Looking over this enormously fruitful field of cardiovascular pharmacology, one is struck by the observation that the truth had been delayed by authoritarian thoughts and dogma, some originating from a high authority. In science, authority can be as much of a hindrance to progress as ignorance.

The importance of receptors in myocardial failure became apparent in 1977, when it was discovered that after several days the inotropic response to norepinepherine and isoproterenol became markedly depressed in dogs with congestive heart failure, while chronotropic and blood pressure response remained unaltered (66). At the same time it was shown that a reduction in norephinephrine stores in the heart muscle was associated with a depressed inotropic response to tyramine in papillary muscle from patients with heart failure. Later it was found that the injection of dobutamine, a beta-1 agonist, resulted in development of tolerance to long-term infusion; tolerance became significant at seventy-two and ninety-six hours (67). This suggested that beta-adrenergic receptors are "desensitized in the failing human heart," possibly by norepinephrine (68). This desensitization was not restricted to the heart muscle. Colucci, for example, found that density of beta-adrenergic receptors on lymphocytes of patients treated with a beta-adrenergic agonist was significantly depressed as compared with that of untreated patients with heart failure of comparable severity. Apparently tolerance can develop in areas other than heart muscle. It is likely that clinically relevant concentrations of administered sympathomimetic agents can affect beta-adrenergic receptor density (69). Other reports soon confirmed this. Obviously the burden of proof is on the beta-adrenergic receptor, which through combination with hormone agonists stimulates the enzyme adenylate cyclase to form cyclic AMP, which in turn promotes transmembrane calcium flux. In 1986 a selective downgrading of beta-1 as compared to beta-2 receptors was found in the failing ventricle (70).

The question arose as to the cause of this selective downgrading. Increased exposure to norepinephrine, which has a very high affinity for beta-receptors, may be responsible for selective beta-1 downgrading. It is known that the failing human heart is exposed to a high concentration of norepinephrine and that selective myocardial beta-1 receptor downregulation in the number of beta-adrenergic receptors appears to be chamber-specific; patients with primary right ventricular failure show a greater reduction in beta-receptor numbers in the right ventricle than in the left, whereas patients with biventricular failure show an equivalent degree of beta-adrenergic receptor downregulation in both ventricles (71, 72). Postsynaptic myocardial alpha-1 receptors exist in most mammalian species, including humans. They mediate a positive inotropic response without notably affecting heart rate (71). This positive inotropic mechanism is not related to the accumulation of cyclic AMP and the stimulation of adenylate cyclase. Selective myocardial alpha-1 adrenergic stimulation may provide effective inotropic support in congestive heart failure even if beta-receptor density is markedly reduced (73). Enhanced vasocontriction, which is a hallmark of congestive heart failure, may result in part from increased alpha-1 adrenoceptor activity in peripheral arterial smooth muscle (74). The mechanism by which cardiac alpha-1 adrenergic receptors increase the force of myocardial contraction is not completely understood, but their inotropic effect may be mediated by receptor-mediated hydrolysis of phosphoinositides to diacyglyceride (75) or more important by inositol triphosphate, which opens intracellular calcium channels. It has been speculated that the loss of inhibition of norepinephrine release in congestive heart failure contributes to the elevation in synaptic and plasma catecholamine levels in congestive heart failure.

From a clinical viewpoint it seemed logical to counteract the downgrading of beta-1 receptor in the myocardium by treatment with beta-1 adrenergic agonists. Several beta-agonists have been proposed that might accomplish this goal. But treatment of downgrading of beta-receptor with beta-1 adrenergic blockers appears more promising; there have been reports that beta-adrenergic blocking agents are of benefit in congestive heart failure. Treatment with beta-1 blockers such as propranolol in patients with congestive heart failure appears to increase the number of beta-1 receptors (76). In a U.S. multicenter trial, the use of carvedilol, a nonselective beta-blocker with adrenergic blocking properties, was stopped prematurely because of a significant reduction in mortality in patients receiving this compound (77). Whether beta-blockers can be considered as a proven therapeutic modality in chronic heart failure is not certain. Additional large-scale well-controlled studies are needed. However, there is reason to believe that beta-blockers will emerge as part of the therapy of chronic congestive heart failure.

Biochemistry of Myocardial Failure and Contractile Proteins

The preceding discussion indicated that studies dealing with congestive heart failure were primarily descriptive or clinical. At the beginning of this century, there occurred a definite shift: knowledge from the fundamental sciences, physics, chemistry, and molecular biology, biochemistry, and electromicroscopy began to influence the approaches to myocardial failure (78).

Coronary sinus catheterization, begun in the mid-1940s, was among the early studies on myocardial failure (78). By introducing a catheter into the coronary sinus and simultaneously sampling arterial and coronary sinus blood, the coronary arteriovenous differences not only of oxygen, but also of nutrients such as glucose, lactate, pyruvates, amino acids, ketone bodies, and fatty acids could be determined. Congestive heart failure was recognized as a disturbance of energy production rather than energy utilization since there was no change in myocardial extraction of either oxygen or substrates. It is not the scope of this historical review to detail current knowledge of the biochemical basis of heart function and contractile failure. The reader is referred to recent reviews on this subject (78, 79, 80, 81).

Recent developments in fundamental knowledge of myocardial failure are concerned with (1) calcium movements, membrane function of mitochondria, subcellular organelles (cytoplasmic reticulum), and (2) contractile machinery of the heart, the contractile proteins.

The pioneering figure in the field of contractile proteins is Albert Szent-Györgyi (Fig. 10.4). Szent-Györgyi received the Nobel prize in medicine and physiology for his discoveries in connection with the biological combustion process and the catalysis of fumaric acid, leading to the discovery of vitamin C. Unquestionably Szent-Györgyi was one of the most colorful and creative scientists of our age. He was born in 1893 in Budapest, Hungary, and his early career was intimately connected with the fate of his native land. He published an autobiographical note in the *Annual Review of Biochemistry* (82):

> I finished school in feudal Hungary as the son of a wealthy land owner and I had no worries about my future. A few years later I find myself working in Hamburg, Germany with a slight hunger edema. In 1942 I find myself in Istanbul involved in secret diplomatic activity, with a setting fit for a cheap and exciting spy story. Shortly after, I get a warning that Hitler had ordered the Governor of Hungary to appear before him, screaming my name at the top of his voice and demanding my delivery. Arrest warrants were passed out even against members of my family. In my pocket I find a Swedish passport, having been made a full Swedish citizen on the order of the King of Sweden—I am "Mr. Swenson," my wife, "Mrs. Swenson." Sometime later I find myself in Moscow being

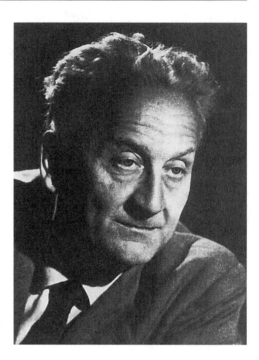

Figure 10.4. Albert Szent-Györgyi. *(Courtesy of the New York Academy of Medicine)*

treated in the most royal fashion by the government (with caviar three times per day), but it does not take long before I am declared a "traitor of the people" and I play the role of the villain. At the same time I am refused entrance to the USA for my Soviet sympathies. Eventually, I find peace at Woodshole, Massachusetts, USA working in a solitary corner of the Marine Biological Laboratory. After some nerve-wrecking complications, due to McCarthy, things straighten out, but the internal struggle is not completely over. I am troubled by grave doubts about the usefulness of scientific endeavor and have a whole drawer filled with treatises on politics and their relation to science, written for myself with the sole purpose of clarifying my mind completely and finding an answer to the question: will science lead to the elevation or destruction of man, and has my scientific endeavor made any sense?

What may lend additional interest to his story is that it reflects the turbulence of our days. This is not very different from the story of Copernicus who lived in the sixteenth century and whose life was influenced and darkened by the turmoil of his times. Szent-Györgyi was a rebel and an unruly genius. In science he fought what he called "accepting things without evidence" and he believed that we were living in the middle of the transition from the prescientific to the scientific thinking, hence the "tumult." As a child he described himself as dull and his uncle, a noted histologist, believed that he was not promising enough to go on to medical school, but suggested that he go into cosmetics. Later his uncle admitted the possibility of his becoming a proctologist. So his first scientific paper, written in the first year of medical studies, dealt with the epithelium of the anus. As he says, "I started science at the wrong end, but soon I shifted to the vitreous body." Later in his career he became fascinated by succinohydrogenase and citrocodehydrogenase. He believed that these enzymes should have some general catalytic role and he demonstrated that once the succinodehydrogenase was inactivated, which could be done by malonic acid, respiration stopped. This proved that succinic acid and citric acid had some general catalytic activity and could not be simple metabolites as thought before. This idea was later confirmed by Krebs and became the foundation of the so-called Krebs cycle. It was partly this discovery of the C4 dicarboxylic acid catalysis for which Szent-Györgyi was honored by the Nobel prize.

At the same time Szent-Györgyi became interested in vegetable respiration because as he expressed it, "there is no basic difference between man and the grass he mows." Eventually, he was able to isolate a reducing agent crystallized from oranges, lemons, cabbages, and the adrenal gland. He knew that it was related to sugars, but he did not know which. He called this compound "Ignose." The editor of the biochemical journal to whom he submitted the article reprimanded him for being flippant. Thereupon Szent-Györgyi changed the name of this sugar to "Godnose," but this was not more successful. Finally he called the new substance hexuronic acid since it had six carbons and was acid. To get more material he moved to the Mayo Clinic, where there was ample adrenal tissue available. Returning to Hungary and the University of Szeged, he found that hexuronic acid was identical to vitamin C. As he wrote "we (that is Hayworth and I) rebaptized hexuronic acid to ascorbic acid" (82).

Szent-Györgyi then turned to the biochemistry of muscle. As he wrote, "with its valiant, physical, chemical and dimensional changes, muscle is an ideal material to study." With his associates he discovered a new protein, "actin," which was isolated by his pupil Straub. By complexing actin and myosin he found a contractile protein, actomyosin, which contracted upon the addition of adenosine triphosphate (ATP). As Szent-Györgyi wrote, "to see these fibers contract for the first time, and to have reproduced in vitro one of the oldest signs of life, motion, was perhaps the most thrilling moment of my life." Szent-Györgyi concludes his autobiographical sketch:

> to me, science in the first place is the society of men which knows no
> limits in time and space. I am living in such a community, in which
> Lavoisier and Newton are my daily companions; an Indian or Chinese
> scientist is closer to me than my own milkman. The basic moral rule
> of this society is simple: Mutual respect, intellecutal honesty, and good
> will (82).

Based on Albert Szent-Györgyi's discovery, the knowledge of the role of contractile proteins in normal and failing hearts has explanded (79, 80). It has been found that reconstituted actomyosin exhibits the salient properties of muscle. It was Huxley who first proposed the sliding model, in which actin and myosin molecules slide by each other during shortening of the muscle (83). Actin has been found to consist of two portions, F and G actin. Tropomyosin and troponin are found with actin on the thin filament (84). In the myofibril, the thin filament surrounds the thick filament and interacts by overlapping. Actin forms a macromolecule to comprise a thin filament (84). Troponin and trypomyosin are known to play a regulatory role in the interaction of actin and myosin and an additional protein (C-protein) has also been identified in cardiac muscle (79). Actin-myosin forms cross-bridges and shortens against mechanical load at the expense of the chemical energy contained in the high-energy phospate bond in ATP. The tropomyosin and troponin proteins confirm calcium sensitivity on the contractile machinery. Troponin-C is the subunit that binds Ca^{2+} and troponin 1 (79, 80, 81).

Another important development concerns the phosphorylation of cardiac contractile proteins (85). Phosphorylation of proteins by protein kinase is a reversible process. Aside from the regulation of cardiac contractility through changes in intracellular concentration of calcium ions, phosphorylation of cardiac contractile proteins also plays a considerable role. When hearts are stimulated with catecholamines, troponin-I and C-protein are rapidly phosphorylated in response to increased intracellular concentration of cyclic AMP.

Molecular biology has also been applied in an attempt to understand myocardial failure. It is now apparent that the well-known changes in gross and histological structure, and in the ultrastructure of the failing heart, extend to the molecular level. Hypertrophy of the overloaded myocardium is accompanied by complex changes in the expression of the genes that encode key myocardial proteins. For example, in the pressure-overloaded rodent ventricle, preferential synthesis of a "slow" isoform of the myosin heavy chain helps ventricular function adapt to a chronic increase in the rate of energy expenditure. This occurs because the slow myosin reduces the rate of energy expenditure while, at the same time, increasing efficiency (84). While these abnormalities are not seen in the human ventricle, changes in myosin gene expression similar to those in the rat ventricle have been documented in overloaded human atria (86, 87).

The changes in myosin described above represent but one example of a growing number of alterations in the composition of the overloaded, hypertrophied heart (88). A reduction in the density of calcium pump ATPase molecules in the sarcoplasmic reticulum of the hyperthrophied human heart has also been described (89), in this case, without a change in the protein itself. Additionally, myocardial infarction profoundly affects regulatory light chain phosphorylation in the myocardium, leading to a diminution in myocardial contractility (90).

A pattern that emerges is that there is a preferential synthesis of fetal isoforms of several proteins in the failing heart. This appearance of fetal isoforms may be related to the accelerated growth that occurs in cardiac hypertrophy. It is well known that the cells of the adult myocardium, which are unable to divide, normally synthesize protein at only a very slow rate. In order for the overloaded myocardium to initiate rapid protein synthesis, it appears that isoforms of many newly synthesized proteins revert to those seen earlier in development, during fetal life. The functional significance of this reversion to primitive isoforms is not well understood, but may result in myocardial cells that "wear out" at an accelerated rate, and so may contribute to the deterioration of the myocardium that is largely responsible for the poor prognosis in patients with heart failure (see Chapter 13).

Other possible mechanisms that may contribute to the deterioration of the failing heart relate to the signal transduction pathways that mediate the growth response to overload. These pathways are adaptive, in that they provide additional sarcomeres which, in an overloaded or damaged heart, improve hemodynamic function. At the same time, however, activation of these growth-promoting pathways appears to initiate a maladaptive response that shortens the survival of the damaged heart (91). The nature of the deleterious consequences of the hypertrophic response to overload remains unclear; one factor may be related to cell elongation, a change in cardiac myocyte phenotype that causes "remodeling," the progressive dilatation of a damaged heart. Other consequences of this growth response include architectural and molecular changes that contribute to a state of "energy starvation" in the failing heart (92), and stimulation of apoptosis (programmed cell death) (91). The importance of these maladaptive features of the hypertrophic response to overload lies in their ability to explain the large number of surprising findings that have come from recent clinical heart failure trials. These center on several classes of drugs which, although they improve symptoms over the short term, had to be abandoned because they worsened prognosis over the long term (91). These drugs include a number of inotropic agents (93, 94, 95), vasodilators (96, 97, 98) and antiarrhythmic drugs (99). These counterintuitive findings indicate that even though we start from a seemingly high level of knowledge about heart failure, our understanding of this syndrome remains incomplete.

Calcium and Myocardial Failure

Several studies have indicated that altered calcium cycling may play a dominant role in disturbed myocardial function in end-stage human heart failure. (1) Myothermal studies have demonstrated that the amount and rate of evolution of tension-independent heat is significantly reduced in failing human myocardium at a stimulation rate of 60 beats per minute (37°C). This indicates that the total amount of calcium cycling and the rate of calcium removal are reduced (100). (2) Systolic free calcium concentration was shown to be reduced when FURA-2 was used to measure free intracellular calcium concentrations in isolated myocytes from failing human hearts (101). (3) It was shown that alteration of calcium transients depends on the frequency of stimulation. Using the photoprotein aequorin to evaluate calcium transients in isolated muscle strip preparations it was observed that the frequency-dependent rise of the calcium transients is blunted and that even an inversion of the calcium-frequency relation occurs in most ventricular muscle strip preparations from end-stage failing human hearts (102). (4) Postrest potentiation of calcium transients was diminished, suggesting decreased sarcoplasmic reticulum calcium accumulation (103). (5) Regarding diastolic function, studies in isolated myocytes and ventricular muscle strip preparations indicated that diastolic calcium levels are elevated and that calcium transients are prolonged in failing compared to nonfailing human myocardium (101, 104).

Transsarcolemmal Calcium Influx

Calcium entry through voltage-gated L-type calcium channels is the key event causing the transition from the resting state of the myocardium to contraction (105). Several studies have been performed to evaluate abundance of the L-type calcium channel subunit in failing and nonfailing human myocardium. Takahashi et al. reported a significant decrease in mRNA levels encoding the dihydropyridine receptor as well as a decrease in dihydropyridine binding sites in failing human hearts with dilated and ischemic cardiomyopathy (106). However, this is in contrast to findings by Rasmussen et al., which indicate that dihydropyridine binding sites are not significantly altered in the human ventricular tissue from hearts with end-stage dilated cardiomyopathy (107).

Unaltered levels of the subunit of L-type calcium channels would be consistent with functional measurements indicating that calcium current densities, measured during basal conditions, are similar in isolated myocytes from failing hearts with dilated cardiomyopathy as compared to nonfailing hearts (108, 109). In addition, measurements by Piot et al. recently suggested that function of L-type calcium channels may be altered in human heart failure (110).

Sarcoplasmic Reticulum and Calcium
Ryanodine Receptors and Calcium Release

The calcium-sensitive ryanodine receptor (RyR), which is located in the immediate vicinity of the L-type calcium channel, is activated by a local increase in calcium subsequent to transsarcolemmal calcium influx (111). Once activated, the channel opens and releases calcium for activation of contractile proteins. This process is termed calcium-induced calcium release (105).

Several groups have studied mRNA expression of the RyR in human heart failure, but results have not been consistent. While Brillantes et al. observed decreased mRNA levels in ischemic but not in dilated cardiomyopathy, Go et al. described a reduction of RyR mRNA levels in both ischemic and dilated cardiomyopathy (112, 113). In three studies, a radioligand binding assay was used. Go observed that high-affinity binding sites for [^{3}H]ryanodine were decreased by about 30 percent in left ventricular myocardium from failing human hearts (113). Schumacher et al. noted no differences in [^{3}H]ryanodine binding between failing and nonfailing hearts (114), while Sainte Beuve observed an increase of RyRs in failing hearts (115). At the level of the protein, no change in RyR levels between failing and nonfailing hearts was consistently observed (115, 116). From the findings of unchanged protein levels but increased [^{3}H]ryanodine binding in failing hearts, Sainte Beuve et al. calculated that ryanodine binding properties may be affected in failing myocardium reflecting altered channel activity (115).

Calsequestrin and calreticulin are calcium-binding proteins located within the lumen of the SR (117–119). Calsequestrin, a high-capacity moderate affinity calcium-binding protein, is primarily responsible for the calcium storage capacity of the SR in cardiac muscle. Studies in failing human myocardium consistently showed unchanged mRNA and protein levels of calsequestrin as compared to nonfailing myocardium (106, 116, 120, 121). Similarly, calreticulin protein levels were shown to be unchanged in the failing human hearts (116). This suggests that the capacity of the SR to bind calcium is unchanged.

Calcium transport into the SR occurs by SR-Ca^{2+}-ATPase, which transports two calcium ions per molecule of high-energy phosphate hydrolyzed against a high free calcium gradient of intracellular 100 nM to 10 M into the SR with ~1mM (117, 122). The SR competes for calcium with the sarcolemmal Na$^+$-Ca^{2+}-exchanger. As a consequence, increased activity of the Na$^+$-Ca^{2+}-exchanger may reduce SR calcium accumulation and the amount of calcium available for systolic activation of contractile proteins. With respect to diastolic calcium concentration and thus diastolic function, the SR-Ca^{2+}-ATPase and the Na$^+$-Ca^{2+}-exchanger work in concert.

The SR-Ca^{2+}-ATPase is regulated by phospholamban (118, 122). Dephosphorylated phospholamban is an inhibitor of the SR-Ca^{2+}-ATPase activity. The inhibition has been suggested to involve direct protein-protein interaction followed by conformational changes in the SR-Ca^{2+}-ATPase, resulting in a decrease in the affinity of the calcium pump for calcium (123, 124). Several studies indicated that SR calcium uptake or SR-Ca^{2+}-ATPase activity is reduced in the failing human myocardium (125–127).

It has been reported that mRNA levels of SR-Ca^{2+}-ATPase are reduced in the failing compared to the nonfailing human heart (125, 128–130), while findings on protein levels have been controversial (116, 121, 125, 128, 129, 130). A significant correlation between SR calcium uptake and SR-Ca^{2+}-ATPase protein levels has been observed (126). Furthermore, there was a significant correlation between SR-Ca^{2+}-ATPase protein levels and myocardial function. This indicates that a wide variation in protein levels of SR-Ca^{2+}-ATPase within the group of failing hearts (protein levels differed by a factor of 4); this variation in protein levels reflects differences in myocardial function. Therefore in a subgroup of failing hearts SR-Ca^{2+}-ATPase protein levels are similar to those in nonfailing hearts with preserved myocardial systolic function (126).

Previous work in transgenic mice showed that the stoichiometry between SR-Ca^{2+}-ATPase and phospholamban is crucial for SR-Ca^{2+}-ATPase activity and myocardial function (131). Accordingly, it is important to evaluate alterations in SR-Ca^{2+}-ATPase levels in relation to alterations in phospholamban levels. While a decrease in phospholamban mRNA levels has been consistently observed in failing human myocardium (125, 130, 132), only one study (116) showed a small decrease in phospholamban protein levels relative to total protein in failing dilated cardiomyopathy (121, 125, 130). However, when phospholamban was normalized to calsequestrin, no difference existed between failing and nonfailing myocardium (116). Meyer et al. observed that in the failing myocardium SR-Ca^{2+}-ATPase protein levels were decreased to a greater proportion than protein levels of phospholamban (116). Accordingly, if we assume that the relation of phospholamban to SR-Ca^{2+}-ATPase determines the level of SR-Ca^{2+}-ATPase inhibition, this finding indicates that in the basal low phosphorylated state inhibition of SR-Ca^{2+}-ATPase is more pronounced in the failing human myocardium (131).

In summary, there is considerable evidence that the capacity of the SR calcium pump system to accumulate calcium into the SR is significantly reduced in the failing human heart. In addition, altered expression and function of the Na$^+$-Ca^{2+}-exchanger may further compromise SR calcium accumulation (see below).

Sarcolemmal calcium transport is dominated by activity of the Na$^+$-Ca^{2+}-exchanger, whereas the sarcolemmal calcium pump does not contribute quantitatively to beat calcium elimination and myocardial relaxation (133). The Na$^+$-Ca^{2+}-exchanger extrudes one calcium ion for three sodium ions using the electrochemical sodium gradient (134, 135). In the outward mode, it produces a net movement of charge, resulting in a net inward current. The Na$^+$-Ca^{2+}-exchanger is also voltage-dependent and can reverse its mode during the action potential (134, 135). Under experimental conditions in the presence of high intracellular sodium levels, the Na$^+$-Ca^{2+}-exchanger can promote calcium influx sufficiently to induce excitation-contraction coupling (136).

Studer et al. showed that mRNA as well as protein levels are significantly increased in the failing human heart (129). This finding was confirmed by Flesch et al. (137). Accordingly, it was shown that Na^+-Ca^{2+}-exchange activity is increased in myocardium from failing hearts (138). Functional relevance of increased Na^+-Ca^{2+}-exchanger expression is evident from a recent study showing that diastolic performance of failing human myocardium correlates inversely with protein levels of Na^+-Ca^{2+}-exchanger (139).

Surgical Attempts to Treat Myocardial Failure

Cardiac surgery has begun to make inroads in the treatment of severe myocardial failure. Examples are dynamic cardiomyoplasty introduced in 1985 by the French surgeon Carpentier in which after dissection, the latissimus dorsi muscle is wrapped around the heart in a clockwise position (140). During the first two weeks following the operation, the muscle is not electronically stimulated in order to allow for the healing process. After three months the muscle is stimulated with every second heart beat (2:1 mode) (140).

Another procedure still to be evaluated is partial left ventricular resection. This procedure was introduced by the Brazilian surgeon Batista in 1996 (141). In this operation a portion of the left ventricular muscle is resected between the anterior and posterior papillary muscle from the apex of the heart to the mitral annulus. The operation is based on the relationship between wall tension radius and pressure as defined by the Law of La Place.

The purpose of these operations is to tie the patients with New York Heart Association class III heart failure until transplantation is feasible and after conservative medical treatment has failed (see Chapter 5).

Coda

It is clear, therefore, that we must continue the processes of discovery reviewed in this chapter. Knowledge of this history will be invaluable in the process because an appreciation of history helps both in understanding the present and predicting the future. As Winston Churchill wrote: "The longer you look back, the farther you can look forward. This is not a philosophical or political argument—any oculist can tell you it is true" (142).

References

1. Jarcho, S. The Concept of Heart Failure from Avicenna to Albertini. Cambridge, MA, Harvard University Press, 1980, p. 407.
2. Husain ibn 'Abd Allah, (Abu 'Ali) called Ibn Sina or Avicenna. On the Signs [of Suffocation and Angina] (Bk 3, Gen 9 treatise 1, chap. 9). Quoted by Jarcho (1), op. cit., p. 4.

3. Mercatus, L. (Luiz Mercado). De internorum morborum curatoine. Frankfurt: Palthemius, 1619–20, Bk 2, chap. 1, pp. 160–161. Quoted by Jarcho (1), op. cit., p. 91.

4. Piso, C. (Charles le Pois). Selectiorum observationum et consiliorum de praetervisis hactenus morbis affectibusque praeter naturam, ab aqua seu serosa colluviae et diluvie ortis Pont-à-Mousson, 1618. Quoted by Jarcho (1), op. cit., p. 113.

5. Harvey, W. Exercitatio anatomica de motu cordis et sanguinis in animalibus. Francoforti, Sumpt. Guilielmi Fitzeri, 1628.

6. Malpighi, M. De pulmonibus. Bologna, 1661.

7. Malpighi, M. et Jo. Mariae Lancisii. Consultationum medicorum, Venezia. Corona, 1747. Tr., in part, by Jarcho (1), op. cit., pp. 190–209.

8. Baglivi, G. Opera omnia medico-practica, et anatomica. Lugduni, Anisson, J. Posuel, 1704.

9. Vieussens, R. Traite nouveau de la structure et des causes du mouvement naturel du coeur. Toulouse, Guillemette, 1715. Quoted by Jarcho (1), op. cit., p. 243.

10. Sten, N. De musculis et glandulis observationum specimen Cum epistolis duabus anatomicis. Ludg. Batav., 1683. Hafniae, Lit. Matt. Godicchenii, 1664 [OT].

11. Lower, R. Tractatus de corde. London, J. Allestry, 1669.

12. Senac, J.B. Traité de la structure du coeur, de son action, et de ses maladies. 2 vols. Paris, Chez Braisson, 1749, p. 1246.

13. Haller, A. Deux mémoires sur le mouvement du sang; et sur les effets de la siagnée; fondes sur des expériences faites sur des animaux. Lausanne, Mark-Mic Bousquet Comp, 1756, p. 342.

14. Albertini, I. F. Animadversiones super quibusdam difficilis respirationis vitiis a laesa cordis et praecordiorum structura pendentibus. In: De Bononiensi Scientiarum et Artium Instituo atque Academia Commentarii, 1:382–404, 1731, reprinted in 1748. Translated in (1).

15. Laennec, R.T.H. A Treatise on the Diseases of the Chest in which they are Described According to their Anatomical Characters and their Diagnosis Established as a New Principle Means of Acoustic Instrument. Book 3, Chapter 1, Section 290. Translated by John Forbes. Philadelphia, Janus Webster, 1823.

16. Morgagni, J.B. The Seats and Causes of Diseases Investigated by Anatomy, in Five Books, 1769. Alexander B., London, Millar & Cadell. (Reprinted 1983 by the Classics of Medicine Library, Gryphon Ed. Ltd., Birmingham, AL.)

17. Corvisart, J.N. An Essay on the Organic Diseases and Lesions of the Heart and Great Vessels. Gates, J. Boston, Bradford & Read, 1812. (Reprinted 1984 by the Classics of Medicine Library, Gryphon Ed. Ltd., Birmingham, AL.)

18. Schroetter, L. Diseases of the heart substance. In: Practice of Medicine. Vol. 6. Diseases of the Circulatory System, Ziemssen, H. (ed.). New York, Wood, 1876.

19. Paul, C. Diseases of the Heart. New York, Wood, 1884.

20. Osler, W. The Principles and Practice of Medicine. New York, Appleton, 1892. (Reprinted 1978 by the Classics of Medicine Library, Gryphon Ed. Ltd., Birmingham, AL.)

21. Hales, S. Statical Essays, Containing Haemostaticks. Vol. 2. London, W. Innys & R. Manby, 1733.

22. Bernard, C. Lecons sur la chaleur Animale. Paris, Bailliere, 1876.

23. Chaveau, A., and J. Marey. Determination graphique des rapports du choc du coeur avec les mouvements des oreillettes et des ventricules: experience faite a l'aide d'un appareil enregistreur (syphygmographe). C.R. Acad. Sci. (Paris), 53:622–625, 1861.

24. Ludwig, K. Beitraege zur Kenntnis des Einflusses der Respirationsbewegungen auf den Blutlauf im Aortensysteme. Arch. Anat. Physiol. Wiss. Med., 242–302, 1847.

25. Vierodt, K. Die bildliche Darstellung des menschlichen Arterienpulses. Arch. Physiol. Heilk., 13:284–287, 1854.

26. Basch, S.S. von. Ein Metall-Sphygmomanometer. Wien. Med. Wschr., 33:673–675, 1883.

27. Potain, M. Theorie du bruit de galop. C.R. de L'Assoc. Francaise pour L'Advancement des Sciences, pt. 1, 14:201–203, 1885.
28. Fick, A. Ueber die Messung des Blutquantums in den Herzventrikeln. S.B. Phys. Med. Ges. Wuerzburg, 1870, p. 16.
29. Forssmann, W. Die Sondierung des rechten Herzens. Klin. Wschr., 8:2085–2087, 1929.
30. Cournand, A. Cardiac catheterization. Development of the technique, its contributions to clinical medicine and its initial applications in man. Acta Med. Scand. Suppl., 579, 1975.
31. Mackenzie, J. Abnormal inception of the cardiac rhythm. Quart. J. Med., 1:39, 1907.
32. Krikler, D.M. Sir James MacKenzie. Clin. Cardiol., 11:193–194, 1988.
33. Hope, J. A Treatise on the Diseases of the Heart and Great Vessels. London, Kidd, 1832.
34. Mackenzie, J. Diseases of the Heart. London, Henry Frowde, 3rd ed., 1913.
35. Stead, E.A., Jr., J.V. Warren, and E.S. Brannon. Cardiac output in congestive heart failure. An analysis of the reason for lack of close correlation between the symptom of heart failure and the resting cardiac output. Am. Heart J., 35:529–541, 1948.
36. McMichael, J. Circulatory failure studied by means of venous catheterization. Adv. Intern. Med., 2:64–101, 1947.
37. Merrill, A.J. Edema and decreased renal blood flow in patients with chronic congestive heart failure. Evidence of "forward failure" as the primary cause of edema. J. Clin. Invest., 25:389–400, 1946.
38. Frank, O. In: Circulation of the Blood: Men and Ideas, Fishman A.P., and D.W. Richards (eds.), New York, Oxford University Press, 1964, pp. 111–113.
39. Patterson, S.W., and E.H. Starling. On the mechanical factors which determine the output of the ventricles. J. Physiol., 48:357–379, 1914.
40. Patterson, S.W., H. Piper, and E.H. Starling. The regulation of the heart beat. J. Physiol., 48:465–513, 1914.
41. Sarnoff, S.J., and E. Berglund. Ventricular function. I. Starling's law of the heart studied by means of simultaneous right and left ventricular function curves in the dog. Circulation, 9:706–718, 1954.
42. Sonnenblick, E.H., and S.E. Downing. Afterload as a primary determinant of ventricular performance. Am. J. Physiol., 204:604–610, 1963.
43. Franciosa, J.A., N.H. Guiha, C.J. Limas, E. Rodriguerqa, and J.N. Cohn. Improved left ventricular function during nitroprusside infusion in acute myocardial infarction. Lancet, 1:650–654, 1972.
44. Mommaerts, W.F.H.M. Chapter III: Heart muscle. In: Circulation of the Blood: Men and Ideas, Fishman A.P., and D.E. Richards (eds.). New York, Oxford University Press, 1964, pp. 127–198.
45. Hill, A.V. The design of muscles. Brit. Med. Bull., 12:165–166, 1956.
46. Szent-Györgyi, A. Chemical Physiology of Contraction in Body and Heart Muscle. New York, Academic Press, 1953.
47. Fozzard, H.A., E. Haber, R.B. Hennings, A.N. Katz, and H.E. Morgan (eds.). The Heart and Cardiovascular System: Scientific Foundation. New York, Raven Press, 1986.
48. Abelmann, W.H. The dilated cardiomyopathies: experimental aspects. Cardiol. Clin., 6:219–231, 1988.
49. Katz, A.M. Regulation of myocardial contractility, 1958–1983: an odyssey. J. Am. Coll. Cardiol., 1:42–51, 1983.
50. Parmley, W.W. Pathophysiology and current therapy of congestive heart failure. J. Am. Coll. Cardiol., 13:771–785, 1989.
51. Wever, K.T. (ed.). Heart Failure: Current Concepts and Management. Cardiol. Clin., 7, 1989.

52. Williams, J.F., Jr. Evolving concepts in congestive heart failure. Mod. Concepts Cardiovasc. Dis., 59:43–48, 49–53, 1990.

53. Alhquist, R.P. A study of the adrenotropic receptors. Am. J. Physiol., 153:586–600, 1948.

54. Koelle, G.B. Reflections on the pioneers of neurohumoral transmission. Perspect. Biol. Med., 28:434–439, 1985.

55. Blaschko, J. Dihydroxyphenylserine (DOPS) as a therapeutic agent: reflections on pure and applied science. J. Appl. Cardiol., 3:429–432, 1988.

56. Von Euler, U.S. A specific sympothomimetic ergone in adrenergic nerve fibers (sympathin) in its relations to adrenaline and noradrenaline. Acta Physiol. Scand., 12: 73–97, 1946.

57. Cannon, W., and A. Rosenblueth. Studies on conditions of activity in endocrine organs, XXIX. Sympathin E and Sympathin I. Am. J. Physiol., 104:557–574, 1933.

58. Ahlquist, R.P. Adrenergic receptors: a personal and practical view. Perspect. Biol. Med., 17:119–122, 1973.

59. Ahlquist, R.P. Present state of alpha and beta adrenergic drugs. II. The adrenergic blocking agents. Am. Heart J., 92:804–807, 1976.

60. Ahlquist, R.P. Development of the concept of alpha and beta adrenotropic receptors. Ann. N.Y. Acad. Sci., 139:549–552, 1967.

61. Black, J.W. Ahlquist and the development of beta-adrenoreceptor antagonists. Postgrad. Med. J., 52(Suppl. 4):11–13, 1976.

62. Langley, J.N. On the reaction of cells and of nerve-endings to certain poisons, chiefly as regards the reaction of striated muscle to nicotine and to curari. J. Physiol., 33: 374–413, 1905–6.

63. Elliott, T.R. The action of adrenalin. J. Physiol., 32:401–467, 1905.

64. Powell, C.E., and I.H. Slater. Blocking of inhibitory adrenergic receptors by a dichloro analog of isoproterenol. J. Pharm. Exp. Ther., 122:480–488, 1958.

65. Black, J.W., A.F. Crowther, T.G. Shanks, L.H. Smith, and A.C. Dornhost. A new adrenergic beta-receptor antagonist. Lancet, 1:1080–1081, 1964.

66. Newman, W.H. A depressed response to left ventricular contractile force to isoproterenol and norepinephrine in dogs with congestive heart failure. Am. Heart J., 93: 216–221, 1977.

67. Unverferth, D.V., M. Blanford, R.E. Kates, and C.V. Leier. Tolerance to dobutamine after a 72 hour continuous infusion. Am. J. Med., 69:262–266, 1980.

68. Thomas, J.A., and B.H. Marks. Plasma norepinephrine in congestive heart failure. Am. J. Cardiol., 41:233–243, 1978.

69. Colucci, W.S., W. Alexander, G.H. Williams, R.E. Rude, B.L. Holman, M.A. Konstam, H. Wynne, G.H. Mudge Jr., and E. Braunwald. Decreased lymphocyte beta-adrenergic-receptor density in patients with heart failure and tolerance to the beta-adrenergic agonist pirbuterol. N. Engl. J. Med., 305:185–190, 1981.

70. Bristow, M.R., R. Ginsburg, V. Umans, M. Fowler, W. Minobe, R. Rasmussen, P. Zera, R. Menlove, P. Shah, S. Jamieson, and E. Stinson. β-1 and β-2-adrenergic receptor subpopulations in nonfailing and failing human ventricular myocardium: coupling of both receptor subtypes to muscle contraction and selective β-1-receptor down-regulation in heart failure. Circ. Res., 59:297–309, 1986.

71. Ruffolo, R.R., Jr., and G.A. Kopia. Importance of receptor regulation in the pathophysiology and therapy of congestive failure. Am. J. Med., 80: 67–72, 1986.

72. Bristow, M.R., R. Ginsburg, W.A. Minobe, D.C. Harrison, B.A. Reitz, and E.B. Stinson. Beta-adrenergic receptor measurements in normal and failing human right and left ventricle (abstr). Circulation Suppl., II-207, 1982.

73. Chang, H.Y., R.M. Klein, and G. Kunos. Selective desensitization of cardiac beta receptors by prolonged in vivo infusion of catecholamines in rats. J. Pharmacol. Exp. Ther., 221:784–789, 1982.

74. Forster, C., S.L. Carter, and P.W. Armstrong. α-1-adrenoreceptor activity in arterial smooth muscle following congestive heart failure. Can. J. Phys. Pharmacol., 67:110–115, 1989.

75. Wald, M., E.S. Borda, and L. Sterin-Borda. α-adrenergic supersensitivity and decreased number of α-adrenoceptors in heart from acute diabetic rats. Can. J. Phys. Pharm., 66:1154–1157, 1988.

76. Bristow, M.R., J.A. Laser, W. Minobe, R. Gisburg, M.B. Fowler, and R. Rasmussen. Selective down regulation of beta-adrenergic receptors in failing human heart (abstr.). Circulation Suppl., II–67, 1974.

77. Sackner-Bernstein, J.D., and D.M. Mancini. Rationale for treatment of patients with chronic heart failure with adrenergic blockage. JAMA, 274:1462–1467, 1995.

78. Bing, R.J. Metabolism of the heart. Harvey Lectures, 50:27–70, 1954–55.

79. Dhalla, N.S., I.M.C. Dixon, and R.E. Beamish. Biochemical basis of heart functions and contractile failure. J. Appl. Cardiol., 6:7, 1991.

80. Katz, A.M. Physiology of the Heart. New York, Raven Press, 1977. 2nd ed., 1992.

81. Kako, K., and R.J. Bing. Contractility of actomyosin bands prepared from normal and failing human hearts. J. Clin. Invest., 37:465–470, 1958.

82. Szent-Györgyi, A. Lost in the twentieth century. Annual Review of Biochemistry, 32:1–14, 1963.

83. Huxley, A.F. Muscular contraction. J. Physiol., 243:1–43, 1974.

84. Hamrell, B.B., and N.A. Alpert. Cellular basis of the mechanical properties of hypertrophied myocardium In: The Heart and Cardiovascular System, Fozzard, H., E. Haber, A. Katz, R. Jennings, and H.E. Morgan (eds.). New York, Raven Press, 1986.

85. England, P.J. Phosphorylation of cardiac contractile proteins. Chapter 16. Handbook of Physiology. Baltimore, Williams & Wilkens, 1977.

86. Tsuchimochi-H., M. Sugi, M. Kuroo, S. Ueda, F. Takau, S. Furuta, T. Shirai, and Y. Yazaki. Isozymic changes in myosin of human atrial myocardium induced by overload. Immunohistochemical study using monoclonal antibodies. J. Clin. Invest., 74:662–665, 1984.

87. Mercardier, J.J., D. dela-Bastie, P. Menasche, A. N-Guyen-Van-Cao, P. Bouveret, P. Lorente, A. Piwnica, R. Slama, and K. Schwartz. Alpha-myosin heavy chain isoform and atrial size in patients with various types of mitral valve dysfunction: a quantitative study. J. Am. Coll. Cardiol., 9:1024–1030, 1987.

88. Katz, A.M. Cardiomyopathy of overload. A major determinant of prognosis in congestive heart failure. N. Engl. J. Med., 322:100–110, 1990.

89. Mercardier, J.J., A.M. Lompre, P. Duc, K.R. Boheler, J.B. Fraysse, C. Wisnewsky, P.D. Allen, M. Komajda, and K. Schwartz. Altered sarcoplasmic reticulum Ca^{2+}-ATPase gene expression in the human ventricle during end stage heart failure. J. Clin. Invest., 85:305–309, 1990.

90. Akiyama, K., G. Akopian, P. Jinadasa, T.L. Gluckman, A. Terhakopian, B. Massey, and R.J. Bing. Myocardial infarction and regulatory myosin light chain. J. Mol. Cell. Cardiol., 29:2641–2652, 1997.

91. Katz, A.M. The cardiomyopathy of overload: an unnatural growth response in the hypertrophied heart. Ann. Intern. Med., 121:363–371, 1994.

92. Katz, A.M. Is the failing heart an energy-starved organ? (editorial) J. Cardiac. Failure, 2:267–272, 1996.

93. The Xamoterol in Severe Heart Failure Group. Xamoterol in severe heart failure. Lancet, 2:1–6, 1990.

94. Packer M., J.R. Carver, R.J. Rodeheffer, R.J. Ivanhoe, R. DiBianco, S.M. Zeldis, G.H. Hendrix, W.J. Bommer, U. Elkayam, M.L. Kukin, G.I. Mallis, J.A. Soliano, J. Shannon, P.K. Tandon, and D.L. De Mets. Effect of oral milrinone on mortality in severe heart failure. New Engl. J. Med., 325:1468–1475, 1991.

95. Feldman, A., J. Young, R. Bourge, P. Carson, B. Jaski, D. DeMets, B.G. White, and

J.N. Cohn for the Ves T Investigators. Mechanism of increased mortality from ves-narinone in the severe heart failure trial (VesT) (abstr.). J. Am. Coll. Cardiol., 29: 64A, 1997.

96. Packer, M., J. Rouleau, K. Swedberg, et al. Effect of flosequinan on survival in chronic heart failure: preliminary results of the profiles study (abstr.). Circulation, 88:I–301, 1993.

97. Califf, R.M., K.F. Adams, P.W. Armstrong, et al. Flolan international randomized survival trial (first): final results. J. Am. Coll. Cardiol., 27:143A, 1996.

98. Goldstein, R.E., S.J. Boccuzzi, D. Cruess, and S. Nattel. The Adverse Experience Committee and The Multicenter Diltiazem Postinfarction Research Group. Dilti-azem increases late-onset congestive heart failure in postinfarction patients with early reduction in ejection fraction. Circulation, 83:52–60, 1991.

99. The Cardiac Arrhythmia Suppression Trial [CAST] Investigators. Effects of en-cainide and flecainide, imipramine and moricizine on mortality in a randomized trial of arrhythmia suppression after myocardial infarction. New Engl. J. Med., 321: 406–410, 1989.

100. Hasenfuss, G., L.A. Mulieri, B.J. Leavitt, P.D. Allen, J.R. Haeberle, and N.R. Alpert. Alteration of contractile function and excitation-contraction coupling in dilated cardiomyopathy. Circ. Res., 70:1225–1232, 1992.

101. Beuckelmann, D.J., M. Nabauer, and E. Erdmann. Intracellular calcium handling in isolated ventricular myocytes from patients with terminal heart failure. Circulation, 85:1046–1055, 1992.

102. Pieske, B., B. Kretschmann, M. Meyer, C. Holubarsch, J. Weirich, H. Posival, K. Mi-nami, H. Just, and G. Hasenfuss. Alterations in intracellular calcium handling asso-ciated with the inverse force-frequency relation in human dilated cardiomyopathy. Circulation, 92:1169–1178, 1995.

103. Pieske, B., M. Sutterlin, S. Schmidt-Schweda, K. Minami, M. Meyer, M. Olschew-ski, C. Holubarsch, H. Just, and G. Hasenfuss. Diminished post-rest potentiation of contractile force in human dilated cardiomyopathy. Functional evidence for alter-ations in intracellular Ca^{2+} handling. J. Clin. Invest., 98:764–776, 1996.

104. Gwathmey, J.K., L. Copelas, R. MacKinnon, F.J. Schoen, M.D. Feldman, W. Gross-man, and J.P. Morgan. Abnormal intracellular calcium handling in myocardium from patients with end-stage heart failure. Circ. Res., 61:70–76, 1987.

105. Fabiato, A. Calcium-induced release of calcium from the cardiac sarcoplasmic retic-ulum. Am. J. Physiol., 245:C1–C14, 1983.

106. Takahashi, T., P.D. Allen, R.V. Lacro, A.R. Marks, A.R. Dennis, F.J. Schoen, W. Grossman, J.D. Marsh, and S. Izumo. Expression of dihydropyridine receptor (Ca^{2+} cannel) and calsequestrin genes in the myocardium of patients with end-stage heart failure. J. Clin. Invest., 90:927–935, 1992.

107. Rasmussen, R.P., W. Minobe, and M.R. Bristow. Calcium antagonist binding sites in failing and nonfailing human ventricular myocardium. Biochem. Pharmacol., 39: 691–696, 1990.

108. Beuckelmann, D.H., and E. Erdmann. Ca^{2+}-currents and intracellular $(Ca^{2+})_i$-tran-sients in single ventricular myocytes isolated from terminally failing human my-ocardium. Bas. Res. Cardiol., 87(Suppl. I):235–243, 1992.

109. Mewes, T., and U. Ravens. L-type calcium currents of human myocytes from ven-tricle of non-failing and failing hearts and from atrium. J. Mol. Cell. Cardiol., 26:1307–1320, 1994.

110. Piot, C., S. Lemaire, B. Albat, J. Seguin, J. Nargeot, and S. Richard. High fre-quency-induced upregulation of human cardiac calcium currents. Circulation, 93:120–128, 1996.

111. Cheng, H., W.J. Lederer, and M.V. Cannell. Calcium sparks: elementary events un-derlying excitation-contraction coupling in heart muscle. Science, 262:740–744, 1993.

112. Brillantes, A.M., P. Allen, T. Takahashi, S. Izumo, and A.R. Marks. Differences in cardiac calcium release channel (ryanodine receptor) expression in myocardium from patients with end-stage heart failure caused by ischemic versus dilated cardiomyopathy. Circ. Res., 71:18–26, 1992.

113. Go, L.O., M.C. Moschella, J. Watras, K.K. Handa, B.S. Fyfe, and A.R. Marks. Differential regulation of two types of intracellular calcium release channels during end-stage heart failure. J. Clin. Invest., 95:888–894, 1995.

114. Schumacher, C., B. Konigs, M. Sigmund, B. Kohne, F. Schondube, M. Vob, B. Stein, J. Weil, and P. Hanrath. The ryanodine binding sarcoplasmic reticulum calcium release channel in nonfailing and in failing human myocardium. Naunyn-Schmiedebergs Arch. Pharm., 353:80–85, 1995.

115. Sainte Beuve, P.D. Allen, G. Dambrin, F. Rannov, I. Marty, P. Trouvé, V. Bors, A. Pavie, I. Gandgjbakch, and D. Charlemagne. Cardiac calcium release channel (ryanodine receptor) in control and cardiomyopathic human hearts: mRNA and protein contents are differentially regulated. J. Mol. Cell. Cardiol., 29:1237–1246, 1997.

116. Meyer, M., W. Schillinger, B. Pieske, C. Holubarsch, C. Heilmann, H. Posival, G. Kuwajima, K. Mikoshiba, H. Just, and G. Hasenfuss. Alterations of sarcoplasmic reticulum proteins in failing human dilated cardiomyopathy. Circulation, 92:778–784, 1995.

117. Lytton, H., and D.H. MacLennan. Sarcoplasmic reticulum. In: The Heart and Cardio-vascular System, Fozzard, H.A., R.B. Hennings, E. Haber, and A.M. Katz (eds.). New York, Raven Press, 1991, pp. 1203–1222.

118. MacLennan, D.H., and P.T.S. Wong. Isolation of a calcium sequestering protein from sarcoplasmic reticulum. Proc. Natl. Acad. Sci. USA, 68:1231–1235, 1971.

119. Michalak, M., R.E. Milner, K. Burns, and M. Opas. Calreticulin. Biochem. J., 285:681–692, 1992.

120. Arai, M., N.R. Alpert, D.H. MacLennan, P. Barton, and M. Periasamy. Alterations in sarcoplasmic reticulum gene expression in human heart failure: a possible mechanism for alterations in systolic and diastolic properties of the failing myocardium. Circ. Res., 72:463–469, 1993.

121. Movsesian, M.A., M. Karimi, K. Green, and L.R. Jones. Ca^{2+}-transporting ATPase, phospholamban, and calsequestrin levels in nonfailing and failing human myocardium. Circulation, 90:653–657, 1994.

122. Bers, D.M.. Possible sources and sinks of activator calcium. In: Excitation-Contraction Coupling and Cardiac Contractile Force, Bers, D. M. (ed.). Dordrecht, Boston, London, Kluwer Academic Publishers, Developments in cardiovascular medicine, 1991, 122:33–48.

123. Kim, H.W., N.A.E. Steenaart, D.G. Ferguson, and E.G. Kranias. Functional reconstitution of the cardiac sarcoplasmic reticulum Ca^{2+}-ATPase with phospholamban in phospholipid vesicles. J. Biol. Chem., 265:1702–1709, 1990.

124. Voss, J., L.R. Jones, and D.D. Thomas. The physical mechanism of calcium pump regulation in the heart. Biophys. J., 67:190–196, 1994.

125. Schwinger, R.H., M. Böhm, U. Schmidt, P. Karczewski, U. Bavendiek, M. Flesch, E.G. Krause, and E. Erdmann. Unchanged protein levels of SERCA II and phospholamban but reduced Ca^{2+} uptake and Ca^{2+}-ATPase activity of cardiac sarcoplasmic reticulum from dilated cardiomyopathy patients compared with patients with nonfailing hearts. Circulation, 92:3220–3228, 1995.

126. Hasenfuss, G., H. Reinecke, R. Studer, M. Meyer, B. Pieske, J. Holtz, C. Holubarsch, H. Posival, H. Just, and H. Drexler. Relation between myocardial function and expression of sarcoplasmic reticulum Ca^{2+}-ATPase in failing and nonfailing human myocardium. Circ. Res., 75:434–442, 1994.

127. Limas, C.J., M.T. Olivari, I.F. Goldenberg, T.B. Levine, D.G. Benditt, and A. Simon Calcium uptake by cardiac sarcoplasmic reticulum in human dilated cardiomyopathy. Cardiovasc. Res., 21:601–605, 1987.

128. Mercadier, J.J., A.M. Lompre, P. Duc, K.R. Boheler, J.B. Fraysse, C. Wisnewsky, P.D. Allen, M. Komajda, and K. Schwartz. Altered sarcoplasmic reticulum Ca^{2+}-ATPase gene expression in the human ventricle during end-stage heart failure. J. Clin. Invest., 85:305–309, 1990.

129. Studer, R., H. Reinecke, J. Bilger, T. Eschenhagen, M. Böhm, G. Hasenfuss, H. Just, J. Holtz, and H. Drexler. Gene expression of the cardiac Na$^+$-Ca^{2+}-exchanger in end-stage human heart failure. Circ. Res. 75:443–453, 1994.

130. Linck, B., P. Bokník, T. Eschenhagen, F.U. Müller, J. Neumann, M. Nose, L.R. Jones, W. Schmitz, and H. Scholz. Messenger RNA expression and immunological quantification of phospholamban and SR-Ca^{2+}-ATPase in failing and nonfailing human hearts. Cardiovasc. Res., 31:625–632, 1996.

131. Koss, K.L., I.L. Grupp, and E.G. Kranias. The relative phospholamban and SERCA2 ratio: a critical determinant of myocardial contractility. Basic Res. Cardiol., 92 (Suppl. 1):17–24, 1997.

132. Feldman, A.M., P.E. Ray, C. Silan, J.A. Mercer, W. Minobe, and M.R. Bristow. Selective gene expression in failing human heart. Quantification of steady-state levels of messenger RNA in endomyocardial biopsies using the polymerase chain reaction. Circulation, 83:1866–1872, 1991.

133. Bers, D.M. Ca transport during contraction and relaxation in mammalian ventricular muscle. Basic Res. Cardiol., 92(Suppl. I):1–10, 1997.

134. Schulze, D.H., and W.J. Lederer. Advances in the molecular characterization of the Na$^+$/Ca^{2+} exchanger. In: Molecular Biology of Cardiovascular Disease, Marks, A.R., and M.B. Taubman (eds.). New York, Marcel Dekker, 1997, pp. 275–290.

135. Philipson, K.D. The cardiac Na$^+$-Ca^{2+}-exchanger. In: Calcium and the Heart, Langer, G.A. (ed.). New York, Raven Press, 1990, pp. 85–108.

136. Bers, D.M., D.M. Christensen, and T.X. Nguyen. Can Ca^{2+} entry via the Na$^+$-Ca^{2+}-exchanger directly activate cardiac muscle contraction? J. Mol. Cell. Cardiol., 20: 405–414, 1988.

137. Flesch, M., R.H.G. Schwinger, F. Schiffer, K. Frank, M. Südkamp, F. Kuhn-Regnier, G. Arnold, and M. Böhm. Evidence for functional relevance of an enhanced expression of the Na$^+$-Ca^{2+} exchanger in failing human myocardium. Circulation, 94: 992–1002, 1996.

138. Reinecke, H., R. Studer, R. Vetter, I. Holtz, and H. Drexler. Cardiac Na$^+$/Ca^{2+} exchange activity in patients with end-stage heart failure. Cardiovasc. Res., 31:48–54, 1996.

139. Hasenfuss, G., M. Preuss, S. Lehnart, J. Prestle, M. Meyer, and H. Just. Relationship between diastolic function and protein levels of sodium-calcium-exchanger in end-stage failing human hearts. Circulation, 94 (Suppl. I):433, 1996.

140. Carpentier, A., and J.C. Chachques. Myocardial substitution with a stimulated skeletal muscle: first successful clinical case. Lancet, 8440:1267, 1985.

141. Batista, R.J.V., J.L.V. Santos, N. Takeshita, L. Bocchino, P.N. Lima, and M.A. Cunha. Partial left ventriculectomy to improve left ventricular function in end-stage heart disease. J. Card. Surg., 11:96–97, 1996.

142. Churchill, W.C. Cited by Manchester, W. in Winston Spencer Churchill. The Last Lion. Boston, Little, Brown, 1983.

Chapter 11   Valvular Surgery

R. HEIMBECKER
T. DAVID
R.J. BING

CARDIOPULMONARY BYPASS WAS the long path that made valvular surgery effective. A look at the history of medicine with the retrospectroscope reveals costly, often futile, slow graspings for solutions until a breakthrough drastically changes the situation. This happened in surgery of cardiac valves with the introduction of cardiopulmonary bypass. It is easy for a Monday morning quarterback to judge yesterday's football game; it is difficult for the players in the midst of a game to foresee if and when a touchdown will occur. Players must painfully advance yard by yard until a sudden spurt by a particular player brings victory. Nevertheless, there is heroism in the steady plodding, pioneering work with difficult inch-by-inch advance.

The history of valvular surgery started with a suggestion concerning treatment of mitral stenosis. Sir Lauder Brunton, in 1902, was motivated like many others by a particular patient's suffering (1; Fig. 11.1). He wrote, "mitral stenosis is not only one of the most distressing forms of cardiac disease, but in its severe form it resists all treatment by medicine." He continued: "I was much impressed by the case of a man under middle age whom I had under my care at St. Bartholomew's hospital. For no fault of his own, but simply because of his disease, this man was really exiled from his family, one might almost say imprisoned for life in as much as he could only live in a hospital ward or a work house infirmary. It occurred to me that it was worthwhile for such a patient to run a risk and even a greater risk in order to obtain such improvement as might enable him at least to stay at home. But no one would be justified in attempting such a dangerous operation as dividing a mitral stenosis on a fellow-creature without having

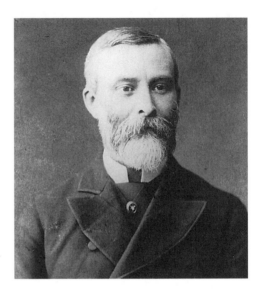

Figure 11.1. Sir Lauder Brunton. (*Courtesy of the New York Academy of Medicine*)

first tested its practicability and perfected its technique by previous trials on animals."

Brunton accordingly performed experiments of dividing stenosed valves in diseased hearts from the postmortem theater, operated on the hearts of cats, and tried operations on the dead animal. He continued: "I therefore think that it may be worthwhile to write the preliminary note, especially as, after all, if the operation is to be done in man it will be surgeons who will do it and they must of course make their own preliminary experiments, however fully the operation may be described by others and each must find out for himself the methods which he will employ in each particular case."

Brunton suggested use of a tenotomy knife "but some which I had made of ladies bonnet pins, were too thin and flexible for stenosed valves, although they were sufficiently strong to divide the normal valves in the hearts of cats." He mentioned that the main part of the valve could be divided with comparative ease, but that the thickened edge resisted the knife. He wrote that he had not yet decided on the best form of knife and he believed that this would depend on whether the surgeon approached the valve from the atrium or the ventricle. He suggested that in the living heart the knife should be used during diastole only, as one was less likely to wound the opposite wall of the ventricle. One sentence in particular is worth noting: "The good results that have been obtained by surgical treatment of wounds in the heart emboldens one to hope that before very long similar good results may be obtained in cases of mitral stenosis."

Brunton's fame does not rest entirely on his suggestion for operation on the mitral valve. Introduction of the use of amylnitrite in the treatment of angina

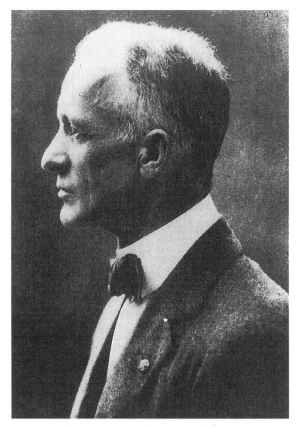

Figure 11.2. Harvey Cushing. *(Courtesy of the New York Academy of Medicine)*

pectoris was certainly another important Brunton contribution to medicine. In 1876 he also reported results of his studies on the use of nitroglycerin in animal experiments. But he found the headache induced by nitroglycerin so severe in man that he delayed its use. It was Murrell who first advocated the use of nitroglycerin in patients with angina pectoris (2).

In 1908 Harvey Cushing and J.R.B. Branch, from the Johns Hopkins Hospital in Baltimore, published some notes on the experimental and clinical approach to chronic valvular lesions in the dog and the possible relation to future surgery of the cardiac valves (3; Fig. 11.2). (This was prior to Cushing's main interest in neurosurgery.) In his paper in the *Journal of Medical Research*, Cushing described the clinical history and the autopsy findings on animals with valvular heart disease. He mentions that "Our interest in these observations was researched in the spring of this year by the admission to the laboratory of another animal with symptoms the counterpart of those which were present in the patient whose malady first suggested these investigations." A large Newfoundland dog was brought to the Hunterian Laboratory of the Johns Hopkins Hospital in 1905 suffering from general anasarca, ascites, and other sequelae of passive congestion due to tricuspid insufficiency with compensatory failure, resulting in advanced chronic endocarditis. Autopsy on that animal disclosed a thickened mitral valve, a dilated and hypertrophied heart showing tricuspid insufficiency, together with an unusually marked degree of venous congestion. Being interested in experimental surgery, Cushing then proceeded to produce this condition experimentally (3).

Cushing's was the first successful attempt to produce valvular lesion by an intrathoracic exposure of the heart with subsequent recoveries. He paid particular attention to anesthesia and mentioned the fact that the desired intrapulmonary pressure could be readily achieved by inflation of the lung through an opening in the trachea as commonly used in a physiological laboratory. He wrote, "I have twice in a human subject given artificial respiration by this method with immediate closure of the tracheal wound without drainage. These were cases of temporary respiratory failure due to an intracranial pressure. Both patients recovered and in both the cervical wound healed without reaction."

Cushing used a valvulotome to produce mitral insufficiency by dividing one mitral valve leaflet with a cutting hoop, introducing the instrument through the apex of the left ventricle. He mentioned the difficulty of producing serious mitral insufficiency in the dog since the heart is able to compensate rapidly for the lesion; he thought it might be necessary for the operation to be done in successive stages in order to reproduce conditions of compensatory failure such as occurs in chronic endocarditis resulting from disease of the valves. "During the course of our observation our attention was called by Futcher to a recent note in the *Lancet* by Sir Lauder Brunton which puts the matter from a physician's point of view so forcibly that his words may well be used to express our own feeling in regard to these measures should it ever prove justifiable to transfer the experiments to man."

From the same Johns Hopkins laboratory, B.M. Bernheim repeated most of Cushing's experiments, confirming that "We have not as yet been able to reproduce the typical presystolic murmur of the usual symptoms characteristic of the 'button hole' stenosis in man" (4). Cushing and his group believed that in order to proceed with the surgical treatment of valvular disease the condition had to first be reproduced in the dog.

In 1914 in New York, a particularly ingenious approach to the treatment of pulmonary stenosis was introduced by the French surgeons Theodore Tuffier and Alexis Carrel of the Rockefeller Institute for Medical Research (5). (Carrel's pioneering work has been repeatedly noted in these pages, particularly in regard to blood vessel surgery.) Carrel and Tuffier sought to develop a technique to enlarge the pulmonary orifice. The operation involved suturing a venous patch to the anterior side of the pulmonary orifice, permitting an increase in the circumference of the orifice after the arterial wall had been incised. Eight experiments on dogs were carried out. The authors concluded that it is possible to perform an operation aimed at increasing the circumference of the pulmonary orifice without involving much danger to the life of the animal. The pulmonary valve itself was incised by the long blade of specially constructed scissors. Once the instrument had been used and the valve incised, the surgeon compressed the flap against the opening, thus arresting hemorrhage. Then the lower side of the flap was rapidly united to the cardiac wall by means of continuous suture. Tuffier and Carrel predicted that operations of this type might be employed in the treatment of pulmonary artery stenosis in man. In 1913 Tuffier operated on a twenty-six-year-old man with severe aortic stenosis. The patient survived and was reported to be improved and alive twelve years later (6). As Lindblom writes, "This must be regarded as the first successful surgical approach to valvular heart disease" (7). Another attempt, by Allen and Graham, using a cardioscope with a knife attachment for widening the orifice of cardiac valves was destined for failure (8). One wonders about the use of the cardioscope since obviously visualization of the valve through the cardioscope did not contribute to the technique's success. Allen and Graham's method was a valiant attempt, but the big step forward was operation under direct vision made possible by cardiopulmonary bypass.

In the 1920s the idea of incising the valve by an appropriate instrument was vigorously pursued by Elliot Cutler and his group from the Harvard Medical School. In the *Boston Medical and Surgical Journal* of 1923, Cutler and S.A. Levine described the first operation on a patient, carried out on May 20, 1923 (9). A valvulotome, an instrument that they likened to a tenotome or a slightly curved tonsil knife, was plunged into the left ventricle at a point about one inch from the apex and away from the branches of the descending coronary artery. The knife was then pushed upward about two and one-half inches until it encountered "what seems to us, must be the mitral orifice." Two cuts were then made on opposite sides of the valve. Cutler was so proud of the results that "the patient was brought to the large amphitheatre and presented before the reunion group of doctors and nurses the fourth day after the operation."

Alas, this success could not be duplicated. Cutler and C.S. Beck (Beck would later make important contributions to cardiac surgery) reported such operations on a total of seven patients at the Peter Bent Brigham Hospital in Boston (10). Only one patient survived; six died following the operation. In another paper by Beck and Cutler, the cutting instrument was described in detail (11). The instrument actually excised a segment from the mitral orifice and removed this from the blood stream.

The persistence and optimism of these pioneers is to be admired. The situation

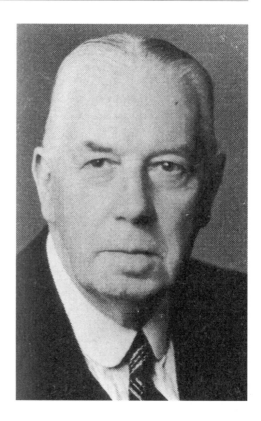

Figure 11.3. H.S. Souttar. (*Courtesy of the New York Academy of Medicine*)

was not dissimilar to that at the onset of cardiac transplantation, when the mortality rate was also extremely high.

In 1925 a great step forward was made by H.S. Souttar at the London hospital using a method noteworthy for its simplicity and directness (12; Fig. 11.3). Souttar had the good sense not to employ sharp cutting instruments, but merely his finger to open the mitral valve. He furthermore used the atrial approach and applied a curved clamp, strikingly similar to the Pott's clamp, to occlude the atrial appendage. The clamp was then withdrawn and the appendage was drawn over the finger like a glove by means of sutures. As Souttar wrote, "the whole inside of the left auricle could now be explored with facility. It was immediately evident from the rush of blood against the finger that gross regurgitation was taking place, but there was not so much thickening of the valves as had been expected. The finger was passed into the ventricle through the orifice of the mitral valve without encountering resistance and the cusp of the valve could be easily felt and the condition estimated."

How much simpler this was than the use of a cardioscope. He continued: "As however the stenosis was of such moderate degree, and was accompanied as a little thickening of the valves, it was decided not to cut out the valve section which had been arranged, but to limit intervention to such dilatation as could be carried out by the finger. It was felt that an actual section of the valve might only make matters worse by increasing the degree of regurgitation, while the breaking down of adhesions by the finger might improve the condition as regards to both regurgitation and stenosis."

The patient made an uneventful recovery, being kept in bed for six weeks according to the surgical practice at that time. Souttar concluded his article in the *British Medical Journal:* "it appears to me that the method of digital exploration through the auricular appendage cannot be surpassed for simplicity and directness. I could not help being impressed by the mechanical nature of these lesions and by the practicability of their surgical relief" (12).

Souttar was an extraordinary surgeon (13). He participated in World War I as surgeon in chief of a field ambulance and wrote a book on his experience, *A Surgeon in Belgium*. He mentions how, at a time when things were in complete chaos in Belgium, he felt reassured when he saw the First Lord of the Admiralty, Winston Churchill, quietly eating breakfast at a local hotel.

Souttar was particularly interested in physics, which helped him play a leading part in the development of radium therapy. When radium was first discovered, he traveled to Paris to meet the Curies and he may have been the first Englishman to see the new element, radium. His obituary, published in *Lancet* in 1964, mentions that his interest may well have been further stimulated by meeting Madame Curie during his war work in Belgium (13). Souttar's interest in physics extended to construction of a private planetarium. Souttar, who died at the age of eighty-eight in 1964, was evidently twenty years ahead of his time. Twenty years passed before Charles P. Bailey of Philadelphia, using Souttar's atrial approach, divided the mitral valve at the fused commissures under digital control, a procedure that he called "commissurotomy" (14; Fig. 11.4).

In 1948 Horace G. Smithy from Charleston, South Carolina, had attempted a surgical approach to aortic stenosis with an aortic valvulotome (15, 16, 17, 18). His failure to successfully treat this condition was particularly tragic since Smithy himself succumbed to this disease. In 1950 Smithy persuaded Alfred Blalock, from the Johns Hopkins Hospital, to operate on him using his method. Smithy's method consisted of division of one or more valvular leaflets by approaching the valve through the wall of the left ventricle, using a valvulotome. Like most other attempts with valvulotomes, this one also failed. Smithy described the operative results in seven patients with a high mortality (17). In one of the patients the aortic valve apparently had not been cut at all.

In most of his papers, Smithy was concerned with the frequency of arrhythmias that occurred in these patients during the operation (16). This also was the cause of his own death! He tried various means to overcome this difficulty, such

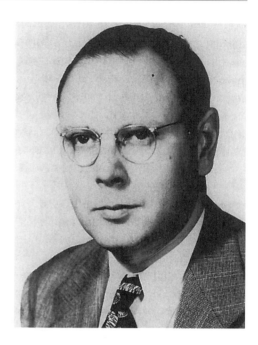

Figure 11.4. Charles Bailey. *(Courtesy of the New York Academy of Medicine)*

as epicardial application of procaine, infiltration of procaine beneath the epicardium and into the myocardium, intravenous procaine, or infiltration of the intraventricular septum with procaine. He also administered quinidine sulfate intravenously in a fifth group of experimental animals. These procedures were not of particular value when it came to surgery on aortic valves with markedly hypertrophied left ventricles. As it happened in his own case, a transventricular approach to the aortic valve created fatal arrhythmias that could not be overcome with antiarrhythmic compounds.

It had become clear by that time that blind cutting of the cardiac valves carried with it a considerable mortality. Since pulmonary venous congestion and pulmonary artery hypertension are the main hemodynamic consequences of mitral stenosis, it seemed appropriate to attempt to decompress pulmonary veins by creating a shunt between these vessels and the low pressure venous circulation—for example, the superior vena cava or the azygos vein. The first such operation was experimentally performed on dogs by Henry Swan in 1948 (19). He proved that in dogs the shunt is technically feasible if an end-to-end anastomosis of the azygos and pulmonary veins is carried out using a vitallium tube.

R.H. Sweet, working with E.F. Bland, carried the shunt idea further by constructing an anastomosis between the dorsal segment branch of the right inferior pulmonary vein to the azygos vein (20, 21). The first report described the results in five patients (20). Considerable improvement in the first three patients was noted. The authors admit that this operation is "a compromise and not a cure." In 1949 Sweet and Bland presented their findings to the American Surgical Association (21). The report published in the *Journal of Thoracic Surgery* contains an interesting discussion by Blalock. He also mentioned the possibility of creating a shunt between the left atrium and ventricle, thus bypassing the stenotic mitral valve using a vein graft. Another suggestion made was the creation of an intraatrial defect already accomplished by him and Hanlon several years before.

John H. Gibbon's pioneering work was the breakthrough in cardiac surgery that made blind approaches to the cardiac valves obsolete. Gibbon wrote a paper with J.Y. Templeton in 1944 (22) concerned with the future when "eventually a practical method of oxygenating large quantities of blood outside the body will permit operation in the open human heart." Gibbon undertook experiments to determine whether grafted tissue could be used to replace a portion of the cardiac valve. A cusp of the tricuspid valve of dogs was replaced by grafts of vein or pericardium sutured in position. The results were good: seven of the dogs survived in apparent good health. Several years later, in 1950, Murray, from Toronto, transplanted an aortic valve segment as replacement of a diseased aortic valve with good results (23).

In the late 1940s considerable progress was made toward the treatment of cardiac valvular disease by C.P. Bailey and Dwight E. Harken. These improvements made prior to the introduction of cardiopulmonary bypass remained limited in scope.

In 1949 Bailey presented his procedure of surgical treatment of mitral stenosis before the American College of Chest Physicians (24). After briefly referring to the success of manual dilatation of the valve reported by Souttar, Bailey presented his conclusions on the surgical treatment of mitral stenosis: approach through the left atrial appendage is the most satisfactory with less chance of arrhythmias, greater ease of entering the valve, and better ability to control hemorrhage; extensive cutting of the anterior cusp of the mitral valve is dangerous since it results in the production of mitral insufficiency, which is poorly tolerated; the accurate placement of an instrument to divide a mitral valve depends on actually palpating the valve from within at the time of operation. A considerable variety of instruments may be employed for commissurotomy. We, so he wrote, "now prefer a backward cutting punch and a scalpel with a hooked blade." In contrast to others who had used cutting instruments, one of Bailey's approaches was to attach the commissurotomy knife to the right index finger between two layers of gloves.

Bailey presented several operative cases; some cases of mitral stenosis showed gratifying postoperative results. He concluded that the operation of commissurotomy had great value in certain cases of mitral stenosis. Later in 1954, Bailey and co-workers presented procedures for the treatment of mitral insufficiency by grafting pericardial tissue to the valve orifice (25).

Bailey also tackled the problem of surgical treatment of aortic insufficiency and aortic stenosis. He quoted two papers of Hufnagel in his bibliography. Following the example of Hufnagel, Bailey's paper also describes a valvular prosthesis that was made of nylon and silicon rubber. Bailey concluded that the rather remarkable immediate improvement obtained in some of his patients encouraged him to feel that he was at least on the right course. Perhaps, he wrote, it will soon be possible to add aortic insufficiency to the growing list of cardiac lesions readily responsive to surgical intervention.

Concerning the treatment of aortic stenosis, Bailey mentioned that his interest in this disease was aroused by a discussion he had with Smithy in June 1958. Bailey applied the principle of commissurotomy which he had successfully used in the treatment of mitral stenosis to the problem confronting him in aortic stenosis (26). He wrote that it is occasionally necessary to bend or redirect a guidewire inserted through a valve. Initially, the actual mortality rate was high. There was no further mortality in nine patients using the new instrument. Six of these patients were subjected to simultaneous commissurotomy procedures for coexisting mitral stenosis.

In 1948 Harken and his group published a report in which they described their approach to the surgery of mitral stenosis by a procedure which they called "valvuloplasty" (27; Fig. 11.5). The main principles were as follows: access to the mitral valve should be from the atrial side; surgical enlargement of the stenotic orifice should be planned so that there is minimal restoration of valvular function by "valvuloplasty," and undue acceleration of the heart rate should be prevented.

Harken and Black expanded on this theme in 1955 (28). They wrote that there was now a technique that assured complete separation of the commissures out to the annulus and mobilization of the valve leaflet by freeing restricting fused chordae and papillary muscles. Harken did not shy away from using the finger alone, if a fracture of the valve could easily be obtained (29). Harken and co-workers also addressed the problem of mitral and aortic prosthesis in the shape of bottle to be inserted into the orifice of an incompetent valve (30). Twenty-four terminal patients with proven mitral insufficiency were operated on using this procedure, with seven postoperative and seven late deaths. The high mortality was explained to be correlated with inconsistency of the position of the baffle. Harken believed he could overcome this mortality using a spindle baffle by anchoring both ends of the baffle.

For the treatment of aortic insufficiency, Harken and his group used a circumcluding suture to reduce the aortic valve area (31). Of eleven patients, five survived and improved. Later, after the introduction of cardiopulmonary bypass, Harken and co-workers used as a prosthesis a caged ball valve (32). By that time the breakthrough perfection of cardiopulmonary bypass had been made.

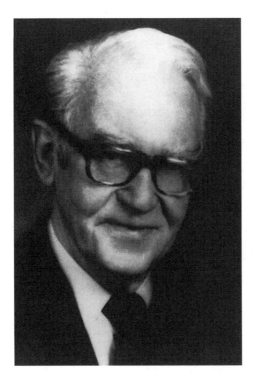

Figure 11.5. Dwight Harken. (*With permission from Alden H. Harken, M.D.*)

The new era of cardiac valvular surgery dawned with the introduction of cardiopulmonary bypass by Gibbons, followed by the work of C. Walton Lillehei and others. The first patient operated on by Gibbons had an atrial septal defect. Lillehei used cardiopulmonary bypass for surgery on aortic stenosis (1956) and on mitral stenosis (1958) (33).

With the introduction of cardiopulmonary bypass, the aspects of valvular surgery changed. New issues arose—for example, whether to produce cardiac arrest, or retroperfuse the coronary sinus, or initiate hypothermia to avoid global myocardial ischemia, or utilize techniques of reconstructing diseased valves, or replace diseased valves with prostheses.

Lillehei and co-workers pioneered in the field using a simple heart-lung machine for cardiopulmonary bypass (Fig. 11.6; see Chapter 3). They operated on patients with aortic and mitral stenosis and aortic and mitral insufficiency. A particularly difficult problem was the initiation and maintenance of cardiac arrest. Lillehei used both potassium chloride and acetylcholine; acetylcholine was finally preferred. For the treatment of mitral insufficiency, they used what they called annuloplasty, consisting in part of selective suturing of the annulus fibrosus to reduce its circumference, reminiscent of the efforts of Bailey and of Harken. Direct vision of the valve rendered cutting by valvulotomes unnecessary. Lillehei

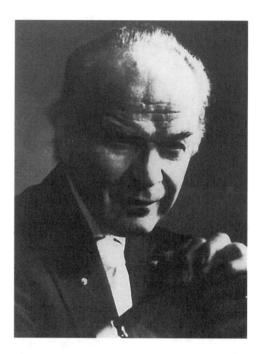

Figure 11.6. C. Walton Lillehei.
(Courtesy of the New York Academy of Medicine)

attempted aortic valve replacement in aortic insufficiency with a prosthesis. As he wrote, "clearly the abnormal leaflet had to be replaced by a space-occupying prosthesis, which would provide sufficient substance." The procedures consisted of a compressed polyvinyl plastic sponge (ivalon) together with one annuloplasty stitch.

A major step forward was the introduction of a prosthetic valve by Charles Hufnagel in 1952. He performed the first implantation of an artificial heart valve in a patient with severe aortic regurgitation. The prosthesis was a caged-ball valve implanted in the descending aorta, thus preventing some regurgitation. Hufnagel (1914–89) was a remarkably inventive surgeon. The son of a physician surgeon, he graduated from Harvard with the M.D. degree in 1941 and received his surgical training at the Peter Bent Brigham Hospital and a year at Children's Hospital under Robert Gross. He participated with Gross in the early pioneering work on coarctation of the aorta.

In 1944 Hufnagel was appointed director of the surgical research laboratory at Harvard, where his investigation of vascular replacement with plastic material originated. Another pioneering venture in which he participated was the first kidney transplant in 1947 by David Hume. He assisted in this epochal operation at the Brigham Hospital (34). Hufnagel thus participated in and witnessed two truly history-making events: the surgical treatment of coarctation of the aorta and the first human kidney transplant; the latter work resulted in a Nobel prize more than forty years later.

In 1950 Hufnagel was appointed professor of experimental surgery at Georgetown University, where he became associated with cardiologist Proctor Harvey who furnished clinical expertise to the team. The first insertion of a valve in the descending aorta was carried out on a thirty-year-old patient with advanced aortic regurgitation. She recovered promptly after the operation and returned to an active life. An unfortuante byproduct of the plastic ball valve was a disturbing click, particularly when the patient opened her mouth. This was soon controlled by altering the composition of the valve. In addition, Hufnagel anchored the prosthesis in the aorta by use of multiple perforations, eliminating the use of sutures. The procedure could be carried out at that time because it did not necessitate use of a cardiopulmonary bypass. The valve was further modified, eventually leading to a trileaflet type and later to a disc valve. Hufnagel implanted the valve in more than two hundred individuals. The valve, on display at the Smithsonian Institute, is part of an exhibit on the development of heart surgery.

Hufnagel also followed Alexis Carrel's example by developing methods of preserving arterial grafts by freezing and use of orlon prostheses. It is not surprising that he had a particular interest in cataloging and editing papers by Alexis Carrel, which are stored in a special portion of the Georgetown library. Another vignette in the life of Hufnagel was his appointment by Judge Sirica of Watergate fame to examine former President Richard Nixon, to determine whether Nixon was medically fit to testify at the Watergate trial. (The former president was considered to be medically unfit to appear.) Hufnagel died of heart disease and renal failure, two of the areas of his main research interest.

The caged ball concept was later developed by Harken and Birtwell. This resulted in the first clinically used caged ball valve on March 10, 1960, and the second on June 6, 1960. The first patient, Mary Richardson, lived for thirty years, finally succumbing to carcinoma of the esophagus. The second patient also survived to succumb to another cardiac operation for mitral valve disease. Of importance is the fact that the same dimensions that were defined in those valves for the height of the cage and for the ratio of the ball to the annulus set the standards in the development of subsequent caged ball valves (34).

Albert Starr, also building on the work of Hufnagel, in association with M. Lowell Edwards (an engineer), developed the Starr–Edwards prosthetic cardiac valves that are, even today, the "gold standard" of valve prostheses. Starr, who later became the chairman of the Division of Thoracic Surgery at the University of Oregon, organized and performed the necessary research and practical applications of these valves. In 1960 Starr published his mitral valve replacement experiments in animals, and one year later reported his clinical work in patients (35). It is remarkable that he was successful since the canine is prone to hypercoagulation. Starr tried many replacement variations and decided that the model using a ball valve was the best. He developed the technique of valve replacement and fixation in the heart; he also recognized the problem of thrombosis. "Thrombosis is a major problem; it first appears at the zone of fixation to the mitral annulus and extends over the valve ring despite changes in the materials used and despite anticoagulant drugs. This always interferes with leaflet function but is less likely to interfere with a ball valve" (35).

Albert Starr's clinical success with mitral valve replacement was remarkable. "While early satisfactory results were obtained in some patients, survival beyond three months has not been reported to now" (36). He reported twelve cases with one operative and three late deaths due to infection.

During the past three decades, numerous prosthetic heart valves have been developed, used, and discarded. With them vanished the hope for an easy solution. The Starr–Edwards silastic ball valve has proven to be the most durable. Pyrolitic carbon disc valves are most often chosen by surgeons today as a mechanical valve for valve replacement. Currently, the St. Jude Medical bileaflet valve is the most frequently implanted mechanical valve in the United States. Other currently available mechanical valves are the Medtronic-Hall, the Omniscience, the monostrut Bjork–Shiley, and the bileaflet Carbomedics (the latter two were not yet available in the United States at time of publication).

Of the well-known late complications of mechanical valve implantation, perhaps the convexo-concave 70° tilt valve of Bjork–Shiley was associated with the most dramatic events. It was developed in 1976 (37) with a larger opening angle to 70° as a means of reducing the transvalvular gradient. The high incidence of devastating late strut fractures caused it to be withdrawn from the market. Since then the Bjork–Shiley monostrut valve has been developed. By 1989 there were more than 53,000 such implants worldwide without a single mechanical complication (38). All the other advantages of such a valve have been retained. This model has now been approved by the FDA.

Aortic valve replacement with antibiotic-sterilized aortic valve homografts was described by Donald Ross from England in 1962 (39), and Sir Brian Barrat-Boyes from New Zealand in 1964 (40). Raymond Heimbecker of Canada had previously reported the replacement of the mitral valve by an antibiotic-sterilized aortic valve homograft (41). Some enthusiasm for this procedure was generated after these reports, but it became popular in only a few centers around the world. With the development of cryopreservation for aortic valve homografts and the encouraging report from Mark O'Brien from Australia (42), however, interest in this operation grew to such a degree that an adequate supply of homografts became the limiting factor in its increased usage. Cryopreservation keeps the aortic valve fibroblasts viable, but it is still not known whether they remain viable after implantation.

Glutaraldehyde-preserved porcine aortic bioprostheses were introduced in the late 1960s by Alain Carpentier from France. Warren Hancock made them commercially available in 1970. This type of bioprosthesis has been extensively used for replacement of aortic, mitral, and tricuspid valves. Thromboembolism is uncommon with this type of bioprosthesis (43). The main problem with this valve is tissue degeneration; at the end of ten years, 20 percent to 25 percent of patients required reoperation because of structural failure (43). A large percentage of valves are probably already calcified at ten years. Tissue degeneration occurs very rapidly in children and slowly in elderly patients. Mechanical stress plays an important role in the degeneration of tissue valves. It has been shown that the durability of the aortic valve homograft is significantly shortened when it is mounted in an artificial stent before being implanted in a patient (44). Based on this clinical observation and other experimental information, Tirone David from Canada postulated that the aortic root was the best stent for aortic valve leaflets, a concept that formed the basis of the development of his stentless glutaraldehyde preserved porcine aortic valve replacement (45). This valve has now been used for a decade in Toronto and tissue degeneration remains a problem. However, its hemodynamic performance is similar to that of aortic homografts and allows for complete left ventricular remodeling in most patients after aortic valve replacement. This restoration of ventricular function has had a beneficial effect in long-term survival.

There has been a renewed interest in aortic valve replacement with pulmonary autograft. In this operation, the patient's diseased aortic valve is replaced with the normal pulmonary valve. Instead of only replacing the aortic valve leaflets, most surgeons replace the entire aortic root with the pulmonary root. This procedure is ideally suited for children and young adults. It may cure the aortic valve disease permanently but because a pulmonary homograft is implanted in the right side of the circulation, reoperations may still be necessary (46).

The anatomy and function of the mitral valve and of the left ventricle are interrelated. Interactions between these two structures are complex and not yet entirely understood. The attachments between the mitral annulus and the ventricular wall are important for left ventricular geometry and function. Lillehei and colleagues were the first to point out the importance of preserving the chordae tendineae during mitral valve replacement (47). This method of mitral valve replacement did not become popular until David and associates published their data on the importance of the mitral apparatus in left ventricular function (48, 49). Understanding of the interactions between the mitral valve and the left ventricle has been greatly improved by the work of Craig Miller from Stanford University (50). Miller and his group established the fact that the papillary muscles with their chordae tendineae not only prevent leaflet prolapse and mitral regurgitation during systole, but also serve as a working structural element of the contractile ventricle to enhance left ventricular systolic pump performance.

Reconstruction of the aortic valve is possible in only a small percentage of patients who need aortic valve surgery. The senile calcific aortic stenosis in the older population can be successfully debrided, but the long-term results have been disappointing. Reconstruction of the incompetent aortic valve is also possible, particularly when the leaflets are normal and distortion of the aortic sinuses is the cause of valve dysfunction. Aortic valve repair is not as easily reproducible as mitral valve repair and should be judiciously performed.

Until the perfect artificial heart valve is created, the diseased native valve should be repaired—but only as long as the results are better than with valve replacement.

The decade of the 1980s was a time of further consolidation and improvement of devices and techniques. Heart transplantation under cyclosporin has been a very worthwhile answer in advanced multivalvular disease with associated myocardial damage. Many centers, including Stanford, Pittsburgh, and London (Canada), report a five-year survival rate of over 80 percent with a return to a normal way of life (51, 52).

The classical paper by Charles T. Dotter and Melvin P. Judkins on dilating atherosclerotic lesions was published in 1964. In their original work, the authors did not use balloon-equipped catheters but successfully dilated atherosclerotic obstructive lesions of the femoral and popliteal arteries using catheters of increasing diameter, the largest being about 0.2 inches (outer diameter). A spring catheter guide was first inserted.

Dotter and Judkins were able to successfully treat six of eleven patients with marked occlusion of the femoral artery. In all their patients amputation had been the only remaining option. They wrote, "we are satisfied that percutaneous transluminal recanalization is the treatment of choice for many lesions of the femoral and popliteal arteries. . . . No doubt the interest and ingenuity of others will lead to refinements of technique as well as the clarification of the role of this attack on arteriosclerotic obstruction" (53). They answered the criticism of some surgeons that coexistent disease in distal branches may defeat the purpose of the procedure by stating that "even a rusty sprinkler may prove capable of doing a creditable job once the faucet is fully opened."

This pioneering venture led to the development of a new technical specialty for nonoperative treatment of obstructive vascular disease including coronary disease. In European countries the procedure of transluminal recanalization of an artery is often referred to as "Dotterize."

Charles Dotter (1920–85) was a true pioneer in the field of the use of balloon-equipped catheter to dilate vascular obstructive lesions (Fig. 11.7). Other procedures also originated from his fertile mind, among them the technique for

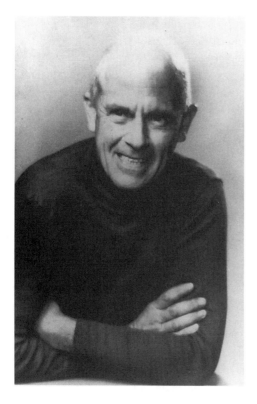

Figure 11.7. Charles Dotter. *(Courtesy of Dotter Interventional Institute, University of Oregon, Portland)*

percutaneous catheterization, which was introduced in 1958, and the use of guide wires, which he developed jointly with Bill Cook and the safety J-tipped guide wire (53). Dotter also first described a flow-guided catheter, an overlooked predecessor of the Swan–Ganz catheter and a transvascular catheter biopsy. Working with Melvin Judkins, Dotter helped develop today's standard techniques for coronary angiography. Like Mason Sones, Charles Dotter used a direct approach. He went straight to the heart of a problem, with simplicity and directness. Neither Sones nor Dotter could be called sophisticated scientists.

Balloon mitral valvoplasty has been attempted by many authors (54). Transluminal dilatation, for example, was of primary interest to many urologists. The first use of a balloon catheter was by Guthrie in 1834, when a catgut balloon was employed to dilate the urethra (55). It is interesting that Gruentzig in 1974 used a similar instrument. Abele was one of the first to define the theoretical basis underlying balloon dilatation, by defining "dilating force" and basing it on the law of LaPlace (56). This law defined the extension of a balloon to stretch and separate at its circumference when inside pressure was applied. Identical pressures will produce more force in larger balloons than in smaller ones. For identical

pressures, the dilating force is proportional to the radius. Abele related the dilating force to the balloon pressure, stenosis size, degree of stenosis, material used,
and balloon length. Finally, he related burst pressure to the inflation time. Abele's
conclusion based on Poiseuille's Law was that in a tight stenosis, a very small difference in size can make a very large difference in flow. He suggested that it is
preferable to dilate to the physiological requirement under conditions of reactive
or pharmacologically induced hyperemia.

Following Dotter's original publication in 1964 it took more than fifteen years
to apply his principle to various stenosed vascular beds. Tegtmeyer applied balloon dilatation to the renal artery (57), Gruentzig to the coronary artery (58),
Lock to the pulmonary arteries (59) and to coarctation of the aorta (60). Kan used
percutaneous transluminal dilatation for congenital pulmonary stenosis (61).
McKay and Palacios used this method in the treatment of calcified mitral stenosis
(62, 63). McKay also treated calcific aortic stenosis with this technique (64).
Lababidi (65) and Cribier (66) applied it to the stenosed aortic valve. The first
percutaneous balloon valvulotomy of a stenosed triscupid valve was reported by
Zaibag (67). For mitral valve surgery J.E. Lock (68) used the antegrade transep-
tal approach while U.U. Babic et al. (54) used a long guide wire transversing the
vascular system from femoral vein to femoral artery to control the position of the
balloon catheter advanced retrogradely across the mitral valve. In 1990 C. Stefanadis et al. reported success in ten adult patients (69). All patients had a significant reduction in valve gradient together with an increase in valve area
and were without serious complications. This encouraging report must be judged
against the fact that many mitral commissures are heavily scarred and can be very
difficult to split, even under direct vision and even with a very forceful surgical
transventricular dilator. Obviously careful selection of cases is of paramount importance. Fatal ventricular perforation is the most feared of the many complications of the procedure (70).

Pulmonary valve stenosis is another area in which there has been considerable success, beginning with Serub et al. in 1979 and further developed by Kan
in 1982. Because of a low morbidity and mortality the field has since grown. Some
centers now report that 10 percent of all catheterizations are for the correction
of pulmonary stenosis (71).

Aortic stenosis has been similarly managed in pediatric group cases beginning with Lababidi in 1983. S. Perry et al. report (72) 111 balloon valvotomies
for congenital aortic stenosis, with patients ranging from one day to thirty-nine
years of age. In neonates it is considered an urgent palliative procedure, with
a mortality of six in sixteen. In the ninety-three other patients, the majority
achieved a 60 percent increase in valve area; only a minority developed severe
regurgitation that required open heart surgery.

Carpentier used four basic techniques either individually or in association depending upon the valvular lesions in mitral insufficiencies: (1) annulus remodeling with a prosthetic ring, (2) leaflet tissue resection and repair, (3) chordal shortening, and (4) chordal fenestration and resection (73). The breakthrough in reconstructive mitral valve surgery, according to Carpentier, was the recognition that mitral insufficiency is almost never the result of one lesion, but of multiple lesions that affect the various components of the mitral apparatus.

Responsible for this progress in this field has been examinations by two-dimensional mode and color flow Doppler echocardiography. These techniques have been helpful in demonstrating the advantage of commissurotomy with preservation of the chordae, and with an assessment of balloon valvuloplasty versus operation by direct vision. For example, Rozich et al. (74) have calculated fractional shortening, muscle cross-sectional area, left ventricular volumes, and end-systolic stress and concluded that mitral valve replacement with preservation of chordae tendineae was highly preferable to standard mitral valve replacement. Preservation of chordae resulted in smaller ventricular size, reduced end-systolic stress, and preservation of ejection performance. They concluded that every effort should be made to preserve the chordae tendineae with the aim of minimizing or eliminating a postoperative decline in left ventricular systolic function. Goldman and his associates (75) also stressed the advantage of the operation of mitral valve repair versus valve replacement. They found significant global and regional ventricular dysfunction immediately after removal of the papillary muscles. Therefore mitral valve reconstruction, when technically feasible, is the procedure of choice for degenerative or ischemic mitral regurgitation because of significantly lower mortality and late valve-related events (76). Additionally, mitral valve reconstruction was associated with a significantly shorter postoperative hospital stay than was mitral valve replacement.

In the field of aortic stenosis, Doppler ultrasonography has made it possible to accurately estimate the severity of aortic stenosis; it enables an accurate assessment of transvalvular gradient and the area of the aortic valve (77). The increase in velocity across the stenosed area detected by the Doppler technique can be translated into a pressure gradient. Velocity also can be used in the continuity equation to estimate aortic valve area. Currie et al. produced the Doppler-determined estimate of systolic pressure gradient across the aortic valve as calculated by the modified Bernoulli equation to assess the severity of calcific aortic stenosis (78). This measurement greatly assists in the noninvasive assessment of adults with suspected aortic valvular stenosis.

Balloon aortic valvotomy for adult-acquired aortic stenosis is not recommended. Otto found that long-term survival after balloon aortic valvuloplasty is poor with a low survival rate of only 55 percent because of early restenosis and recurrent hospitalization (79). In contrast, percutaneous balloon mitral valvuloplasty provides good mechanical relief that usually results in prolonged benefit

(77, 80). This has also been confirmed by Reyes (81), who suggested that mitral balloon valvuloplasty should be considered for all patients with favorable mitral valve anatomy.

An important development was the finding that prognosis of surgery of aortic stenosis, even in the octogenarian, is excellent in the absence of coexisting illness (77).

References

1. Brunton, Sir L. Preliminary note on the possibility of treating mitral stenosis by surgical methods. Lancet, 1:352, 1902.
2. Murrell, W. Nitroglycerine as a remedy for angina pectoris. Lancet, 1:80, 113, 151, 225, 1879.
3. Cushing, H., and J.R. Branch. Experimental and clinical notes on chronic valvular lesions in the dog and their possible relation to a future surgery of the cardiac valves. J. Med. Res., 17:471–486, 1908.
4. Bernheim, B. Experimental surgery of the mitral valve. Johns Hopkins Hosp. Bull., 20:107–110, 1909.
5. Tuffier, T., and A. Carrel. Patching and section of the pulmonary orifice of the heart. J. Exp. Med., 20:3–8, 1914.
6. Tuffier, T. Etat actuel de la chirurgie intrathoracique. London, Trans. XVII Int. Cong. Med., Section VII:316–317, 1913.
7. Lindblom, D. Heredity and Mortality after Heart Valve Replacement. Stockholm, Carolinska Medico Chiruska Institute, 1987.
8. Allen, D., and E. Graham. Intracardiac surgery—a new method. JAMA, 79:1028–1030, 1922.
9. Cutler, E., and S.A. Levine. Cardiotomy and valvulotomy for mitral stenosis. Experimental observations and clinical notes concerning an operated case with recovery. Boston Med. Surg. J., 188:1023–1027, 1923.
10. Cutler, E., and C. Beck. The present status of the surgical procedures in chronic valvular disease of the heart. Arch. Surg., 18:403–416, 1929.
11. Beck, C.S., and E. Cutler. A cardiovalvulotome. J. Exp. Med., 40:375–379, 1924.
12. Souttar, H.S. The surgical treatment of mitral stenosis. Br. Med. J., 2:603–606, 1925.
13. Greenwood, J. Obituary Notices. Br. Med. J., 2:1335–1336, 1964.
14. Bailey, C.P. The surgical treatment of mitral stenosis (mitral commissurotomy). Diseases of the Chest, 15(4):377–397, 1949.
15. Smithy, H.G., H.R. Pratt-Thomas, and H.P. Deyerle. Aortic valvulotomy experimental methods and early results. Surg. Gyn. Obstet., 86:513–523, 1948.
16. Smithy, H.G. The control of arrhythmias occurring during operation upon the valves of the heart: experimental and clinical observations. The Southern Surgeon, 14:611–618, 1948.
17. Smithy, H.G., J.A. Boone, and J.M. Stallworth. Surgical treatment of constrictive valvular disease of the heart. Surg. Gyn. Obstet., 90:175–192, 1950.
18. Smithy, H.G., and E.F. Parker. Experimental aortic valvulotomy. Surg. Gyn. Obstet., 84:625–628, 1947.
19. Swan, H. Mitral stenosis: an experimental study of pulmonary-azygos venous anastomosis. Am. Heart J., 367–375, 1948.
20. Bland, E.F., and R.H. Sweet. A venous shunt for advanced mitral stenosis. JAMA, 140:1259–1265, 1949.
21. Sweet, R.H., and E.F. Bland. The surgical relief of congestion in the pulmonary circulation in cases of severe mitral stenosis. Ann. Surg., 130:384–397, 1949.

22. Templeton, J.Y., III, and J.H. Gibbon Jr. Experimental reconstruction of cardiac valves by venous and pericardial grafts. Ann. Surg., 129:161–176, 1949.
23. Murray, G. Homologous aortic valve segment transplants as surgical treatment for aortic and mitral insufficiency. Angiology, 7:466–471, 1956.
24. Bailey, C.P., and W. Likoff. The surgical treatment of aortic insufficiency. Ann. Intern. Med., 42:388–416, 1955.
25. Bailey, C.P., W.L. Jamison, A.E. Bakst, H.E. Bolton, H.T. Nichols, and W. Gemeinhardt. The surgical correction of mitral insufficiency by the use of pericardial grafts. J. Thor. Surg., 28:551–603, 1954.
26. Bailey, C.P., R. Ramirez, and H.B. Larzelere. Surgical treatment of aortic stenosis. JAMA, 150:1647–1652, 1952.
27. Harken, D.E., L.B. Ellis, P.F. Ware, and L.R. Notman. The surgical treatment of mitral stenosis. I. Valvuloplasty. N. Engl. J. Med., 239:801–809, 1948.
28. Harken, D.E., and H. Black. Improved valvuloplasty for mitral stenosis. N. Engl. J. Med., 253:669–678, 1955.
29. Ellis, L.B., and D.E. Harken. Closed valvuloplasty for mitral stenosis. N. Engl. J. Med., 270:643–650, 1964.
30. Harken, D.E., H. Black, L.B. Ellis, and L. Dexter. The surgical correction of mitral insufficiency. J. Thor. Surg., 28:604–627, 1954.
31. Taylor, W.J., W.B. Thrower, H. Black, and D.E. Harken. The surgical correction of insufficiency by circumclusion. J. Thor. Surg., 35:192–205, 1958.
32. Harken, D.E., H.S. Soroff, W.J. Taylor, A.A. Lefemine, S.K. Gupta, and S. Lunzer. Partial and complete prostheses in aortic insufficiency. J. Thor. Cardiovasc. Surg., 40: 744–762, 1960.
33. Lillehei, C.W., V.L. Gott, R.A. DeWall, and R.L. Varco. The surgical treatment of stenotic or regurgitant lesions of the mitral and aortic valves by direct vision utilizing a pump-oxygenator. J. Thor. Surg., 35:154–190, 1958.
34. Hufnagel, C.A. Basic concepts of cardiac and vascular reconstruction. Georgetown Med. Bull., 14:88–96, 1988.
35. Starr, A. Total mitral valve replacement: fixation and thrombosis. Surg. Forum, 11: 258–260, 1960.
36. Starr, A., and M.L. Edwards. Mitral replacement: clinical experience with a ball-valve prosthesis. Ann. Surg., 154:725–740, 1961.
37. Björk, V.O. The improved Bjork–Shiley tilting disc valve prosthesis. Scand. J. Thorac. Cardiovasc. Surg., 12:81–84, 1978.
38. Björk, V.O. Development of mechanical heart valves: past, present and future. Can. J. Cardiol., 5:64–73, 1989.
39. Ross, D.N. Homograft replacement of the aortic valve. Lancet, 2:487, 1962.
40. Barrat-Boyes, B.G. Homograft aortic valve replacement in incompetence and stenosis. Thorax, 19:131–150, 1964.
41. Heimbecker, R.O., R.J. Baird, T.Z. Lajos, A.T. Varga, and W.F. Greenwood. Homograft replacement of the human mitral valve. Can. Med. Assoc. J., 86:805–809, 1962.
42. O'Brien, M.F., E.G. Stafford, M.A.H. Gardner, P.G. Pohlner, and D.C. McGiffin. A comparison of aortic valve replacement with viable cryopreserved and fresh allograft valves, with a note on chromosomal studies. J. Thorac. Cardiovasc. Surg., 94:812–823, 1987.
43. Magilligan, D.J., M.W. Lewis, P. Stein, and M. Alam. The porcine bioprosthetic heart valve: experience at 15 years. Ann. Thorac. Surg., 48:324–330, 1989.
44. Angell, W.W., J.H. Oury, J.J. Lamberti, and J. Koziol. Durability of the viable aortic allograft. J. Thorac. Cardiovasc. Surg., 98:48–56, 1989.
45. David, T.E., C. Pollick, and J. Bos. Aortic valve replacement with stentless porcine aortic bioprosthesis. J. Thorac. Surg., 99:113–118, 1990.
46. David, T.E., C.M. Feindel, J. Bos, Z. Sun, H.E. Scully, and H. Rakowski. Aortic valve

replacement with a stentless porcine aortic valve. A six-year experience. J. Thorac. Cardiovasc. Surg., 108:1030–1036, 1994.

47. Lillehei, C.W., M.J. Levy, and R.C. Bonnabeau. Mitral valve replacement with preservation of papillary muscles and chordae tendineae. J. Thorac. Cardiovasc. Surg., 47: 532–543, 1964.

48. David, T.E., D.H. Strauss, E. Mesher, M.J. Anderson, J.L. MacDonald, and A.J. Buda. Is it important to preserve the chordae tendineae and the papillary muscles during mitral valve replacement? Can. J. Surg., 24:236–239, 1981.

49. David, T.E., D.E. Uden, and H.D. Strauss. The importance of the mitral apparatus in left ventricular function after correction of mitral regurgitation. Circulation, 68 (Supp. II):II76–II82, 1983.

50. Sarris, G.E., J.I. Fann, M.A. Niczyporuk, G.C. Derby, C.E. Handen, and D.C. Miller. Global and regional left ventricular systolic performance in the in situ ejecting canine heart. Importance of the mitral apparatus. Circulation, 80 (Suppl. I):I24–I42, 1989.

51. Devineni, R., R.N. McKenzie, W.J. Kostuk, R.O. Heimbecker, et al. Cyclosporine in cardiac transplantation: observations on immunological monitoring, cardiac histology and cardiac function. Heart Transplantation, vol. 11, 3–219, May 1983.

52. Heimbecker, R.O., N. McKenzie, C. Stiller, W.J. Kostuk, and M.D. Silver. Heart and lung transplantation. J. Critical Care, 13:11–14, 1984.

53. Riosch, J., H.L. Abrams, and W. Cook. Charles Theodore Dotter Memorials. Am. J. Roentgenol., 144:1321–1323, 1985.

54. Babic, U.U., P. Pejcic, Z. Djurisic, et al. Percutaneous transarterial balloon valvuloplasty for mitral valve stenosis. Am. J. Cardiol., 57:1101–1104, 1986.

55. Guthrie, G.J. On the Anatomy and Diseases of the Neck of the Bladder and the Urethra. London, Burgess & Hill, 1834.

56. Abele, J.E. Balloon catheters and transluminal dilation: technical considerations. Am. J. Roentgenol., 135:901–906, 1980.

57. Tegtmeyer, C.J., R. Dyer, C.D. Teates, R.M. Carey, H.A. Wellons, and L.W. Stanton. Percutaneous transluminal dilatation of the renal arteries: techniques and results. Radiology, 135:589–599, 1980.

58. Gruentzig, A.R., A. Senning, and W.E. Siegenthaler. Nonoperative dilatation of coronary artery stenosis: percutaneous transluminal angioplasty. N. Engl. J. Med., 301:61–68, 1979.

59. Lock, J.E., W.R. Castaneda-Zuniga, B.P. Fuhrman, and J.L. Bass. Balloon dilatation angioplasty of hypoplastic and stenotic pulmonary arteries. Circulation, 67:962–967, 1983.

60. Lock, J.E., T. Niemi, B.A. Burke, S. Einzig, and W.R. Castaneda-Zuniga. Transcutaneous angioplasty of experimental aortic coarctation. Circulation, 66:1280–1285, 1982.

61. Kan, J.S., R.I. White, S.E. Mitchell, and T.J. Gardner. Percutaneous balloon valvuloplasty: A new method for treating congenital pulmonary artery stenosis. N. Engl. J. Med., 307:540–542, 1982.

62. McKay, R.G., J.E. Lock, J.F. Keane, R.D. Safian, and J.M. Aroesty. Percutaneous mitral valvuloplasty in an adult patient with calcific rheumatic mitral stenosis. J. Am. Coll. Cardiol., 7:1410–1415, 1986.

63. Palacios, I.F., J.E. Lock, J.F. Keane, and P.C. Block. Percutaneous transvenous balloon valvotomy in a patient with severe calcific mitral stenosis. J. Am. Coll. Cardiol., 7:1416, 1986.

64. McKay, R.G., R.D. Safian, J.E. Locke, V.S. Mandell, R.L. Thurer, S.J. Schnitt, and W. Grossman. Balloon dilatation of calcific aortic stenosis in elderly patients: postmortem, intraoperative, and percutaneous valvuloplast studies. Circulation, 74:119–124, 1986.

65. Lababidi, Z., W. Jiunn-Ren, and J.T. Walls. Percutaneous balloon aortic valvuloplasty; results in 23 patients. Am. J. Cardiol., 53:194–197, 1984.
66. Cribier, A., T. Savin, N. Sauudi, P. Rocha, J. Berland, and B. Letac. Percutaneous transluminal valvuloplasty of acquired aortic stenosis in elderly patients: an alternative to valve replacement? Lancet, 1:63–67, 1986.
67. Zaibag, A.L., M. Ribeiro, and S.A. Al-Kasab. Percutaneous balloon valvotomy in triscupid stenosis. Br. Heart. J., 57:51–53, 1987.
68. Lock, J.E., M. Khalilullah, S. Shrivastavca, and J.F. Keane. Percutaneous catheter commissurotomy in rheumatic mitral stenosis. N. Engl. J. Med., 313:1515–1518, 1985.
69. Stefanadis, C., C. Kourouklis, C. Stratos, C. Pitsavos, C. Tentolouris, and P. Toutouzas. Percutaneous balloon mitral valvuloplasty by retrograde left atrial catheterization. Am. J. Cardiol., 65:650–654, 1990.
70. Butany, J., G. D'Amati, D. Charlesworth, L. Schwartz, L. Daniel, A. Adelmen, and M. Silver. Fatal left ventricular perforation following balloon mitral valvuloplasty. Can. J. Cardiol., 6:343–347, 1990.
71. Beekman, R.H., A.P. Rocchini, and A. Rosenthal. Therapeutic cardiac catheterization for pulmonary valve and pulmonary artery stenosis. Cardiol. Clin., 7:331–340, May 1989.
72. Perry, S.B., B. Zeevi, J.F. Keane, and J.E. Lock. Interventional catheterization of left heart lesions, including aortic and mitral valve stenosis and coarctation of the aorta. Cardiol. Clin., 7:341–347, 1989.
73. Carpentier, A., J.N. Fabiani, J. Relland, Cl. d'Allaines, and A. Piwnica. Reconstructive surgery of mitral valve incompetence. J. Thorac. Cardiovasc. Surg., 79:338–348, 1980.
74. Rozich, J.D., B.A. Carabello, B.W. Usher, J.M. Kratz, A.E. Bell, and M.R. Zile. Mitral valve replacement with and without chordal preservation in patients with chronic mitral regurgitation. Mechanisms for differences in postoperative ejection performance. Circulation, 86:1718–1726, 1992.
75. Goldman, M.E., F. Mora, T. Guarino, V. Fuster, and B.P. Mindich. Mitral valvuloplasty is superior to valve replacement for preservation of left ventricular function: an intraoperative two-dimensional echocardiographic study. JACC, 10:568–575, 1987.
76. Akins, C.W., A.D. Hilgenberg, M.J. Buckley, G.J. Vlahakes, D.F. Torchiana, W.M. Daggett, and W.G. Austen. Mitral valve reconstruction versus replacement for degenerative or ischemic mitral regurgitation. Soc. Thorac. Surg., 58:668–676, 1994.
77. Carabello, B.A., and F.A. Crawford Jr. Valvular heart disease. N. Engl. J. Med., 337:32–41, 1997.
78. Currie, P.J., J.B. Seward, G.S. Reeder, R.E. Vlietstra, D.R. Bresnahan, J.F. Bresnahan, H.C. Smith, D.J. Hagler, and A.J. Tajik. Continuous-wave Doppler echocardiographic assessment of severity of calcific aortic stenosis: a simultaneous Doppler-catheter correlative study in 100 adult patients. Circulation, 71:1162–1169, 1985.
79. Otto, C.M., M.C. Mickel, J.W. Kennedy, E.L. Alderman, T.M. Bashore, P.C. Block, J.A. Brinker, J. Diver, J. Ferguson, D.R. Holmes, Jr., C.T. Lambrew, C.R. McKay, I.F. Palacios, E.R. Powers, S.H. Rahimtoola, B.H. Weiner, and K.B. Davis. Three-year outcome after balloon aortic valvuloplasty. Insights into prognosis of valvular aortic stenosis. Circulation, 89:642–650, 1994.
80. Wilkins, G.R., A.E. Weyman, V. M. Abascal, P.C. Block, and I.F. Palacios. Percutaneous balloon dilatation of the mitral valve: an analysis of echocardiographic variables related to outcome and the mechanism of dilatation. Br. Heart J., 60:299–308, 1988.
81. Reyes, V.P., B. Soma Raju, J. Wynne, L.W. Stephenson, R. Raju, B.S. Fromm, P. Rajagopal, P. Mehta, S. Singh, D.P. Rao, P.V. Satyanarayana, and Z.G. Turi. Percutaneous balloon valvuloplasty compared with open surgical commissurotomy for mitral stenosis. N. Engl. J. Med., 331:961–967, 1994.

Hypertension and Hypertensive Heart Disease

Chapter 12

R.J. BING

Franklin delano roosevelt, president of the United States, died on April 12, 1945, in Warm Springs, Georgia, of cerebral hemorrhage resulting from hypertension. In 1970 his cardiologist Howard G. Bruenn published clinical notes on the illness and death of the president (1). Bruenn, an officer in the Navy, became Roosevelt's physician and accompanied the president on most of his voyages including Yalta. Bruenn mentioned that he first saw the president in March 1944 while working at the U.S. Naval Medical Hospital in Bethesda, Maryland. It is well known that the president had suffered from poliomyelitis since 1921 with severe and permanent impairment of the muscles of both lower extremities to the hips. On physical examination, Bruenn found a blood pressure of 186/108. In general the examination, as it was common at that time, was restricted to auscultation and percussion of the heart, an electrocardiogram, and a chest x-ray. Bruenn found a blowing systolic murmur at the apex, and the second aortic sound was loud and booming. Using only one precordial electrode, ST segment depression was present. Fluoroscopy and x-ray showed a considerable increase in the size of the heart.

How was the hypertension of the president treated? It was suggested that he be placed on bed rest for two weeks with nursing care, that he be digitalized with digitalis leaf and receive potassium chloride as salt substitute (1). However, this regimen was rejected because of the demands of the presidency. Instead he was placed on modified bed rest and received cough syrup. But of course the hypertension persisted and later, signs of congestive heart failure were noted when his condition seemed to worsen. The president was placed on phenobarbital, a treatment for high blood pressure and his cigarette smoking was curtailed. But in April 1944 his blood pressure had risen to 222/118. The president was advised to take a rest. Despite his illness the president later traveled to the Pacific, and then following his inauguration for a fourth term, to his rendezvous with Churchill and Stalin at Yalta. The trip was strenuous. At Yalta, the president showed pulsus alternans, a sign of congestive heart failure. Bruenn mentions that the president was quite well despite persistent hypertension. On one day of the Conference he was greatly fatigued, but he seemed to recover and his mood was excellent and he seemed to enjoy Russian food. The president died of a stroke in 1945 (1).

A series of articles have appeared after Roosevelt's death on the state of his health, particularly his hypertension. Averell Harriman, the president's friend and ambassador to Moscow, who saw Roosevelt at Yalta wrote, "I was terribly shocked at the change since our talks in Washington after the November election" (2). "Some people claim that he sold out to the Soviet Union at Yalta. If this were true, it is difficult to understand why the Soviet Union has gone to such lengths to violate the Yalta understandings" (3). Messerli mentioned that it is unlikely that the president had essential hypertension, but believed that it was renovascular disease complicated by heavy smoking which resulted in hypertension (4). He noted that although no autopsy on Roosevelt was performed the embalmer noted that "the arteries were so severely clogged with plaques that the pump serving to inject formaldehyde strained and stopped."

In general, the treatment of the president followed therapeutic nihilism expressed by Paul D. White in 1937, that the treatment of hypertension itself is a difficult and almost hopeless task in the present state of knowledge, and that in fact "hypertension may be an important compensatory mechanism which should not be treated even if it could be controlled" (5).

A diagnosis of hypertension is not possible without accurate determination of blood pressure. Initially, measurement of blood pressure was unavailable, although observations of the pulse were recorded 4,500 years ago (6). O'Brien and Fitzgerald mention that the emperor of China, Huang-Ti, was aware of the importance of change in characteristics of the pulse four thousand years ago; the Ebers Papyrus of 1500 B.C., from ancient Egypt shows that the Egyptians were aware of pulsation in different parts of the body (6). In 1733 Stephen Hales, a minister, recorded blood pressure directly and demonstrated that it rose to a height of eight feet, three inches in a glass tube placed in the artery of a horse. This observation remained unnoticed for nearly a hundred years until in 1828 Jean Leonard Marie Poiseuille reported the measurement of blood pressure with a mercury sphygmomanometer. Following this demonstration the pace quickened and in 1847 the German physiologist Karl Ludwig recorded the blood pressure using a revolving smoked drum and a kymograph. In 1855 Karl Vierordt and Herisson devised an instrument that consisted of a mercury reservoir covered by a rubber membrane from which a graduated glass column arose (6). The sphygmograph by Marey was widely used but was replaced by an invention of Robert Ellis Dudgeon, a homeopath, who in 1882 constructed a lightweight device that could be carried in the pocket, and which incorporated the principles of Marey's instrument. Frederick Akhbar Mahomed also modified Marey's sphygmograph with the aid of a local watchmaker, making it much lighter and more responsive. While a medical student, Mahomed described these improvements and mentioned results obtained with his modified sphygmograph in a variety of patients. In 1874 he pointed to the relationship between renal disease and hypertension (7).

Great progress was made with the invention of arterial and limb occluding devices (6). The first arterial occluding device was developed by von Basche, who devised a sphygmomanometer; the compressing medium was water, which was enclosed in a rubber bulb that had a thin membrane on one side. The most important advance was made by Riva Rocci, who in 1896 used an arm cuff, consisting of an inflatable rubber bladder enclosed in leather encircling the upper arm. In principle this instrument is used today.

What was still lacking was the independent measurement of systolic and diastolic blood pressures. This was accomplished in 1905 by a Russian surgeon, Nicolai Sergeevich Korotkov, who reported his findings to the Imperial Military Academy in St. Petersburg (6). William Dock commented that "the most remarkable fact about the Korotkov sound is that it was discovered" (8); what he was referring to was the fact that Korotkov's paper would have languished in obscurity had it not been for two other Russians, Krilov and Yanovski (6). Krilov published a paper entitled "On Measuring the Blood Pressure with the Sound Method of Korotkov" in which he described elaborate experiments to elucidate the mechanism of the Korotkov sounds (9). Interpretation of Korotkov's sounds still remains disputed—for example, whether the muffling or the disappearance of sound should be taken as the diastolic pressure (6).

Measurement of blood pressure was not available when Morgagni, at the age of eighty, in his *De Sedibus et Causis Morborum per Anatomen Indagatis,* published in Venice in 1761 observed what was probably a case of hypertension (10). "The father of Zani died of apoplexy and his grandfather of bladder stone, when he was more than seventy. He was corpulent, flabby with a very large short neck, a very red face and led a sedentary life devoted to literary studies and generous meals, as it is convenient for a noble person, who is already forty, when he first started making stones, which he passed with the urine." At sixty-three, the patient complained of "tremendous headaches, owing to which his senses became dull, and the movement of the right side of his body feeble." Morgagni continued: "during the autumn his feet became edematous and from the right foot a large quantity of limpid liquid came out, since the skin had corroded. Afterwards, he was found without the use of speech and with the right side of his body almost unmovable." The patient died five days later. Morgagni concluded that "Zani was affected by twofold disease which was hereditary: bladder stone disease and apoplexy." The patient was also afflicted by atherosclerosis, as suggested by the anatomic finding of "Cartilaginous Plaques" in several of his arteries. Morgagni also mentioned an enlarged heart.

Richard Bright in 1827 pointed to an association of renal disease with heart disease, when he described patients with abnormal urinary findings, associated with ascites and peripheral edema (dropsy) (11). In his article on "Cases on Observations, Illustrative of Renal Disease Accompanied with the Secretion of Albuminous Urine" he stressed the importance and extensive prevalence of "that form of disease which, after it has continued for some time, is attended by the peculiar changes in the structure of the kidney." He related that not less than five hundred died of it annually in London. Since Bright was unable to determine blood pressure, he was unaware of the connection between high blood pressure and renal disease. But he did emphasize the relation of kidney disease to scarlet fever and mentioned the physical signs of renal disease now called Bright's disease. He asked the question, "Do we always find such lesions of the kidney as to bear us out in the belief, that the peculiar condition of the urine, to which I have already referred, shews that the disease, call it what we may, is connected necessarily and essentially with a derangement of that organ?" (11).

The early phase of the study of experimental hypertension has been described by Gordon (12). Ludwig Traube was the first to relate high arterial pressure to kidney disease (13). In 1856 he associated diseases of the kidneys to hypertrophy of the heart—more specifically, of the left ventricle. He believed that shrinkage of the kidney resulted in a reduction of blood flow, thereby reducing the total flow from arterial to venous circulation, causing a reduction in the amount of fluid secreted in the urine. As a result, the mean systemic arterial pressure rose and this opposed the outflow of blood from the left ventricle, which as a consequence at first dilated and then hypertrophied.

Ophthalmoscopic evidence of general arterial disease has been found since 1892, when Gunn demonstrated changes in retinal fundus in which "high arterial tension suggested the probability of changes in the arteries usually associated with chronic renal disease. . . . Where an artery, even a small twig passes over a retinal vein, the circulation in the latter is much impeded" (14). Gunn presented case histories with remarkable illustrations of the retina. He believed that retinal arterial changes were associated with a more general arterial disease, particularly of the kidneys and brain; he thought that these changes had prognostic value and suggested that ophthalmoscopic observation should be used for early detection of important arterial changes. In 1975 pathogenesis of hypertensive retinopathy was investigated by Garner and associates (15). They subjected monkeys to bilateral procedures aimed at reducing, but not preventing renal blood flow. With development of hypertension, retinal angiograms using fluorescin were taken. They also examined retinal capillaries by means of electron microscopy.

They concluded that the arterioles constrict as pressure rises, leading to occlusion of the precapillary arterioles followed by dilatation and progressive plasma insudation into the vessel wall (15).

The first experimental work on animals dealing with the role of the kidney and hypertension was performed by two physicians, Paul Grawitz and Oscar Israel, who in 1879 published a paper on the relation between kidney disease and cardiac hypertrophy (16). They occluded renal arteries of rabbits, usually on one side, for a period of several hours. This temporary ischemia led to a deterioration of the injured kidney, but not to cardiac hypertrophy. Grawitz and Israel wrote, "In not a single case did the later second measurement [of blood pressure] give even minimal pressure increase." Working on dogs in 1880, Ludwig Lewinski narrowed the renal artery, but failed to measure blood pressure; nevertheless, he "decided on the blood pressure from the wall thickness of the left ventricle" (17). In some animals the heart showed moderate hypertrophy of the left ventricle. The German clinician Leyden was correct when he concluded from these experiments that "for him who has had some practice in pulse feeling, no doubt can occur, that in contracted kidney disease (Bright's disease) the tension in the aortic system is elevated" (18).

The basis for today's knowledge of hypertension was the discovery of renin by Tigerstedt and Bergman (19). Tigerstedt, professor of physiology in the Karolinska Institute in Stockholm, and his young colleague Bergman who had been a pupil of Ludwig, examined the effects of renal extracts on blood pressure (Fig. 12.1). They showed that the watery extract of rabbit kidneys raised the blood pressure, that the activity could be extracted by glycerin, and that it was stable at 56°C but was destroyed by boiling. They also demonstrated that renal vein blood raised the blood pressure when injected into nephrectomized animals and that renal extract mixed with blood also raised the blood pressure. Since they found that the pressor effects caused by renal extracts were of quicker onset and shorter duration than with renin itself, they also may have demonstrated the activity of angiotensin for the first time.

These studies formed the background for the work of Harry Goldblatt almost fifty years later (20; Fig. 12.2). He realized that narrowing of the arteries and arterioles of the kidney was an almost invariable accompaniment of high blood pressure. Goldblatt made his discovery by limiting the renal circulation without causing significant damage to the kidneys or any obvious impairment of renal excretory function. Goldblatt's studies were of fundamental importance for further research and furnished stimulus for modern research on hypertension. His research showed that moderate constriction of the renal arteries produced benign hypertension. Many of his hypertensive dogs lived for years. He also demonstrated that greater constriction of the renal arteries produced malignant hypertension. Goldblatt wrote in his retrospective statement in 1975 entitled "Reflections,"

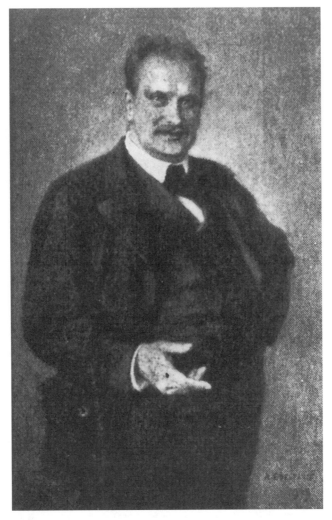

Figure 12.1. Robert A. Tigerstedt. *(Courtesy of the New York Academy of Medicine)*

"As resident in surgery 1916, I witnessed a tragic event which made me realize however that uremia alone is certainly not a sufficient condition for the elevation of the blood pressure (21). In a middle-aged woman, a kidney was removed, presumably for a tumor. It proved to be a congenital anomalous kidney, there was no tumor and therefore no other kidney. The patient survived six days, and I had the opportunity to follow the fatal course. She died in pronounced uremia but at no time was there any elevation of blood pressure"; he continued: "Contrary, therefore, to what I had been taught, I began to suspect that the vascular disease

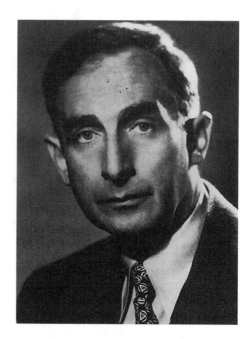

Figure 12.2. Harry Goldblatt. *(Courtesy of the New York Academy of Medicine)*

comes first and, when it involves the kidneys, the resultant impairment of the renal circulation probably, in some way, causes elevation of the blood pressure. . . . I did not know then, nor do I know now, how to produce intrarenal obliterative vascular sclerosis, so I decided to simulate the probably hemodynamic effects of wide-spread intrarenal obliterative vascular sclerosis by producing varying degrees of permanent constriction of the main renal artery of both kidneys in a series of dogs" (21).

Considerable efforts were made to repeat Tigerstedt and Bergman's experiments on the production of renin by the kidneys. But it was not until 1937 that a group in Buenos Aires headed by Braun-Menendez discovered the pressor effects of grafting kidneys into the neck of nephrectomized dogs (22, 23). Houssay, Braun-Menendez, and co-workers had left the University of Buenos Aires during the dictatorship of Peron and worked in a private house, which had been converted into laboratories. In the abstract published in 1939, they called the renal pressor substance hypertensin (23). The material was insoluble in ether, soluble in glacial acetic acid, and was destroyed after three hours of boiling in hydrochloric acid. It was formed on incubating renin with blood serum or a pseudoglobulin fraction of plasma. A more detailed article by Braun-Menendez appeared in 1940 (24).

Braun-Menendez was born in 1903 in Chile, and lived in Buenos Aires; he died in 1959 in a plane crash together with one of his nine children (25; Fig. 12.3).

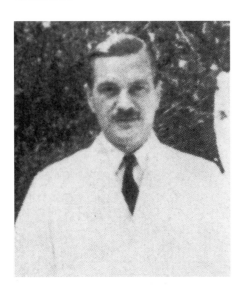

Figure 12.3. Eduardo Braun-Menendez.
(Courtesy of the Fundacion Barcelo, Univer-
sidad de Ciencias de la Salud, Escuela de
Medicina, Buenos Aires, Argentina)

He belonged to a prominent family of landowners in Patagonia and it was to
this southern tip of South America that he was flying when the plane crashed,
killing all fifty-one passengers. I (RJB) visited Houssay and Braun-Menendez
shortly after the fall of Peron, when Houssay was reinstated as professor of physiology at the university before a crowd of twelve hundred, all first-year medical
students!

Simultaneously thousands of miles to the north in Indianapolis, Irvine Page
and O. M. Helmer discovered the same pressor material and called it angiotonin
(26). In contrast to Braun-Menendez, who was quiet and reserved, Page was a
stormy petrel of science (Fig. 12.4); he had drive and originality, and the firm
conviction that he was right, qualities that did not endear him to his superiors.
He graduated from Cornell Medical College and spent two years as a resident at
the Presbyterian Hospital in New York, where he ruffled the feathers of his superiors. Following this, he established a laboratory of brain chemistry at the Kaiser-
Wilhelm Institute for Psychiatry in Munich (now Max-Planck Institute) (27).
Subsequently, he went to the Rockefeller Institute in New York to join Van
Slyke's group. Page returned to Indianapolis, to work at the Lilly Laboratory for
Clinical Research. Here he and Helmer worked on the purification of renin and
demonstrated the existence of angiotonin. By joint agreement, Braun-Menendez
and Page later named the pressor substance angiotensin. Page later moved to the
Cleveland Clinic, where he remained for the rest of his career cooperating with
Bumpus, who later independently followed up these studies at the Cleveland
Clinic. He was never elected to the Association of American Physicians or
the Society of Clinical Investigation, and his name was briefly dropped from

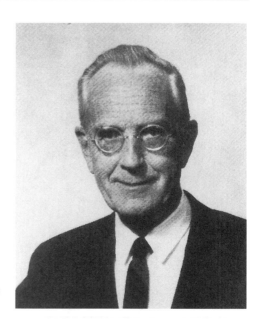

Figure 12.4. Irvine Page. *(Courtesy of the New York Academy of Medicine)*

membership of the American College of Cardiology, because he criticized their national meetings (27). Irvine Page wrote me (RJB) in 1989 when he was almost ninety years old. "I still cannot get into the Young Turks (Society for Clinical Investigation) and the Association of American Physicians. I used to care but no more. I don't even understand most of the papers in the *Journal of Clinical Investigation* and see very little clinical in them" (28). Like most older scientists, he felt that he had been passed by: "I guess each generation looks out after itself and to hell with their predecessors which make their success possible" (28). It is astonishing that he was elected to the National Academy of Science. One of Page's later contributions was the definition of the mosaic nature of hypertension, signifying the multifactorial nature of arterial pressure control and showing that hypertension represents a disregulation among these many factors.

In a moving eulogy his friends Frohlich, Dustan, and Bumpus wrote, "whether we wish to accept it or not, we are all both his legacy and the beneficiaries of his lifetime of scientific quest" (29).

The work of Braun-Menendez and of Page foreshadowed modern antihypertensive therapy, which led from the use of Rauwolfia, ganglionic blocking agents, hydralazine, and veratrum alkaloids to more useful antihypertensive therapy (30), such as thiazide diuretics, beta-blockers, angiotensin-converting enzyme (ACE) inhibitors, centrally acting antihypertensives, and calcium channel blockers.

In 1949 Vakil described one of the early clinical uses of *Rauwolfia serpentina* in treating essential hypertension in India (31). The dried root of *Rauwolfia serpentina* had been on the market in India in tablet form as treatment for hypertension. He writes, " There is hardly a patient with high blood pressure who has not been subjected to its effect in one form or another." The serpentina plant is a large, climbing or twining herb or shrub found in the Himalayas and other parts of the East. The root of the plant has been very popular as an antidote to the stings and bites of insects and poisonous reptiles. Indian workers found several alkaloids in the root that were classified, some of them acting as cardiac, respiratory, and CNS depressants. Vakil's article mentioned a moderate decline in blood pressure in a number of patients.

Chlorothiazide diuretics were described by Karl Beyer in 1982 (32). He mentioned that the discovery of chlorothiazide was a classic example of "designed discovery." He wanted a compound that would increase salt and water excretion safely when administered orally for the relief of edema, hypertension, and pre-eclampsia of pregnancy. He and his team synthesized derivatives of sulfanilamide molecules that were also carbonic anhydrase inhibitors. Beyer writes, "I doubt whether the original new drug application on chlorothiazides could be considered adequate today, as it was considered so at the time. . . . Thank goodness we did not have to prove that lowering blood pressure was good for you, before chlorothiazide could be marketed for that purpose!" It was first used only as a diuretic, but through clinical studies it was finally established that it also lowered blood pressure and was particularly useful as an additive to other antihypertensive therapy.

The development of methyldopa, still a widely used antihypertensive agent, was based on a faulty premise. It was first thought to act through inhibition of decarboxylation of amino acids (33). Sjoerdsma relates that he and Udenfriend discussed the possibility of using dopa decarboxylase inhibitors, a subject that had been previously discussed in the literature by Bing (34). From a number of compounds Udenfriend and Sjoerdsma selected alpha-methyldopa, which had been previously synthesized by Merck and Company. They believed that an effective decarboxylase inhibitor should inhibit the formation of amines. They tried various dopa analogs, but found no pharmacological or biochemical effect on catecholamine activity in the adrenal gland, not surprisingly since decarboxylation is not the rate-limiting step in catecholamine biosynthesis. When methyldopa was eventually given to patients, dramatic results were observed. Later Sjoerdsma and colleagues realized that the site action of methyldopa or one of its metabolites was in the central nervous system. An initially wrong hypothesis had led to the right solution (33).

Bing and Zucker had injected dopa into a kidney made ischemic for several hours. They recorded a marked pressure effect, presumably as a result of the formation of hydroxytyramine (34). Kuchel, on the other hand, believed that "the progression of hypertension is accompanied by a peripheral dopaminergic deficiency and diminished ability to excrete salt" (35).

The development of beta-blockers has been reported in another chapter of this book (see Chapter 10). Black first synthesized pronethalol and propranolol and referred to these agents in terms of Ahlquist's dual-receptor hypothesis (36). Several workers found a carcinogenic potential in pronethalol, which prompted Black and co-workers to look for a less toxic compound, leading to the synthesis of propranolol, which counteracts the beta-adrenergic effects of isoproterenol, adrenaline, and stimulation of the stellate ganglion. Black and Stephenson also showed that pronethalol lowered arterial pressure (37). This was the beginning of a long and successful role of beta-blockers in the treatment of hypertension. The initial report on the antihypertensive effect of beta adrenoreceptor blocking agents appeared in 1964 in a paper by Prichard (38).

There were good reasons for initial opposition to beta-adrenoreceptor blocking agents, since these compounds inhibit myocardial contractility and increase end-diastolic pressure in patients (39). Misgivings about dosage arose from the erroneous concepts of complete beta-adrenoreceptor blockade; a relatively small dose of propranalol blocked the effects of catecholamines (40). In contrast, larger doses are needed for an antihypertensive effect. We know now that beta-adrenoreceptor blocking agents are effective not only in reducing blood pressure, but also in exerting a cardioprotective effect in patients with myocardial infarction. In these individuals, beta-adrenergic-antagonist therapy, begun twenty-eight days after myocardial infarction, significantly reduced mortality for a period of at least two to three years (40).

A far-reaching development in the treatment of hypertension was the direct outcome of the work of Page and Braun-Menendez, involving inhibitions of the formation of angiotensin II. Skeggs demonstrated in 1950 that the blood of hypertensive dogs, when dialyzed and concentrated, contained angiotensin (41). Blood of patients with malignant hypertension contained as much as twenty times the level of angiotensin as compared to normal individuals. Apparently renin and angiotensin were involved in some forms of hypertension (42).

Skeggs and co-workers also purified angiotensin and discovered the existence of two forms of angiotensin, angiotensin I and II (43, 44). They found that the conversion of angiotensin I to angiotensin II occurs readily and is influenced by a protein fraction of plasma. They called this enzyme "angiotensin-converting enzyme" or ACE, which is activated by the chloride ion. Angiotensin I is the product of the action of the enzyme renin on its substrate. It does not raise the blood pressure, whereas angiotensin II is a very powerful pressor substance. It was found that angiotensin-I-converting enzyme is a zinc-metallo cell membrane peptidase, working as an ectoenzyme, with its catalytic site exposed at the extracellular surface. It acts as a dipeptidyl-carboxypeptidase, converting angiotensin I into the active octapeptide, angiotensin II, and degrading bradykinin into inactive peptides by two successive cleavages (45). Historical concepts of renal pressor mechanisms have been summarized by Skeggs (46).

A significant finding was made by Davis, who found in cross-circulation studies in dogs, that a humoral factor was responsible for the release of aldosterone from the adrenal cortex (47). Shortly thereafter it was shown by Laragh that the humoral factor stimulating aldosterone release was angiotensin (48).

It is now recognized that ACE has ubiquitous tissue distribution and can be found in all vascular endothelial cells everywhere (49) after Ng and Vane found it present in the lung (50). For example, it is expressed in smooth muscle cells of the vascular wall, in the adventitia, in the small intestine, and in the kidney proximal convoluted tubules (51, 52). In the CNS it is present in the choroid plexus; it is also found in the prostate and epididymis, macrophages, T-lymphocytes, and fibroblasts (53, 54). ACE is found in basal ganglia and in the striatonigral pathway of the CNS (55). In the heart it is present in valve leaflets, the coronary arteries, and the right atrium. Angiotensin II was also found in the vascular wall and in the adventitial and endothelial layers of the major arteries (56). An interesting finding is the presence of ACE in all cardiac valves, but not in the sino-atrial and atrioventricular nodes (57). Yamada and co-workers found that there is a markedly nonuniform distribution of ACE in the rat heart. In addition, ACE may differ in its properties in the atria and ventricles (56).

By the early 1970s knowledge of the renin angiotensin system led to the development of methods to block the formation of angiotensin (58). Groups from Sao Paolo, Brazil, the Brookhaven National Laboratory on Long Island, and the Royal College of Surgeons in London found that the venom of *Bothrops jaraca* contains enzymes that liberate kinins from plasma kininogen. The venom has two actions: it contains a bradykinin-potentiating factor correlated with the inhibition of kinin-destroying enzymes and it inhibits the peptidase that converts angiotensin I to angiotensin II (59). The converting enzyme and bradykininase inhibitor are the same enzyme (60).

The next step was taken by the pharmacological industry. Ondetti and co-workers from Squibb Laboratory found that a nonapeptide, SQ 20, 881 is a specific and potent inhibitor of angiotensin-converting enzyme in vitro and in vivo, and is also a powerful antihypertensive drug (61). They tested different structural types in their search for a specific inhibitor that would be active when administered orally. It was found that insertion of a mercapto group into the molecule led to a dramatic improvement in inhibitory potency, without any concomitant loss of specificity. They demonstrated that SQ 225, captopril, is a powerful angiotensin-converting enzyme inhibitor in vivo.

Transgenic models have furnished considerable information on the mechanism of hypertension. Numerous candidate genes have been delineated, including the various components of the renin-angiotensin system, endothelin, the components of the adrenergic or muscarinic system, and other peptides in charge of the vasomotricity. Transgenic technology has been successfully applied to the problem and used to decipher the more probable candidates on a more rational basis.

The first candidates to be explored were the various members of the renin-angiotensin-aldosterone system (RAAS), that is, angiotensinogen, renin, or angiotensin-converting enzyme (ACE). The genetic studies so far published have failed to demonstrate any association with renin, but have evidenced a linkage with angiotensinogen and ACE. Transgenic technology has confirmed genetic analysis (62, 63, 64).

Renin is extremely species-specific. Hypertension, and the consecutive left ventricular hypertrophy in the transgenic model in rats, is caused by the overexpression of mice renin. Hypertension in this model is not due to an augmented plasma level of renin, but, in fact, enhanced kinetics of the reaction between mouse renin and rat angiotensinogen; mouse renin reacts more quickly with rat angiotensinogen than rat renin (65). An overexpression of rat or human renin in mice did not result in hypertension (65, 66). Hypertension resulted in rats by overexpressing an entire human angiotensinogen gene, and in mice by overexpressing the entire rat angiotensinogen gene. The plasma levels of both angiotensinogen and angiotensin II were augmented in parallel. In transgenic hypertensive rats, in which hypertension is caused by increased plasma renin, the physiological role of angiotensinogen is a determinant of blood pressure (66, 67).

Two different groups have demonstrated that the best way to obtain a transgenic model of hypertension in mice was to target the simultaneous overexpression of the genes encoding renin and angiotensinogen. This was achieved by cross-mating separate lines of transgenic mice or rats carrying renin or angiotensinogen from either human or rat (68, 69).

The information provided by transgenic technology has so far also been contradictory, since, for example, the knockout of the endothelin-1 gene has resulted in a slight, although significant, increase in blood pressure, and pronounced craniofacial abnormalities, suggesting that the function of the peptide is more related to development than to blood pressure control (70).

Molecular biology and genetics have further elucidated the role of ACE in cardiovascular diseases. As stated by Villard and Soubrier, two forms of the enzyme have been identified, a somatic and a germinal isoform (71). The structure of these isoenzymes has been determined in humans by molecular cloning of the two c-DNAs (72, 73, 74). There is a single ACE gene per haploid genome. It contains twenty-six exons and the somatic and germinal ACE m-RNAs are transcribed from the unique genes by two different promoters (75). It is interesting that the structure of the human ACE gene provides support for the duplication of an ancestral ACE gene. In all mammalian species where the ACE gene

has been cloned, it appears to be duplicated (71). Apparently duplication occurred more than 300 million years ago. A c-DNA coding for an enzyme with
close sequence similarity to ACE has even been cloned in *Drosophila melanogaster*
and expression in mammalian cells showed that it presents similar catalytic activity to the mammalian enzyme (76).

Villard and Soubrier report on the genetic control of plasma ACE, the
insertion/deletion polymorphism of the ACE gene, and ACE gene polymorphism
in cardiovascular diseases (71). This insertion/deletion polymorphism of the ACE
gene may account for the variability in plasma ACE levels (77). Villard and
Soubrier believe that the polymorphism of expression of ACE due to unidenti-
fied etiological variants of the ACE gene may play a role in the predisposition to
various cardiovascular diseases. Polymorphism may increase in conditions where
ACE is induced (71).

ACE can be induced by a series of agents such as cyclic AMP analogs and glu-
cocorticoid hormones (78, 79, 80). After ACE inhibitor treatment, serum ACE
levels and ACE concentration increase (81, 82). In experimental models of heart
failure, both ACE activites and ACE m-RNA are increased in the left ventricular
wall, as well as in the two-kidney, one-clip model of rat hypertension (83).

The presence of ACE in the heart and coronary arteries has broad consequences for hypertension and congestive heart failure (83). In the rat with compensated experimental heart failure induced by coronary artery ligation, Hirsch
et al. found increased cardiac ACE activity possibly as a result of increased local
expression (83).

Several trials have demonstrated that ACE inhibitors have a favorable effect on survival in patients with symptomatic heart failure and reduce morbidity
of heart failure as manifested by the reduction in the number of hospitalizations
and progression of symptoms. ACE inhibitors produced a 20 percent reduction
in death or hospitalization for heart failure and a 30 percent reduction in the
number of patients who developed overt signs of heart failure. At the same time,
ACE inhibitors are also associated with a reduction of ischemic events, and they
are beneficial when administered early after myocardial infarction (84, 85, 86).

One of the advances in the knowledge of hypertension has been the recognition of the existence of an endogenous renin-angiotensin system in the heart.
This system is complete with respect to all the components of the enzymatic
pathway first described in the kidney (87). In the early 1990s it became known that
angiotensinogen, renin, and angiotensin-converting enzyme (ACE) are present
in heart muscle. Equally present are functional angiotensin II receptors (87).
This endogenous renin-angiotensin system in the heart has far-reaching physiological importance as far as coronary vasoreactivity, systolic and diastolic function, and hypertrophy of the heart are concerned. It was found that cardiac ACE
activity and m-RNA are increased in the hypertrophied ventricle and that the

increased rate of angiotensin II production is associated with altered diastolic properties in hypertrophied hearts (88). Ventricular remodeling, as it may occur after myocardial ischemia, is also influenced by the endogenous presence of the renin-angiotensin system. It is likely that remodeling, such as infarct expansion, myocyte hypertrophy, myocyte slippage, and growth of cardiac interstitium, are all influenced by angiotensin II (89). Inhibition of intracardiac angiotensin-converting enzyme also appears to improve diastolic function in patients with left ventricular hypertrophy due to aortic stenosis (89). Equally, ACE inhibitors decrease left ventricular endothelial diastolic pressure, and prevent or attenuate the development of right ventricular and left ventricular hypertrophy and dilatation caused by aortocaval shunt. This action appears to be specific for certain ACE inhibitors (90).

It has been suspected for many years that stretch of the heart muscle is a stimulus for cardiac hypertrophy and the development of myocardial failure. Recent observations have illustrated that stretch of the heart muscle is responsible for the release of angiotensin II; this was first observed in cardiac myocytes in vitro (91). The intracellular signaling mechanism for the production of hypertrophy is the release of angiotensin II. Sadoshima and co-workers working on cultured ventricular cardiac myocytes exposed to uniaxial strain found that stretching cardiomyocytes in vitro causes release of angiotensin II and increases the expression of the angiotensinogen gene. Angiotensin II was also observed in the secretory granule-like structure of ventricular myocytes (91).

Sadoshima as well as Izumo also studied the effects of angiotensin II in primary cultured cardiac myocytes, and found that the hypertrophy of cardiac myocytes and hyperplasia of cardiac nonmyocytes was induced by the expression of a number of genes such as c-fos, c-jun, junB, Egr-1, and c-myc. Production of c-fos also occurs upon stretching of cardiomyocytes (91, 92). Komuro et al. showed that stretching of myocytes stimulated expression of the protooncogene c-fos in a stretch length-dependent manner, and was followed by an increase in amino acid incorporation into proteins (93). c-fos RNA levels were enhanced within fifteen minutes by cardiocyte stretching and peaked at thirty minutes. Apparently angiotensin II directly stimulates protein synthesis and cell growth as demonstrated by Baker (94). The angiotensin II-induced growth response does not result in cellular division but in hypertrophy of individual myocytes (94).

It is interesting that ACE inhibitors and kininogen can significantly increase nitrite production in coronary microvessels, thus reducing oxygen consumption in cardiac muscle slices (95). A reduction in myocardial oxygen demands due to nitric oxide production might benefit ischemia. How nitric oxide, released in response to ACE inhibitors, affects myocardial oxygen consumption remains to be seen.

A genetic background may also influence the development of cardiac hypertrophy (96). In a study, based primarily on the evidence of hypertrophy by electrocardiographic findings, it was found that many individuals with electrocardiographic evidence of left ventricular hypertrophy were normotensive, suggesting that genetics may influence the development of left ventricular hypertrophy. A molecular genetic marker, a deletion polymorphism in intron 16 of the ACE gene, was identified in association with electrocardiographic evidence of left ventricular hypertrophy.

The main focus has been on the role of ACE inhibitors in the treatment of hypertension. It is, however, apparent that complete blockade of the renin-angiotensin system is not achieved with ACE inhibitors alone. In 1988 Urata and co-workers found that the major enzymatic pathway for angiotensin II formation in the myocardium was not suppressed by ACE inhibitors (97). They therefore suspected a dual pathway for angiotensin II formation by the human heart. Definite support for a dual system has come from the work of Wolny (98). In the first place angiotensin II levels returned to normal despite ACE inhibitor therapy (99, 100). Second, a renin inhibitor was more effective than ACE inhibitors. Third, additive blood pressure-lowering effects were reported in hypertensive patients when an angiotensin II receptor blocker was added to an ACE inhibitor (101). ACE inhibitors do not block more than 40 percent of the contraction in human arteries or in human detrusor muscle induced by angiotensin I (102, 103).

These findings suggest new therapeutic approaches to the treatment of cardiac hypertrophy and hypertension. The focal point in this new development is an enzyme, possibly a chymase, a serine protease that is able to form angiotensin II from angiotensin I but is not blocked by ACE inhibitors (97). Chymase is present in human hearts, and is an angiotensin II-forming enzyme (104). Like ACE, chymase is present in many human tissues, particularly blood vessels, lung, kidney, and liver. It is also localized in the cardiac muscle in several cell types, including mast cells and endothelial cells. In contrast to ACE, however, chymase is not present in plasma (97). Furthermore, chymase is secreted by endothelial cells toward the basolateral site, while ACE is located on the luminal suface (98). Wolny has demonstrated the importance of serine protease inhibitors, which significantly inhibit angiotensin II formation (98). This suggests that in left ventricular muscle and in coronary artery homogenates, a serine protease, probably chymase, is the major enzyme converting angiotensin I to angiotensin II. Wolny and co-workers raised the question whether ACE is sufficiently blocked and whether current therapy with ACE inhibitors can be improved (98).

Since the death of President Franklin Delano Roosevelt progress in recognizing, understanding, and treating hypertension has been spectacular. This was primarily due to the recognition of the role of hypertension in the mortality from coronary, cerebral, and peripheral vascular disease (105). Several studies have shown the effectiveness of antihypertensive drugs in reducing morbidity and mortality in hypertensive middle-aged men with sustained elevated blood pressure. Drug treatment produced a significant reduction of morbidity of men with baseline diastolic blood pressure averaging 105 to 114 ml/Hg (106). In the 1970s 85 percent of persons with high blood pressure were inadequately controlled (105). The suggestion was made that a net diastolic blood pressure differences of only 5 mm to 6 mm of Hg should be treated with antihypertensive drugs, and that even this small reduction in blood pressure had great potential for reducing mortality; treatment of even uncomplicated mild hypertension was considered essential. Whether treatment for mild hypertension should be directed only at those with other risk factors is still controversial. But even in uncomplicated patients with a diastolic blood pressure of 90 mm to 94 mm Hg there was substantial benefit from antihypertensive therapy.

The question arises whether success in the treatment of hypertension is the result of fundamental research or of epidemiological or clinical studies. The lion's share must be given to basic research although epidemiological data created the motivation. Pioneers have built the foundation, working with relatively primitive tools. Tigerstedt and Bergman used only aqueous extracts of the kidney to obtain renin. Braun-Menendez and Page used alcohol and ether to extract angiotensin. In contrast, Wolny and associates in 1997, in discovering the importance of a chymase in the formation of angiotonin II, used isotope labeling, high-pressure liquid chromatography, radioimmunoassay, polyclonal antibodies, and ultrasonification, among others. Sophistication of techniques has now limited scientific research to a few well-equipped laboratories. Tigerstedt and Bergman's fundamental experiment may have cost less than $10. Today's pharmacological advances need a budget reaching into the hundred of thousands of dollars with investigators with a high degree of technical sophistication. This has led to dependency on granting agencies or commerical sources. But money can never buy originality and inspiration. Originality and inspiration have been responsible for the fact that the conquest of hypertension has become one of the success stories of modern medicine.

References

1. Bruenn, H.G. Clinical notes on the illness and death of President Franklin D. Roosevelt. Ann. Intern. Med., 72:579–591, 1970.
2. Barach, A.L. Franklin Roosevelt's illness. Effect on course of history. New York State J. Med., 2154–2157, November 1977.
3. Harriman, W.A. Military Situation in the Far East. Hearings before the Committee on Armed Services and the Committee on Foreign Relations, U.S. Senate, 82nd Congress, 1st Session, Part 5—Appendix and Index, U.S. Government. Printing Office, 3330–3331, 3341, 1951.
4. Messerli, F.H. Occasional notes, this day 50 years ago. New Engl. J. Med., 332:1038–1039, 1995.
5. White, P.D. Heart Disease. New York, Macmillan, 2nd ed., 1937.
6. O'Brien, E., and D. Fitzgerald. The history of blood pressure measurement. Journal of Human Hypertension, 8:73–84, 1954.

7. Cameron, J.S. The description of essential hypertension by Frederick Akhbar Mahomed. Nephrology Dialysis Transplant., 10:1244–1247, 1995.
8. Dock, W. Korotkoff sounds. New Engl. J. Med., 302:1264–1267, 1980.
9. Krilov, D.O. On measuring the blood pressure by the sound method of Dr. N.S. Korotkov. Bull. Imperial Mil. Medicine Academy (St. Petersburg), 13:221, 1906.
10. Borsatti, A., M. Rippa-Bonati, and A. Antonello. Familial hypertension in Morgagni's de Sedibus et Causis Morborum per Anatomen Indagatis. American Journal of Nephrology, 14:432–435, 1994.
11. Bright, R. Tabular view of the morbid appearances in 100 cases connected with albuminous urine with observations. Guy's Hospital Reports, 1:380–400, 1836.
12. Gordon, D.B. Some early investigations of experimental hypertension: an historical review. Texas Rep. Biol. Med., 28:179–188, 1970.
13. Traube, L. Ueber den Zusammenhang von Herz- und Nieren-Krankheiten. In: Gesammelte Beitraege zur Pathologie und Physiologie (Collected Contributions to Pathology and Physiology), II:290–353, 1871.
14. Gunn, M. On ophthalmoscopic evidence of general arterial disease. Trans. Ophthalmol. Soc. U.K., 18:356–381, 1898.
15. Garner, A., N. Ashton, R. Tripathi, E.M. Kohner, C.J. Bulpitt, and C.T. Dollery. Pathogenesis of hypertensive retinopathy: an experimental study in the monkey. British Journal of Ophthalmology, 59:3–44, 1975.
16. Grawitz, P., and O. Israel. Experimentelle Untersuchung ueber den Zusammenhang zwischen Nierenerkrankung und Herzhypertrophie. Archiv. fuer Pathologische Anatomie und Physiologie und fuer Klinische Medizin, 77:315–346, 1879.
17. Lewinski, L. Ueber den Zusammenhang zwischen Nierenschrumpfung und Herzhypertrophie. Z. Klin. Med., 1:561–582, 1880.
18. Leyden, E. Klinische Untersuchungen ueber Morbus Brightii. Ueber Nierenschrumpfung und Nierensklerose. Z. Klin. Med., 2:133–171, 1881.
19. Tigerstedt, R., and P.G. Bergman. Niere und Kreislauf. Skand. Arch. Physiol., 8:223, 1898.
20. Goldblatt, H., J. Lynch, R.F. Hanzal, and W.W. Sumerville. Studies on experimental hypertension. 1: The production of persistent elevation of systolic blood pressure by means of renal ischemia. J. Exp. Med., 59:347–379, 1934.
21. Goldblatt, H. Reflections. The urologic clinics of North America. Symposium on management of renovascular hypertension, 2:219–221, 1975.
22. Munoz, J.M., E. Braun-Menendez, J.C. Fasciolo, and L.F. Leloir. Hypertensin: the substance causing renal hypertension. Nature, 144:980, 1939.
23. Peart, W. S. Evolution of renin. Supplement III: Hypertension, 18:100–108, 1991.
24. Braun-Menendez, E., J.C. Fasciolo, L.F. Leloir, and J.M. Munoz. The substance causing renal hypertension. J. Physiol., 98:283–298, 1940.
25. Foglia, V.G. E. Braun-Menendez, 1903–1959. Necrologia. Revista arg. de endocrinologia y metabolismo, 5:57–59, 1960.
26. Page, I.H., and O.M. Helmer. A crystalline pressor substance (angiotonin) resulting from the reaction between renin and renin activator. J. Exp. Med., 71:29, 1940.
27. McBride, G., P. Gunby, W. Check, E. Gonzalez, R. Johnson, and M. Preston. Irvine H. Page, M.D.: Not one man, but many. JAMA, 244:1765–1773, 1980.
28. Page, I.H. Personal letter sent to the author (R.J. Bing), 1989.
29. Frohlich, E.D., H.P. Dustan, and F. M. Bumpus. Irvine H. Page (1901–1991): The celebration of a leader. Hypertension, 18:443–445, 1991.
30. Brest, A.N. Milestones in clinical pharmacology. Antihypertensive drug therapy: A 30-year retrospective. Clinical Therapeutics, 14:78–80, 1992.
31. Vakil, R.J. A clinical trial of Rauwolfia serpentina in essential hypertension. Br. Heart J., 11:350–355, 1949.
32. Beyer, K.H. Chlorothiazide. Br. J. Clin. Pharmacol., 13:15–24, 1982.
33. Sjoerdsma, A. Methyldopa. Br. J. Clin. Pharmacol., 13:45–49, 1982.

34. Bing, R.J., and M.B. Zucker. Renal hypertension produced by an amino acid. J. Exp. Med., 74:235–246, 1941.
35. Kuchel, O.G., and G.A. Kuchel. Peripheral dopamine in pathophysiology of hypertension. Interaction with aging and lifestyle. Hypertension, 18:709–721, 1991.
36. Black, J.W., A.M. Duncan, and R.G. Shanks. Comparison of some properties of pronethalol and propranolol. Br. J. Pharmacol., 25:577–591, 1965.
37. Black, J.W., and J.S. Stephenson. Pharmacology of a new adrenergic beta-receptor-blocking compound (Nethalide). Lancet, 2:311–314, 1962.
38. Prichard, B.N.C. Propanolol and β-adrenergic receptor blocking drugs in the treatment of hypertension. Br. J. Clin. Pharmacol., 13:51–60, 1964.
39. Robin, E., C. Cowan, P. Puri, S. Ganguly, E. DeBoyrie, M. Martinez, T. Stock, and R.J. Bing. A comparative study of nitroglycerin and propanolol. Circulation, 36:175–186, 1967.
40. Hennekens, C.H., C.M. Albert, S.L. Godfried, J.M. Gaziano, and J.E. Buring. Adjunctive drug therapy of acute myocardial infarction—evidence from clinical trials. New Engl. J. Med., 335:1660–1667, 1996.
41. Skeggs, L.T., J.R. Kahn, and N.P. Shumway. The isolation of hypertensin from the circulating blood of normal dogs with experimental renal hypertension by dialysis in an artificial kidney. Circulation, 3:384–389, 1951.
42. Kahn, J.R., L.T. Skeggs, N.P. Shumway, and P.E. Wisenbaugh. The assay of hypertension from the arterial blood of normotensive and hypertensive human beings. J. Exp. Med., 95:523–529, 1952.
43. Skeggs, Jr., L.T., W.H. Marsh, J.R. Kahn, and N.P. Shumway. The purification of hypertensin I. J. Exp. Med., 100:363–370, 1954.
44. Skeggs Jr., L.T., W.H. Marsh, J.R. Kahn, and N.P. Shumway. The existence of two forms of hypertension. J. Exp. Med., 99:275–282, 1954.
45. Ryan, J.W., U.S. Ryan, D.R. Schultz, C. Whitaker, A. Chung, and F.E. Dorer. Subcellular localization of pulmonary angiotensin converting enzyme kininase II. Biochem. J., 146:497–499, 1975.
46. Skeggs, Jr., L.T. Currrent concepts and historical perspectives of renal pressor mechanisms. Journal of Hypertension, 4:S3–S10, 1986.
47. Davis, J.O. Importance of the renin-angiotensin system in the control of aldosterone secretion. In: Hormones and the Kidney, Williams, P.C. (ed.). New York, Academy Press, 1963, pp. 325–329.
48. Laragh, J.H., M. Angers, W.G. Kelly, and S. Lieberman. Hypotensive agents and pressor substances. JAMA, 174:234–240, 1960.
49. Ryan, U.S., J.W. Ryan, C. Whitaker, and A. Chiu. Localization of angiotensin-converting enzyme (kininase II). II. Immunocytochemical and immunofluorescence. Tissue Cell, 8:125–145, 1976.
50. Ng, K.K., and J.R. Vane. Some properties of angiotensin converting enzyme in the lung in vivo. Nature, 225:1142–1144, 1970.
51. Battle, T., J.F. Arnal, M. Challah, and J.B. Michel. Selective isolation of rat aortic wall layers and their cell types in culture—application to converting enzyme activity measurements. Tissue Cell, 26:943–955, 1994.
52. Bruneval, P., N. Hinglais, F. Alhenc-Gelas et al. Angiotensin I converting enzyme in human intestine and kidney. Ultrastructural immunohistochemical localization. Histochemistry, 85:73–80, 1986.
53. Costerousse, O., J. Allegrini, M. Lopez, and F. Alhenc-Gelas. Angiotensin I-converting enzyme in human circulating mononuclear cells: genetic polymorphism of expression in T-lymphocytes. Biochem. J., 290:33–40, 1993.
54. Weinberg, K.S., W.H.J. Douglas, D.R. MacNamee, J.J. Lanzillo, and B.L. Fanburg. Angiotensin I-converting enzyme localization on cultured fibroblasts by immunofluorescence. In Vitro, 18:400–406, 1982.

55. Barnes, K., R. Matsas, N.M. Hooper, A.J. Turner, and A.J. Kenny. Endopeptidase 24.11 is striosomally ordered in pig brain and, in contrast to aminopeptidase N and dipeptidyl dipeptidase, an angiotensin converting enzyme, is a marker for a set of striatal efferent fibers. Neuroscience, 27:799–817, 1988.

56. Yamada, H., B. Fabris, A.M. Allen, B. Jackson, C.I. Johnston, and F.A.O. Mendelsohn. Localization of angiotensin converting enzyme in rat heart. Circ. Res., 68:141–149, 1991.

57. Sun, Y., and K.T. Weber. Tissue angiotensin converting enzyme (TACE) and myocardial remodeling after infarction. In: Abstracts, 15th Meeting of the International Society of Hypertension, Melbourne, March 1994, S187, 1033.

58. Skeggs, L. T., Jr. Historical overview of the renin-angiotensin system. In: Hypertension and the Angiotensin System: Therapeutic Approaches, Doyle, A.E., and A.G. Bearn (eds.). New York, Raven Press, 1984.

59. Ferreira, S.H., L.J. Greene, V.A. Alabaster, et al. Activity of various fractions of bradykinin potentiating factor against angiotensin I converting enzyme. Nature (London), 225:379, 1970.

60. Greene, L.J., C.M. Camargo, E.M. Krieger, et al. Inhibition of the conversion of angiotensin I to angiotensin II and potentiation of bradykinin by small peptides present in Bothrops jararaca venom. Circ. Res., 31:62–71, 1972.

61. Ondetti, M.A., B. Rubin, and D.W. Cushman. Design of specific inhibitors of angiotensin-converting enzyme. New class of orally effective antihypertensive agents. Science, 196:441–444, 1977.

62. Franz, W.M., D. Breves, K. Klingel, G. Brem, P.H. Hofschneider, and R. Kandolf. Heart-specific targeting of firefly luciferase by the myosin light chain-2 promoter and developmental regulation in transgenic mice. Circ. Res., 73:629–638, 1993.

63. Paul, M., and W.M. Franz. Transgenic models for hypertension research. Trends Cardiovasc. Med., 5:108–114, 1995.

64. Corvol, P., and A. Charru (eds.). Génétique des maladies cardiovasculaires. Paris, Bristol-Myers Squibb Cardiovasculaire Pub., 1993.

65. Tokita, Y., R. Franco-Saenz, E.M. Reimann, and P.J. Mulrow. Hypertension in the transgenic rat TGR (mRen-2) 27 may be due to enhanced kinetics of the reaction between mouse renin and rat angiotensinogen. Hypertension, 23:422–427, 1994.

66. Ganten, D., J. Wagner, K. Zeh, M. Bader, J.B. Michel, M. Paul, F. Zimmermann, P. Ruf, U. Hilgenfeldt, U. Ganten, M. Kaling, S. Bachmann, A. Fukamizu, J.J. Mullins, and K. Murakami. Species specificity of renin kinetics in transgenic rats harboring the human renin and angiotensinogen gene. Proceedings of the National Academy of Sciences USA, 89:7806–7810, 1992.

67. Kimura, S., J.J. Mullins, B. Bunnemann, R. Metzger, U. Hilgenfeldt, F. Zimmermann, H. Jacob, K. Fuxe, D. Ganten, and M. Kaling. High blood pressure in transgenic mice carrying the rat angiotensinogen gene. EMBO Journal, 11:821–827, 1992.

68. Fukamizu, A., K. Sugimura, E. Takimoto, F. Sugyama, M.S. Seo, S. Takahashi, T. Hatoe, K-i Yagami, and K. Murakami. Chimeric renin-angiotensin system demonstrates sustained increase in blood pressure of transgenic mice carrying both human renin and human angiotensinogen. J. Biol. Chem., 268:11617–11621, 1993.

69. Ohkubo, H., H. Kawakami, Y. Kahehi, T. Takumi, H. Arai, Y. Yokota, M. Iwai, Y. Tanabe, M. Masu, J. Hata, H. Iwao, H. Okamoto, M. Yokoyama, T. Nomura, M. Katsuki, and D. Nakanishi. Generation of transgenic mice with elevated blood pressure by introduction of the rat renin and angiotensinogen genes. Proceedings of the National Academy of Sciences, 87:5153–5157, 1990.

70. Kurihara, Y., H. Kurihara, H. Suzuki, T. Komada, K. Mamura, R. Nagai, H. Oda, T. Kuwaki, W-H. Cao, N. Kamada, K. Jishage, Y. Ouchi, S. Azuma, Y. Toyoda, T. Ishikawa, M. Kumada, and Y. Yazaki. Elevated blood pressure and craniofacial abnormalities in mice deficient in endothelin-1. Nature, 368:703–710, 1994.

71. Villard, E., and F. Soubrier. Molecular biology and genetics of the angiotensin-I-converting enzyme: potential implications in cardiovascular diseases. Cardiovasc. Res., 32:999–1007, 1996.

72. Soubrier, F., F. Alhenc-Gelas, C. Hubert, et al. Two putative active centers in human angiotensin I-converting enzyme revealed by molecular cloning. Proc. Natl. Acad. Sci. USA, 85:9386–9390, 1988.

73. Lattion, A.L., F. Soubrier, J. Allegrini, C. Hubert, P. Corvol, and F. Alhenc-Gelas. The testicular transcript of the angiotensin I-converting enzyme encodes for the ancestral, non-duplicated form of the enzyme. FEBS Lett., 252:99–104, 1989.

74. Ehlers, M.R.W., E.A. Fox, D.J. Strydom, and J.F. Riordan. Molecular cloning of human testicular angiotensin-converting enzyme: the testis isozyme is identical to the C-terminal half of endothelial angiotensin-converting enzyme. Proc. Natl. Acad. Sci. USA, 86:7741–7745, 1989.

75. Hubert, C., A.M. Houot, P. Corvol, and F. Soubrier. Structure of the angiotensin I-converting enzyme gene. Two alternate promoters correspond to evolutionary steps of a duplicated gene. J. Biol. Chem., 266:15377–15383, 1991.

76. Cornell, M.J., T.A. Williams, L.S. Lamango, D. Coates, P. Corvol, F. Soubrier, J. Hoheisel, H. Lehrach, and R.E. Issac. Cloning and expression of an evolutionary conserved single-domain angiotensin converting enzyme from Drosophila melanogaster. J. Biol. Chem., 270:13613–13619, 1995.

77. Rigat, B., C. Hubert, F. Alhenc-Gelas, F. Cambien, P. Corvol, and F. Soubrier. An insertion/deletion polymorphism in the angiotensin I-converting enzyme gene accounting for half the variance of serum enzyme levels. J. Clin. Invest., 86:1343–1346, 1990.

78. Friedland, J., C. Setton, and E. Silverstein. Angiotensin converting enzyme induction by steroids in rabbit alveolar macrophages in culture. Science, 197:64–65, 1977.

79. Friedland, J., C. Setton, and E. Silverstein. Induction of angiotensin-converting enzyme in human monocytes in culture. Biochem. Biophys. Res. Commun., 83:843–849, 1978.

80. Fishel, R., V. Thourani, S.J. Eisenberg, S.Y. Shai, M.A. Corson, E.G. Nabel, K.E. Bernstein, and B.C. Berk. Fibroblast growth factor stimulates angiotensin converting enzyme expression in vascular smooth muscle cells. J. Clin. Invest., 95:377–387, 1995.

81. Kokubu, T.E., E. Ueda, M. Ono, T. Kawabe, Y. Hayashi, and T. Kan. Effects of captopril (SQ14,255) on the renin-angiotensin-aldosterone system in normal rats. Eur. J. Pharmacol., 62:269–275, 1980.

82. Fyhrquist, F., T. Florslund, I. Tikkanen, and C. Gronhagen-Riska. Induction of angiotensin-converting enzyme in rat lung with captopril. Eur. J. Pharmacol., 67:473–475, 1980.

83. Hirsch, A.T., C.E. Talsness, H. Schunkert, M. Paul, and V.J. Dzau. Tissue-specific activation of cardiac angiotensin converting enzyme in experimental heart failure. Circ. Res., 69:475–482, 1991.

84. Kubo, S.H. Treatment of heart failure with angotensin converting enzyme inhibitors. In: Congestive Heart Failure: From Basic Science to Therapeutics. Puddu, P.E., R.J. Bing, P.P. Campa, and P.A. Poole-Wilson (eds.). Roma, Cardioricerca, 1997, pp. 302–328.

85. Konstam, M.A., M.W. Kronberg, M.F. Rousseau et al. Effects of the angiotensin converting enzyme inhibitor, enalapril, on the long-term progression of left ventricular dilation in patients with asymptomatic systolic dysfunction. Circulation, 88:2277–2283, 1993.

86. Braunwald, E. ACE inhibitors—a cornerstone of the treatment of heart failure. New Engl. J. Med., 20:301–306, 1991.

87. Lindpaintner, K., and D. Ganten. The cardiac renin-angiotensin system: an appraisal of present experimental and clinical evidence. Circ. Res., 68:905–921, 1991.

88. Schunkert, H., V.J. Dzau, S.S. Tang, A.T. Hirsch., C.S. Apstein, and B.H. Lorell. Increased rat cardiac angiotensin converting enzyme activity and mRNA expression in pressure overload left ventricular hypertrophy: effect on coronary resistance, contractility, and relaxation. J. Clin. Invest., 86:1913–1920, 1990.

89. MacDonald, K. Relative effects of alpha adrenergic blockade, converting enzyme inhibitor therapy, and angiotensin II subtype I receptor blockade on ventricular remodeling in the dog. Circulation, 90:3034–3036, 1994.

90. Friedrich, S.P., B.H. Lorell, M.F. Rousseau, W. Hayashida, O.M. Hess, P.S. Douglas, S. Gordon, C.S. Keighley, C. Benedict, H.P. Krayenbuehl, W. Grossman, and H. Pouleur. Intracardiac angiotensin-converting enzyme inhibition improves diastolic function in patients with left ventricular hypertrophy due to aortic stenosis. Circulation, 90:2761–2771, 1994.

91. Sadoshima, J-I, Y. Xu, H.S. Slayter, and S. Izumo. Autocrine release of angiotensin II mediates stretch-induced hypertrophy of cardiac myocytes in vitro. Cell, 75:977–984, 1993.

92. Sadoshima, J.I., and S. Izumo. Molecular characterization of angiotensin II-induced hypertrophy of cardiac myocytes and hyperplasia of cardiac fibroblasts: critical role of the AT, receptor subtype. Circ. Res., 73:413–423, 1993.

93. Komuro, I., T. Kaida, Y. Shibazaki, M. Kurabayashi, Y. Katoh, E. Hoh, F. Takaku, and Y. Yazaki. Stretching cardiac myocytes stimulates protooncogene expression. J. Biol. Chem., 265:3595–3598, 1990.

94. Baker, K.M., and J.F. Aceto. Angiotensin II stimulation of protein synthesis and cell growth in chick heart cells. Am. J. Physiol., 259:H610–H618, 1990.

95. Zhang, X., Y-W. Xie, A. Nasjletti, X. Xu, M.S. Wolin, and T.H. Hintze. ACE inhibitors promote nitric oxide accumulation to modulate myocardial oxygen consumption. Circulation, 95:176–182, 1997.

96. Schunkert, H., H. Hans-Werner, S.R. Holmer, M. Stender, S. Perz, U. Keil, B.H. Lorell, and G.A.J. Riegger. Association between a deletion polymorphism of the angiotensin-converting enzyme gene and left ventricular hypertrophy. New Engl. J. Med., 330:1634–1638, 1994.

97. Urata, H., B. Healy, R.W. Stewart, F.M. Bumpus, and A. Husain. Angiotensin II-forming pathways in normal and failing human hearts. Circ. Res., 66:883–890, 1990.

98. Wolny, A., J.P. Clozel, J. Rein, P. Mory, P. Vogt, M. Turino, W. Kiowski, and W. Fischli. Functional and biochemical analysis of angiotensin II-forming pathways in the human heart. Circ. Res., 80:219–227, 1997.

99. Biollaz, J., H.R. Brunner, I. Gavras, B. Waeber, and H. Gavras. Antihypertensive therapy with MK 421: angiotensin-renin relationships to evaluate efficacy of converting enzyme blockade. J. Cardiovasc. Pharmacol., 4:966–972, 1982.

100. Mento, P.F., and B.M. Wilkes. Plasma angiotensins and blood pressure during converting enzyme inhibition. Hypertension, 9:III42–III48, 1987.

101. Azizi, M., G. Chatellier, T.T. Guyene, D.M. Geoffroy, and J. Menard. Additive effects of combined angiotensin-converting enzyme inhibition and angiotensin II antagonism on blood pressure and renin release in sodium-depleted normotensives. Circulation, 92:825–834, 1995.

102. Lindberg, B.F., L.G. Nilsson, H. Hedlund, M. Stahl, and K.E. Andersson. Angiotensin I is converted to angiotensin II by a serine protease in human detrusor smooth muscle. Am. J. Physiol., 266:R1861–R1867, 1994.

103. Okunishi, H., Y. Oka, N. Shiota, T. Kawamoto, K. Song, and M. Miyazaki. Marked species-difference in the vascular angiotensin II-forming pathways: humans versus rodents. Jpn. J. Pharmacol., 62:207–210, 1993.

104. Kinoshita, A., H. Urata, F.M. Bumpus, and A. Husain. Multiple determinants for the high substrate specificity of an angiotensin II-forming chymase from the human heart. J. Biol. Chem., 266:19192–19197, 1991.

105. Hypertension detection and follow up program cooperative group. Five-year findings of the hypertension detection and follow-up program. 1) Reduction in mortality of persons with high blood pressure, including mild hypertension. JAMA, 242: 2562–2571, 1979.
106. Veterans Administration cooperative study group on antihypertensive agents. Effects of treatment on morbidity in hypertension: III. Influence of age, diastolic pressure, and prior cardiovascular disease; further analysis of side effects. Circulation, 45:991–1004, 1972.

Molecular Biology and Genetics of Cardiovascular Diseases

Chapter 13

R.J. BING
K. SCHWARTZ
G. BONNE

The Beginnings

Progress in molecular biology has been logarithmic. It has taken years to progress from Miescher's discovery of nuclein in 1869 to Kossel's nucleic acid to the DNA of Levene, the transforming role of DNA by Avery, the symmetry of bases by Chargaff, and the double helix of Watson and Crick. Then the floodgates opened and a torrent of discoveries and new techniques appeared. We now deal with a new science that is changing the world (1, 2, 3, 4). A new scientific language has been created.

This chapter begins with an early history of molecular biology; it extends to the discovery of the double helix, a period that might be called the heroic age of molecular biology. Heroic figures bestrode the stage of science. The second period started around 1960 and continues up to the present. It is the period of genetic engineering using methods allowing the isolation and characterization of individual genes. We have now learned to recognize the changes in a gene in individuals afflicted with a certain disease. New technologies have led to molecular genetic tools for use in forensic medicine, molecular diagnostics, and therapy (1). More than four thousand human disorders are known to be caused by genetic defects (1). The science of molecular genetics has also made it possible to alter defective genes and reinsert corrected genes. DNA molecules can be changed and genes can be introduced into certain living organisms by in vivo or ex vivo methods.

Matthew Meselson defined the latest period as the "great dispersal." "The field was like a river hitting sand" (4). Freeland Judson put it in perspective: a

symposium of molecular biologists at Cold Spring Harbor in 1941 had 85 participants and 33 papers. In 1989 in a symposium devoted to immunological recognition alone there were 446 participants and 114 speakers. With growth came
dispersion and increased and more ruthless competition. The development of
technical methods became of paramount interest (4). Clearly, the foundations of
molecular genetics rest on a few massive columns built by a few pioneers.

PROTEINS AS ESSENTIAL GENETIC MATERIAL?

At the onset, proteins were considered the leading candidates for the genetic
material. It took a considerable amount of time to prove that deoxyribonucleic
acid (DNA) was important in the process of reproduction. It began in 1869, just
after Mendel's discovery, when a Swiss scientist, Friedrich Miescher, found that
a substance derived from cell nuclei differed from protein; it contained phosphorus and dissolved in alkali but not in water. Miescher called this substance
nuclein (5). He obtained the material from bandages from surgical wounds that
contained large amounts of pus cells. Later he obtained the material from salmon
sperm.

After Miescher's death it was established that the nucleic material was
acid in nature and it was named nucleic acid. Forty years later a German
chemist, Albrecht Kossel, found that the basic composition of nucleic acid included four nitrogen-containing compounds, the purines adenine and guanine
and the pyrimidines thymine and cytosine. Kossel, a native of Rostock, a university town in the north of Germany, was awarded the Nobel prize in 1910.
He foresaw the biological significance of nucleic acid and felt that the future
would stress the "dynamic rather than the static importance of nucleic acid";
the future would emphasize the dynamic metabolic pathways rather than the
static (chemical) structure (6). He concluded from his physiological studies
that nucleic acids act neither as storage compounds nor as energy sources but
are closely involved in the synthesis of fresh tissues. Later he suggested that
chromatin might be the free acid. He wrote, "the occurrence of nucleic acid is
confined to the cell nucleus, indeed to a part of the nucleus which has been
long known by the name 'chromatin,' on account of its tendency to take up
basic dyes" (3).

ROCKEFELLER INSTITUTE, NEW YORK

The scene now shifted to the Rockefeller Institute in New York City (now the
Rockefeller University), where Phoebus A. T. Levene showed that the sugar in
nucleic acid was a ribose or a deoxyribose. Later deoxyribose (desoxyribose) be-
came deoxyribonucleic acid (DNA) and ribose became ribonucleic acid (RNA).
RNA was distinguished from DNA by one base. Where DNA contains thymine,
RNA contains uracil. Both DNA and RNA have a phosphate group (7). Before

coming to this country Levene had studied with Alexander Borodin, professor of chemistry in Moscow, who was distinguished not only by being an outstanding chemist, but more so as one of the great composers of the nineteenth century. Phoebus A. Levene had come to America in 1891 at the age of twenty-one (3). Afflicted with tuberculosis, he spent some time at a sanatorium, Saranac Lake, where he later worked as a chemist. Simon Flexner, the director at the Rockefeller Institute in New York, invited him to join his staff. In 1929 Levene carried out enzymatic studies that led to the identification of the sugar in thymus nucleic acid as desoxyribose (7). His early experience in Pavlov's laboratory in Moscow was helpful because there he had learned to use techniques, such as the construction of an intestinal fistula in dogs, which made it possible to achieve nucleic acid hydrolysis under controlled conditions by passing thymonucleic acid through the stomach and collecting it from the intestine. He obtained the nucleosides of the two purines and the two pyrimidines and their constituent sugar, which turned out to be a ribose or a deoxyribose (3). Levene, however, mistakenly proposed the idea that each nucleic acid molecule was an aggregation of the four bases (tetranucleotide) and that this aggregation repeated itself in a monotonous fashion (3). Later it was found by the German biophysicist Robert Feulgen, using a dye fuchsin, that DNA is largely present in the nucleus and RNA in the cytoplasm (8).

These findings still did not alter the general belief that proteins were the significant genetic material. This began to change when a medical officer in the British Ministry of Health, Fred Griffith, studied two types of pneumococci, one nonpathogenic with a rough coating, the other pathogenic with a smooth coating and capable of causing the disease (3). In his experiment he mixed live rough with the dead smooth bacteria and injected both into mice. Since the smooth bacteria, which are pathogenic, were dead the mice should not have developed pneumonia. However, the mice died and Griffith found that there were many live smooth pathogenic pneumococci in the animals' systems. He erroneously believed that the harmless rough bacteria had broken up and were "used" by the smooth bacteria (9). Griffith was a civil servant and he was proud of it, "the most English of Englishmen" (3). Being employed by the Ministry of Health to do a specific job, he believed in fulfilling his contract, however frustrating that might be (10). Griffith was killed in the early years of the war.

During Griffith's and Avery's time, pneumonia was the great killer, particularly of older people. This writer (RJB) still remembers that in medical school on rotation through Pathology in the late 1920s during the winter months, many of the people in the autopsy room had died from pneumonia. Pneumonia was called "the captain of the men of death." In order to find a treatment, Rufus Cole, the head of the Rockefeller Hospital, organized teams of investigators to discover antibodies to the various types of pneumonia. It was in this setting that Avery

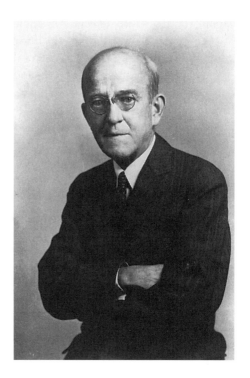

Figure 13.1. Oswald T. Avery. *(Courtesy of the New York Academy of Medicine)*

carried out his work on pneumococcus. When this writer (RJB) was a young physician working at the Rockefeller Institute, resident scientists included Avery, Landsteiner, Carrel, Rous, Bergman, and Levene among others. Over this ingenious but sometimes unruly crowd ruled the director of the Institute, Simon Flexner. Few places in the history of science have had equally illustrious faculty! From the view of this young observer (RJB) Phoebus A. Levene and Oswald T. Avery appeared to be unassuming, modest individuals who did not conform to the popular notion of great scientists.

OSWALD THEODORE AVERY

One of the main contributions that opened the door of science to the new era of molecular biology was the work of Oswald Theodore Avery (1877–1955) (3, 11). Avery was born in 1877 in Halifax, Nova Scotia. In 1877 the family moved to New York City, where he graduated with an M.D. degree from the College of Physicians and Surgeons at Columbia University in 1904. He became a member of the Hoagland Laboratory in Brooklyn, New York, and later assistant and member of the Rockefeller Institute for Medical Research. He died in 1955 in Nashville, Tennessee (3; Fig. 13.1).

Avery's father was a Baptist minister who received an invitation to be pastor of a mission church at Henry Street in New York's Lower East Side. John D. Rockefeller, who endowed the Rockefeller Institute, was deeply interested in the Baptist church and frequently contributed to the church where the elder Avery was pastor. On December 30, 1890, Rockefeller sent the Reverend Avery a Christmas check for $50.00, inviting him to join the Rockefellers at their house on 54th Street for ice skating in the backyard. Part of the letter read: "You will find an entrance on either side of the house, put your hand through the gate and pull the bolt" (11). Oswald Avery was a gifted musician, playing the cornet on the steps of the elder Avery's church on Sunday afternoons. When his father died in 1892, Avery continued as a church musician. In 1893 he left New York to attend Colgate Academy. There he became leader of the brass band and graduated with a major in humanities. Obviously he was not interested in sciences during his college years and took only a few compulsory courses. Avery was admitted to the College of Physicians and Surgeons at Columbia University and obtained his M.D. degree in 1904. He practiced medicine for three years but became frustrated because he could do so little for people with serious diseases (11).

What is the factor which transforms one type of pneumonia into another? Avery's quest for the nature of the transforming factor of pneumococcus observed by Griffith is best stated in his own words, in a letter written to his brother Roy in May 1943 (12). He wrote: "For the past two years, first with MacLeod and now with Dr. McCarty, I have been trying to find out what is the chemical nature of the substance in the bacterial extract which induces the specific change." Maclyn McCarty, who together with MacLeod, was one of Avery's original coworkers, carefully outlined the progress of this study by publishing and reprinting handwritten data from the laboratory experiments (13). These protocols are impressive because of their thoroughness and clarity.

One of Avery's characteristics was his caution in coming to conclusions and his patience in dealing with scientific matters. McCarty states that "during this period I am afraid that both Colin (Colin MacLeod) and I became increasingly impatient with Avery's caution even though we were not unaware of the importance of being sure of our ground. We were just young enough to become convinced more readily" (13). One of his co-workers, René Dubos, characterized Avery by stating "his was not so much a vision as a thread along which all the observations were organized" (14). Avery's co-workers were not all seasoned Ph.Ds; many were medical doctors (3). Everyone who worked with Avery contributed their own intellectual work. Avery never suggested a topic to a young scientist, but all those who came to the Rockefeller Hospital, especially those in the pneumonia service, ended up in his office discussing the pneumococcus (3).

The historical paper entitled "Studies on the Chemical Nature of the Substance Inducing Transformation of Pneumococcal Types" was published in 1944 in the *Journal of Experimental Medicine* (15). The paper is a model in simplicity.

It clearly shows that proteins have nothing to do with the transformation processes and that transformation is not affected by removal of proteins. It was later shown that the DNA from dead smooth bacteria moves into the live rough cell, where it integrated itself so thoroughly into the genetic machinery of the rough cells that it cannot be distinguished from the host DNA.

The question arose whether Avery's findings were peculiar only to bacteria. Hershey and Chase, using radioactive phosphorus and sulfur, showed later that DNA was a universal hereditary agent and was not confined to bacteria (16).

ERWIN CHARGAFF

The most important step leading to Watson and Crick's discovery of the structure of DNA was the work of Erwin Chargaff and Ernst Vischer (17). Erwin Chargaff was born in Vienna; Vischer was Swiss. Chargaff joined the famous group of Hans Clarke's Department of Biochemistry at the College of Physicians and Surgeons at Columbia University, where Rudolph Schoenheimer was also a member (see Chapter 8). The technique that brought Chargaff success was paper chromatography, developed in 1944 (3). Olby relates that Chargaff presented Vischer with a Beckman photometer, filter paper, and nucleic acid (3). The result of this work was the discovery of A:T (adenine:thymine) and G:C (guanine:cytosine) ratios and the overthrow of the tetranucleotide hypothesis. There is an observable difference in the amount of each base among different types of organisms. However, in all organisms the number of adenines always equals that of thymines and the number of guanines equals that of cytosines (17).

MAX DELBRÜCK

A fascinating part of the history of molecular biology was played by Max Delbrück and his group, referred to as the "Phage Group." Phages are viruses that infect only bacteria. Among these scientists, Delbrück was the center and the driving force (Fig. 13.2). Delbrück was originally a physicist and his study with Niels Bohr in Copenhagen did much to formulate his early idea: one can apply orthodox physical principles to biology (3, 18). As Bohr had stated (19), "In every experiment on living organisms, there must remain an uncertainty as regards the physical conditions to which they are subjected." "The existence of life must be considered as an elementary fact that cannot be explained but must be taken as a starting point in biology, in a similar way as the quantum of action" (19). Bohr therefore thought of explaining biological phenomena by principles of quantum physics. Delbrück, Timoféef, a biologist, and Zimmer, a physicist, published a paper in which they wrote about the effect of ionizing radiation (20). Zimmer was interested in the physicochemical changes, the dosimetry; Timoféef performed the genetic analysis (3). Delbrück thought of the effect of radiation as depending on the original arrangements of atoms in the gene. He was certain

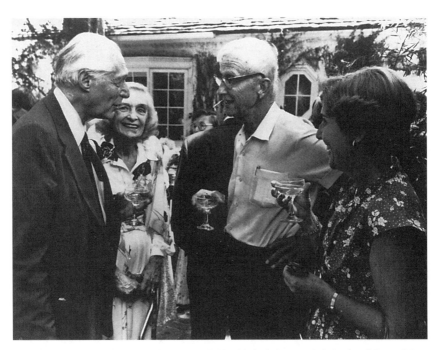

Figure 13.2. Max Delbrück (third from left), (from left to right) Richard Bing, Mary Whipple Bing, and Ingelore Bonner. *(Courtesy of Richard J. Bing)*

that genetics could be related to fundamental physical principles (3): the stability of the gene was due to a quantum jump from one stable configuration over the energy "hump" that separates one configuration from another (3). Delbrück believed that biochemistry had no place in this exploration and that physics could furnish the key to genetics (3).

The "Phage Courses" began at Cold Spring Harbor in 1945 (3). Delbrück became interested in phage when he returned from a camping trip to Caltech and heard that he had missed a presentation by Emory Ellis on phage. As Delbrück said, "I was absolutely overwhelmed that there were such very simple procedures with which you could visualize particles. . . . I mean you could put them on a plate with a lawn of bacteria and the next morning every virus particle would have eaten a macroscopic 1 millimeter hole in the lawn. You could hold up the plate and count the plaques. It seemed to me just beyond my wildest dreams of doing simple experiments on something like atoms in biology" (2). Delbrück conceptualized the riddle of life with the replicating of phage within the black box of the cell.

In the beginning Delbrück opposed approaches by biological chemistry in favor of physics; but the experimental facts proved otherwise. He and Luria finally changed their opinion and by 1950 Luria suggested sending James Watson to Europe to learn nucleic acid chemistry.

Delbrück came from a highly cultured German background (Berlin), his father was university professor of history. He was related to the Bonhöfers, whose opposition to Hitler is one of the most heroic aspects of German history. Delbrück's interests not only covered science, but music and literature; Rainer Maria Rilke was his favorite poet. Delbrück died in 1981 of multiple myeloma.

THE ALPHA HELIX AND THE HYDROGEN BOND

Linus Pauling was born in Portland, Oregon, and graduated from the Oregon State College with a degree in chemical engineering. He then joined the staff at Caltech (3). Together with Robert Corey, Pauling was interested in the structure of protein molecules by submitting them to x-ray analysis (5). Corey had been a research fellow at the Rockefeller Institute in New York, where he took x-ray pictures of porcupine quills. Pauling had for years struggled with the problem of protein structure. In 1948 when he came to Oxford as a visiting professor, he fell ill. After passing away the time reading detective stories, he decided to try to solve the structure of alpha keratin using a pencil and ruler (3). The result of this exercise was the model of the structure of alpha and gamma helices (21). Pauling simply drew a polypeptide chain across a sheet of paper and the alpha C-atom rotated so as to bring all the carbonyl groups on the same side of the chain (3). The result was that in 1948 Pauling had arrived at a rough approximation to the 3.7 residue helix now known as the alpha helix (21). As Pauling wrote in his paper jointly with Corey and Branson in 1951, "hence the only configuration for a chain compatible with our postulate of equivalence of the residues are helical configurations" (21). A couple years later, Pauling suggested that the same might be true of DNA. Meanwhile, Maurice Wilkins in England, using x-ray defraction, found that the DNA molecule strongly resembled a helical structure (22).

Closely related to the structure of proteins was the matter of hydrogen bonding. This concept had been introduced in 1920 by Latimer and Rodebuch, who thought of a hydrogen atom being shared between two oxygen atoms in water, thus forming a weak bridge or bond between neighboring molecules (3). Apparently the idea of a hydrogen bond as a feature of protein structure was already in Pauling's mind in 1936. He attributed the denaturation of proteins to the breakdown of a uniquely folded polypeptide chain by destruction of the hydrogen bond (21).

THE DOUBLE HELIX

The foundations were now laid for Watson and Crick's discovery of the structure of the DNA molecule. In the April 25 issue of *Nature* in 1953 there appeared three papers that changed the course of biology and medicine (23, 24, 25). The first paper was authored by Watson and Crick on the molecular structure of nucleic acid; the second paper was by Wilkins and co-workers on the molecular structure of deoxypentose nucleic acid; and the final paper was by Rosalind E. Franklin and Gosling on the molecular configuration in sodium thymonucleate. The role of Rosalind Franklin in the discovery of the structure of DNA has been the subject of much discussion (3, 4). Particularly remarkable is the careful tone of Watson and Crick's article, which began "We wish to suggest a structure for the salt of deoxyribose nucleic acid (DNA). This structure has novel features which are of considerable biological interest"; in another paragraph they wrote, "It has not escaped our notice that the specific pairing we have postulated immediately suggests a possible copying mechanism for the genetic material." Indeed, this turned out to be true (23).

Gene Therapy in Cardiovascular Diseases

Gene therapy as applied to cardiovascular diseases has brought some of the most promising advances in molecular biology. Some of the applications of gene therapy will be briefly discussed here. Gene therapy is the introduction of normal or modified genes into the somatic cells of a target organism to correct or prevent disease (26). Delivery of genes into cells has been accomplished by both ex vivo and in vivo methods. In the former, transfection of the cells is accomplished in vitro (cell cultures), while in in vivo gene transfection or transduction (when viral vectors are employed) takes place in the organism (27). Both noninfectious and infectious approaches have been used. The noninfectious approaches are mostly based on the use of cationic liposomes, while infectious approaches use viruses such as retroviral vectors or adenovirus or adenovirus-augmented receptors (26, 27, 28). With retroviral vectors, the viral vector integrates into the chromosomal DNA of the target cell, resulting in a change in gene expression (26, 27, 28). Retroviral vectors are frequently used for ex vivo transfer for cardiovascular diseases.

Transduction with adenoviral vectors has been widely used in cardiovascular research. The adenovirus genome is composed of linear, double-stranded DNA of approximately 36 kb in length (29). Adenoviruses have a lytic life cycle characterized by attachment to an adenoviral glycoprotein receptor on mammalian cells and entry into the cell by receptor-mediated endocytosis (28). Cotten presented evidence that viral vector conjugate systems may be applied to vascular gene therapy, including adenovirus-augmented, receptor-mediated gene delivery (30). Several findings suggest that a low level of replication of recombinant virus may perhaps even be responsible for the persistence of gene expression in vivo (27).

In the noninfectious approach, cationic liposomes are used. They are positively charged artificial lipid vesicles that incorporate negatively charged DNA and deliver nucleic acid to the cells through fusion with the cell membrane and receptor-mediated endocytosis (31). Plasmid DNA is then released into the cytoplasm and transported to the nucleus. Consequently, nonviral methods of gene transfer rely on the normal mechanism used by the cells for the uptake of macromolecules (26).

The simplest approach for gene delivery is transfer by unmodified (naked) DNA. It has been used successfully in vivo by intramuscular transfection of genes encoding vascular endothelial growth factor to augment collateral development and tissue perfusion. This may constitute an alternative treatment strategy for patients with extensive peripheral vascular disease in whom the use of intravascular catheter-based gene transfer is compromised and/or prohibited (32).

Gene therapy as applied to cardiovascular diseases has been discussed by a number of authors (26, 27, 28, 33, 34, 35).

ANGIOGENESIS AND GENE TRANSFER

The concept of therapeutic angiogenesis is based on the premise that the existing potential for vascular growth can be utilized to promote the development of new blood vessels by appropriate growth factors (33). This results in either the formation of capillaries, the transformation of preexisting arterioles into small muscular arteries, or the expansion of preexisting collateral vessels. Vascular growth factors are polypeptides originally isolated in studies of tumor growth and found to be responsible for natural as well as pathological angiogenesis (36). Fibroblast growth factor (FGF) and vascular endothelial growth factor (VEGF) are used to induce therapeutic angiogenesis in animals (35). Vascular endothelial growth factor (VEGF) is secreted by intact cells and has affinitive binding sites on endothelial cells; it has no mitogenic effect on smooth muscle cells and fibroblasts. The factor is significantly unregulated by hypoxia in vitro (34).

Several vectors are used to transfer angiogenic factors such as liposomes, viral vectors, and naked DNA. Implanting a stent seeded with cells that have been genetically modified to express vascular endothelial growth factor represents another approach (34, 37, 38). Gene therapy for therapeutic angiogenesis has been reported in patients with peripheral arterial disease (39). Most of these procedures use intravascular catheters (passive diffusion by means of a transfection chamber between two inflated balloons, pressure and mechanical facilitation, and intracoronary stents). Direct myocardial gene delivery has also been attempted (40).

GENE THERAPY TO PREVENT RESTENOSIS
OF CORONARY ARTERY FOLLOWING ANGIOPLASTY

Restenosis occurs after angioplasty as a result of injury to the arterial wall, involving the release of a host of cytokines and growth factors by various cell elements leading to the proliferation primarily of smooth muscle cells and intimal growth. The success of percutaneous transluminal coronary revascularization, introduced by Gruentzig, is frequently jeopardized by restenosis, which occurs in 30 percent to 50 percent of cases (see Chapter 1). It is refractory to all pharmacological therapies (41). Two technical steps in arterial gene therapy for the prevention of restenosis are involved: the delivery system and the vector. Most delivery systems use catheters (42). These include double-balloon catheters (43), catheters with porous and microporous balloons, channel transport and sheath balloons, and hydrogen balloon catheters (42). Catheter-based arterial gene transfer carries the risk of systemic dissemination of the transgene.

A number of vectors have been used. For example, ex vivo gene transfer of porcine endothelial cells expressing the "marker" beta galactosidase gene from a murine amphotropic retroviral vector has been successfully accomplished by directly introducing a catheter into the denuded arteries to deliver the recombinant (virally infected) cells (44). Subsequent studies have employed adenoviral vectors, herpes simplex virus thymidine kinase, antisense oligonucleotide technology, and introduction of a cytostatic protein (41).

A promising approach is the introduction of an inducible gene expression vector together with systemic ganciclovir treatment. Cells expressing the thymidine kinase (TK) become sensitive to anciclovir and its analogs (ganciclovir). Systemic administration of ganciclovir allows killing of the cells targeted with a vector expressing the thymidine kinase. This approach relies on the ability to selectively deliver TK-expressing vectors to a well-defined cell population. In a number of animal models, adenoviral transfer of the gene encoding thymidine kinase coupled with ganciclovir administration has been associated with inhibition of vascular cell proliferation and reduction of neointimal developments (45, 46).

GENETIC TREATMENT OF HYPERLIPIDEMIAS

The genetic treatment of hyperlipidemias has been a tangible result of molecular biology. Familial hypercholesterolemia (FH) is an autosomal dominant disorder caused by defects in the low-density lipoprotein (LDL) receptor gene, which leads to elevated serum LDL (see Chapter 6). Homozygotes with two mutant LDL receptor genes comprise one out of every million individuals in the United States. They exhibit four times the normal plasma cholesterol levels, often develop cutaneous xanthomata and coronary artery disease in childhood, and frequently die before the age of twenty (47). Familial hyperlipidemia heterozygotes comprise about one out of every five hundred individuals in the U.S. population; they have lesser elevation in plasma cholesterol levels and often develop coronary artery disease in their twenties (47). The homozygous form is refractory to therapy except for orthotopic liver transplantation, which has led to complete correction of the hyperlipidemia (48, 49, 50). The success of the liver transplantation suggests that selective reconstitution of hepatic LDL receptor by somatic gene transfer should be sufficient for metabolic corrections (51).

Several methods have been attempted to reduce the hyperlipidemia by in vivo and ex vivo manipulation. Some investigators have used recombinant adeno-viruses containing the LDL receptor gene through hepatic delivery (47, 51). Chowdhury and co-workers have shown long-term improvement of hypercho-lesterolemia in low-density lipoprotein receptor-deficient rabbits (Watanabe) after live-directed gene therapy based on transplantation of autologous hepatocytes that were genetically corrected ex vivo with recombinant retroviruses. This group later performed successful ex vivo gene therapy directed to the liver in a patient with familial hypercholesterolemia (52). Cells from a liver segment were seeded on plates on medium containing the LDL receptor expressing recombinant retro-viruses. The genetically corrected hepatocytes were then harvested and infused through a catheter into the portal bed. Prolonged improvement of dyslipidemia was noted.

Other promising attempts involve, among others, adenovirus-mediated gene transfer of very-low-density lipoprotein receptors (53) and transfer of a gene en-coding cholesterol 7-a hydroxylase (54). The genetic treatment of familial hy-percholesterolemia is of great clinical significance, and the general progress in this field has been encouraging.

GENE THERAPY BY MYOCYTE TRANSPLANTATION

An attempt to replace dead cardiac myocytes with viable, contracting myocytes has been made to treat ischemic heart disease. Adult cardiomyocytes cannot regenerate after injury. Consequently, new viable cardiomyocytes have to be introduced into the still viable heart muscle or into the infarcted sclerotic area. This has been attempted by means of engrafting viable myocytes into the infarcted area. Engrafting has been attempted by means of the use of fetal cells (55, 56). Since the source of fetal donor cardiomyocytes is limited, efforts have been made to use differentiating embryonic stem cells, which can be used as a renewable source of donor cardiomyocytes suitable for cardiac engraftment. Klug et al. found that totipotent embryonic stem cells can be genetically modified to yield highly differentiated and stable cardiomyocytes suitable for the formation of intracardiac grafts (57). Li implanted primary cultured fetal or neonatal rat cardiomyocytes into the fibrous subcutaneous tissue of the adult rat hind limb, to see whether these cells were viable and assumed characteristics of contracting myocardial cells, as checked by echocardiography (58). Suspensions of fetal and neonatal car-diomyocytes were inserted into the subcutaneous tissue of rats. Echocardiography demonstrated that contracting tissue formed as early as seven days after trans-plantation. A large number of experiments were performed to study the effects of transplantation of myocytes into the myocardium (59, 60, 61, 62). Li and co-workers, for example, found that cardiomyocytes isolated from normal fetal and neonatal rat myocardium grew in vitro and contained organized sarcomeres. They contracted regularly, spontaneously, and synchronously. Human fetal cardiomyocytes were equally successful in vitro. Transplanted cardiomyocytes survived and grew when engrafted into connective tissue. Cell transplantation was more successful with fetal cardiomyocytes as compared to neonatal cardiomyocytes.

GENE TRANSFER INTO THE MYOCARDIUM

Leor (63) described the various strategies for gene transfer into the ischemic or infarcted myocardium. Immune reactions against adenovirus have been found to affect the expression of genes delivered by adenoviral vectors. To address this issue, DNA containing the luciferase reporter gene was injected into the ischemic area. Significant levels of luciferase gene expression were obtained in ischemic hearts, showing that ischemic myocardium is capable of taking up and expressing DNA. In another series of experiments, retrovirus carrying the reporter gene lac Z was injected directly into the infarcted area under direct visualization. Infarcted hearts that were injected with retrovirus stained positive for beta-galactosidase. Ischemic or infarcted myocardium can be a target. To assess and measure the efficiency of adenovirus-mediated gene transfer and expression in infarcted myocardium, Leor et al. also injected replication-defective adenovirus vector encoding the bacterial reporter gene product beta-galactosidase into the infarcted area (63); however, beta-galactosidase gene expression was limited to viable myocytes at the border of the myocardial infarction (63).

TRANSPLANTATION OF FIBROBLASTS

An interesting attempt is the implantation of cardiac fibroblasts into the scar of infarcted areas (63). Apparently cardiac fibroblasts can be converted into skeletal muscle cells by forced expression of the MyoD gene. Fibroblasts isolated from rat hearts were infected with retrovirus carrying the MyoD gene. Leor et al. injected infarcts with two retroviruses—one carrying the regulatory gene MyoD and the other encoding for beta-galactosidase. Histochemical analysis with X-gal identified successful transfection in several hearts. In areas of positive beta-galactosidase staining, specific antibody against skeletal fast myosin heavy chain identified rare cells that were stained positive for the myosin heavy chain. This suggests that exogenous transfer of the MyoD gene can result in conversion of cardiac fibroblasts into cells that express skeletal fast myosin heavy chain (63). Murry et al. reported successful transduction in vivo with MyoD gene transfer into myocardial granulation tissue of rats (64). One week after they injected adenovirus carrying the MyoD or beta-galactosidase gene, cells were identified that expressed both myogenin and embryonic skeletal myosin heavy chain (64). They demonstrated MyoD mRNA expression in the injured region of hearts receiving the

MyoD virus. Another effort was the transplantation of skeletal muscle cells into heart muscle in the hope that transplanted skeletal muscle cells can undergo transformation to myocytes (63). Chiu et al. (65) used satellite cells, myogenic cells existing in each mature skeletal myofiber. These cells remain in an undifferentiated state and are activated following skeletal injury, after which they enter the mitotic cycle and later fuse with each other and with injured myofibers to restore continuity and function of skeletal muscle. Chiu et al. showed that cultured satellite cells from skeletal muscle of dogs can be implanted into the injured myocardium of the same animal and can differentiate into "cardiac-like" myocytes and couple to each other by intracellular junctions resembling gap junctions or intercalated discs.

These are interesting attempts to replace poorly functioning cardiomyocytes with new and vigorous cells that can improve at least partially the contractility of the infarcted area of the heart. This work is still in the early stages, but the stakes are high and progress is rapid.

Myosin and Genetic Heart Diseases

Cardiomyopathies are diseases of the heart muscle associated with disturbances in cardiac function. Many different types of cardiomyopathies exist, including dilated, hypertrophic, restrictive, and arrhythmogenic right ventricular cardiomyopathy (66).

FAMILIAL HYPERTROPHIC CARDIOMYOPATHY

Familial hypertrophic cardiomyopathy (FHC) was described in the middle of the last century at the Hospital La Salpetriere in Paris by A. Vulpian (67). It was, however, only in the late 1950s that the unique clinical features of FHC were systematically described. FHC is characterized by left and/or right ventricular hypertrophy, which is usually asymmetric and involves the interventricular septum; there exists no hemodynamic cause of increased cardiac mass (68). Typically, the left ventricular volume is normal or reduced. Systolic gradients are common. Morphological changes include myocyte hypertrophy and disarray surrounding areas of increased loose connective tissues.

This disorder is included in this chapter since it is a familial disease with autosomal dominant inheritance. None of the previous hypotheses of the pathophysiological mechanisms of FHC would have predicted that defects in sarcomeric genes could be one of its possible molecular bases. However, myosin heavy chain was the first disease gene found and mutations in other sarcomeric genes have been described (69, 70).

Myosin is the force generator in striated muscle cells. It transduces energy from the hydrolysis of ATP into directed movement, and by doing so, drives sarcomere shortening and muscle contraction. It is encoded by a multigene family that exhibits tissue-specific, developmental, and physiologically regulated patterns of expression.

Cardiac myosin is a conventional class II myosin that consists of two heavy chains (MyHC) and two pairs of light chains (MLC), referred to as essential (or alkali) light chains (MLC-1s/v) and regulatory (or phosphorylatable) light chains (MLC-2s/v), respectively (71). The myosin molecule is highly asymmetric, consisting of two globular heads joined to a long, rodlike tail. The light chains are apart from the motor domain of the heavy chains. Neither myosin light chain type is required for the adenosine triphosphatase activity of the myosin head, but they probably modulate activity in the presence of actin and contribute to the rigidity of the neck, which may function as a lever arm for generating an effective power stroke.

b-MyHC is the major myosin heavy chain isoform of the human ventricle and of slow-twitch skeletal fibers (71). It is also expressed in the human atria. It is encoded by the *MYH7* gene, which is composed of 40 exons and encompasses approximately 23 kb of DNA. It encodes a protein of 1,935 amino acids (72). The globular amino-terminal part of the molecule corresponds to the motor domain that contains the ATP-binding site and the actin-binding site. Recent studies conducted on a skeletal/smooth chimeric myosin showed that the ATPase cycle rate, the ATP hydrolysis rate or phosphate release rate, is solely determined by the globular head domain (73). The neck region of MyHC, which consists of a long alpha-helix, is associated with the light chains (71). The carboxy-terminal rod, which has a characteristic alpha-helical coiled-coil structure, is responsible for the assembly of myosin into thick filaments. At least fifty mutations were found in *MYH7* in unrelated families with FHC (69, 74–79), and three hot spots for mutations were identified. All but three of these mutations are missense mutations that produce the replacement of one amino acid by another. The missense mutations are located either in the head or in the head-rod junction of the molecule, and twenty-nine have been precisely positioned on the three-dimensional structure of chicken skeletal myosin S1 (80).

Both types of myosin light chains are expressed both in the ventricular myocardium and in the slow-twitch muscles (81). Their removal significantly decreases the velocity of actin movement on skeletal myosin (82). As a matter of fact, their function has been studied more in skeletal muscles than in cardiac muscles. Some data strongly suggest that MLC-1s/v potently produces an inotropic effect through a cooperative mechanism that may involve activation of the entire thin filament (83), and recent studies have showed that the partial transgenic-driven replacement of MLC-2s/v with the skeletal isoform in the mouse ventricle reduces both left ventricular contractility and relaxation (84). MLC-1s/v is encoded by *MYL3*. It is composed of seven exons, six of which encode a polypeptide of 195 amino acids. MLC-2s/v is encoded by MYL2, and five mutations were reported in cardiomyopathy (70, 85). Akiyama and co-workers found that myocardial infarction profoundly affects regulatory myosin light chain phosphorylation and that MLC-2s/v plays a significant part in my-ocardial contractility (86).

The finding of a mutation that cosegregates with FHC in a given pedigree and that is absent from a large number of normal chromosomes (usually a mini-mum of two hundred are tested) is not sufficient to prove that it causes the dis-ease. Several in vivo and in vitro studies strongly suggest a direct link. Two mouse models of FHC were produced by the introduction of the R430QMYH7 mu-tation into the mouse gene that encodes another MyHC cardiac isoform, the a-MyHC (the adult mouse ventricle contains only a-MyHC and no b-MyHC) (87, 88). These transgenic animals exhibited alterations of cardiac structure and function similar to FHC patients and thus provide important model systems for analysis of the pathophysiological mechanisms of FHC. The presence of a mu-tated protein would alter sarcomeric function, resulting first in altered cardiac function, second, in the alteration of the sarcomeric and myocyte structures, and finally in the compensatory response of the heart to develop hypertrophy, the last manifestation observed in the two models. Moreover, several in vitro studies have shown that FHC mutants alter sarcomere function, either by decreasing the translocating filament activity and/or force leading to a reduction of power production by cardiac cells (73, 89–92) or, on the contrary, by increasing in vitro motility rates of filament sliding (70)

FHC is of clinical importance because arrhythmias and premature sudden deaths are constant threats (66). Clinically the disease is more frequent in the general population than previously thought (one in 500) and it afflicts patients of all ages (93). Because of its potential for causing sudden death, the manage-ment of the condition is of great importance (93). In general the treatment con-sists in management of heart failure by means of beta-blockers or verapamil. However, there is no evidence that either of these agents protects patients from sudden death (94). In children, drug treatment may be appropriate since this may reduce the hemodynamic load and improve the clinical course (93). Atrial fibril-lation develops in a large number of adult patients and sudden episodes of atrial fibrillation are particularly hazardous. Treatment with amiodarone is probably the most effective antiarrhythmic agent for the prevention of reoccurrence of atrial fibrillation (95).

In some patients medical therapy fails and surgery is indicated. This applies particularly to patients who have both a large outflow gradient and severe symp-toms of heart failure unresponsive to medical treatment. Surgical treatment consists in removing a small amount of muscle from the basal septum (myotomy-myectomy) (96). Surgery should not be performed in asymptomatic or mildly symptomatic patients. Dual-chamber pacing is another suggested therapy; it has been associated with a substantial decrease in the outflow gradient and symptomatic improvement (97). However, it is possible that a placebo effect may play an important part in the short-term symptomatic improvement. In patients who are considered to be at particularly high risk of life-threatening tachyarrhythmias, amiodarone or the implantable cardioverter-defibrillator are most frequently used (93).

Because of the danger of sudden death due to arrhythmia, clinical indicators of high-risk patients are of great importance. These features include the onset of symptoms in childhood, particularly marked hypertrophy and foremost exercise-induced hypotension (93). There is no evidence that electrophysiological testing plays an important role in identifying the patients who are at high risk for sudden death.

Genetic testing in this condition may be important. A recent approach to assess risk in hypertrophic cardiomyopathy has focused on the impact of genotype on clinical outcome. Several types of mutations appear to be associated with markedly reduced survival. The available data suggest that b-myosin heavy-chain mutations may account for approximately 30 percent to 40 percent of cases of FHC (98). Some myosin mutations are benign (e.g., Val606Met), whereas others are associated with premature death from either heart failure or sudden catastrophic events (98). In families with the Arg403Gln mutation, no more than 50 percent of the affected family members survived past forty-five years of age (99). Cardiac troponin T mutations, in which the cardiac hypertrophy is relatively mild but life expectancy is substantially reduced, are estimated to account for about 10 percent to 20 percent of familial hypertrophic cardiomyopathy (100).

It is interesting to examine the value of our knowledge of the molecular genetics of FHC. In this context, the term "value" can have several meanings; it can signify a better understanding of the mechanisms of this disease or it can demonstrate a therapeutic success. Quite clearly, our understanding of the mechanism of FHC has been tremendously expanded. In contrast there has been no direct spin-off for the treatment of this condition. The reason may well be that the disease is transmitted as an autosomal dominant trait and affected persons have one mutant and one normal allele (93). Since most mutations result in substitution of a single amino acid within the encoded protein, one would have to selectively inactivate the mutated gene, the encoded protein, or both (93). This, however, is not yet in sight.

Coda

A utopian vision of molecular genetics was presented in 1963 at a Ciba Foundation meeting. H.J. Muller advocated measures that would enhance evolutionary selection through molecular genetics. Lederberg predicted that the molecular knowledge of microbes would be applied to the human genome. He further suggested: "The same culture that has uniquely acquired the power of global annihilation must generate the largest quota of intellectual and social insight to secure its own survival." Francis Crick was more realistic. His reservations centered primarily on the feasibility of implementation of biological-social technologies (101).

When we look at these predictions with hindsight, we realize that fortunately we have not yet controlled, selected, or integrated desired genes for eugenic practice. We have made a beginning in defining the human genome, hopefully more for prevention, recognition, and treatment of human diseases than for mental eugenic practices. Controlling future minds genetically is a utopian fallacy. At the present there has been wide application of molecular genetics to forensic medicine and biotechnical developments, where billions of dollars are at stake. Let us not forget that ideas depend on evolutionary changes, which may accelerate or slow; what is useful has a chance to survive.

References

1. Berg, P., and M. Singer. Dealing with Genes: The Language of Heredity. Mill Valley, CA, University Science Books, 1992.
2. Kay, L.E. The Molecular Vision of Life: Caltech, the Rockefeller Foundation and the New Biology. New York, Oxford University Press, 1993.
3. Olby, R. The Path to the Double Helix. Seattle, University of Washington Press, 1974.
4. Judson, H.F. The Eighth Day of Creation: Makers of the Revolution in Biology. Plainview, NY, Cold Spring Harbor Laboratory Press, 1996.
5. Fried, J. J. The Mystery of Heredity, the Frontiers of Science Series. New York, The John Day Co., 1971.
6. Kossel, K.M.L.A. Ueber die Beschaffenheit des Zellkerns. Nobel Lectures Including Presentations, Speeches, and Laureates' Biographies: Physiology or Medicine, 1901–1921. Amsterdam, 1967, pp. 394–405.
7. Levene, P.A., G. Schmidt, and E.G. Pickles. Enzymatic dephosphorylation of desoxyribonucleic acids of various degrees of polymerization. J. Biol. Chem., 127:251–259, 1939.
8. Feulgen, R., and H. Rossenbeck. Mikroskopisch-chemischer Nachweis einer Nucleinsaure vom Typus der Thymonucleinsaure und die darauf beruhende elektive Farbung von Zellkernen in mikroskropischen Preparaten, Hoppe-Seyler's Z. Physiol. Chem., 135:203–248, 1924.
9. Griffith, F. The significance of pneumococcal types. J. Hygiene, 27:113–159, 1928.
10. Elliott, S.D. Letter to Pollock dated March 3 (original with Pollock) As quoted by Olby, 1970. See reference 3.
11. Oswald Avery and the Sugar-coated Microbe. The Rockefeller University Research Profiles, Rockefeller University Archives, New York, Spring 1988, pp. 1–4.
12. Avery, O.T., 1943, letter to Roy Avery, dated May 13. (As published by Hotchkiss in Cairns et al., 1966, pp. 185–187. Original at the University of Vanderbilt Archive.)
13. McCarty, M. A retrospective look: how we identified the pneumococcal transforming substance as DNA. J. Exp. Med., 179:385–394, 1994.

14. Dubos, R.J. The Professor, the Institute, and DNA. New York, The Rockefeller University Press, 1976.

15. Avery, O.T., C.M. Mac Leod, and M. McCarty. Studies on the chemical nature of the substance inducing transformation of pneumococcal types. J. Exp. Med., 79(2):137–158, 1944.

16. Hershey, A.D., and M. Chase. Independent functions of viral proteins and nucleic acid in growth of bacteriophage. J. Gen. Physiol., 36:39–56, 1952.

17. Chargaff, E., E.M. Vischer, R. Doniger, C. Green, and F. Misani. The composition of the desoxypentose nucleic acids of thymus and spleen. J. Biol. Chem., 177:405–416, 1949.

18. Delbrück, M. A physicist's renewed look at biology: twenty years later (Nobel lecture). Science, 168:1312–1315, 1970.

19. Bohr, N. Light and life. Nature, 131:421–423, 1933.

20. Timoféef-Ressovsky, N.W., K.G. Zimmer, and M. Delbrück. Ueber die Natur der Genmutation und der Genstruktur. Nachr. Ges. Wiss. Gottingen, math-phys. Kl. Fachgr, 6(1):189–245, 1935.

21. Pauling, L., R.B. Corey, and H.R. Branson. The structure of proteins: two hydrogen-bonded helical configurations of the polypeptide chain. Proc. Natl. Acad. Sci. USA, 37:205–211, 1951.

22. Wilkins, M.H.F., W.E. Seeds, A.R. Stokes, and H.R. Wilson. Helical structure of crystalline deoxypentose nucleic acid. Nature, 172:759–762, 1953.

23. Watson, J.D., and F.H.C. Crick. Molecular structure of nucleic acids. Nature, 171:737–738, 1953.

24. Wilkins, M.H.F., A. R. Stokes, and H.R. Wilson. Molecular structure of deoxypentose nucleic acids. Nature, 171:738–740, 1953.

25. Franklin, R.E., and R.G. Gosing. Molecular configuration in sodium thymonucleate. Nature, 171:740–741, 1953.

26. Buttrick, P.M. Gene therapy in the cardiovascular system: current strategies and practical limitations. American College of Cardiology Current Journal Review, May–June: 17–21, 1997.

27. Mulligan, R.C. The basic science of gene therapy. Science, 260:926–932, 1993.

28. Nabel, E.G. Gene therapy for cardiovascular disease. Circulation, 91:541–548, 1995.

29. Graham, F.L., and L. Prevec. Adenovirus-based expression vectors and recombinant vaccines. In: Vaccines: New Approaches to Immunological Problems, Ellis, R.W. (ed). Boston, MA, Butterworth-Heinemann, 1992, pp. 363–390.

30. Cotten, M., E. Wagner, K. Zatloukal, S. Phillips, D.T. Curiel, and M.L. Birnstiel. High-efficiency receptor-mediated delivery of small and large (48 kilobase) gene constructs using the endosome-disruption activity of defective or chemically inactivated adenovirus particles. Proc. Natl. Acad. Sci. USA, 89:6094–6098, 1992.

31. Felgner, P.L., T.R. Gadek, M. Holm, R. Roman, H.W. Chan, M. Wenz, J.P. Northrop, G.M. Ringold, and M. Danielsen. Lipofection: a highly efficient, lipid-mediated DNA-transfection procedure. Proc. Natl. Acad. Sci. USA, 84:7413–7417, 1987.

32. Tsurumi, Y., S. Takeshita, D. Chen, M. Kearney, S.T. Rossow, J. Passeri, J.R. Horowitz, J.F. Symes, and J.M. Isner. Direct intramuscular gene transfer of naked DNA encoding vascular endothelial growth factor augments collateral development and tissue perfusion. Circulation, 94:3281–3290, 1996.

33. Safi, J., Jr., T.R. Gloe, T. Riccioni, I. Kovesdi, and M.C. Capogrossi. Gene therapy with angiogenic factors: a new potential approach to the treatment of ischemic diseases. J. Mol. Cell. Cardiol., 29:2311–2325, 1997.

34. Lewis, B.S., M.Y. Flugelman, A. Weisz, I. Keren-Tal, and W. Schaper. Angiogenesis by gene therapy: a new horizon for myocardial revascularization? Cardiovas. Res., 35:490–497, 1997.

35. Melillo, G., M. Scoccianti, I. Kovesdi, J. Safi, T. Riccioni, and M.C. Capogrossi. Gene therapy for collateral vessel development. Cardiovas. Res., 35:480–489, 1997.
36. Shing, Y., J. Folkman, J. Sullivan, R. Butterfield, J. Murray, and M. Klagsbrun. Heparin-affinity purification of a tumor-derived capillary endothelial cell growth factor. Science, 223:1296–1299, 1984.
37. Van der Gissen, W.J., P.W. Serruys, W.J. Visser, P.D. Verdouw, W.P. van Schalkwijk, and J.F. Jongkind. Endothelialization of endovascular stents. J. Intervent. Cardiol., 1:109–120, 1988.
38. Dichek, D.A., R.F. Neville, J.A. Zwiebel, S.M. Freeman, M.B. Leon, and W.F. Anderson. Seeding of intravascular stents with genetically engineered endothelial cells. Circulation, 80:1347–1353, 1989.
39. Isner, J.M., K. Walsh, J. Symes, A. Pieczek, S. Takeshita, J. Lowry, S. Rossow, K. Rosenfield, L. Weir, E. Brogi, and R. Schainfeld. Arterial gene therapy for therapeutic angiogenesis in patients with peripheral artery disease. Circulation, 91:2687–2692, 1995.
40. Feldman, L.J., and G. Steg. Optimal techniques for arterial gene transfer. Cardiovas. Res., 35:391–404, 1997.
41. Feldman, L.J., O. Tahlil, and G. Steg. Perspectives of arterial gene therapy for the prevention of restenosis. Cardiovasc. Res., 32:194–207, 1996.
42. Brieger, D., and E. Topol. Local drug delivery systems and prevention of restenosis. Cardiovasc. Res., 35:405–413, 1997.
43. Jorgenson, B., K.H. Tonnesen, J. Bulow , J.D. Nielson, M. Jorgensen, P. Holstein, and E. Andersen. Femoral artery recanalization with percutaneous angioplasty and segmentally enclosed plasminogen activator. Lancet, 1:1106–1108, 1989.
44. Nabel, E.G., G. Plautz, F.M. Boyce, J.C. Stanley, and G.J. Nabel. Recombinant gene expression in vivo within endothelial cells of the arterial wall. Science, 244:1342–1344, 1989.
45. Chang, M.W., T. Ohno, D. Gordon, M.M. Lu, G.J. Nabel, E.G. Nabel, and J.M. Leiden. Adenovirus-mediated transfer of the herpes simplex virus thymidine kinase gene inhibits vascular smooth muscle cell proliferation in neointima formation following balloon angioplasty of the rat carotid artery. Mol. Med. 1:172–181, 1995.
46. Guzman, R.J., E.A. Hirschowitz, S.L. Brody, R.G. Crystal, S.E. Epstein, and T. Finkel. In vivo suppression of injury-induced vascular smooth muscle cell accumulation using adenovirus-mediated transfer of herpes simplex thymidine kinase gene. Proc. Natl. Acad. Sci. USA, 91:10732–10736, 1994.
47. Li, J., B. Fang, R.C. Eisensmith, X.H.C. Li, I. Nasonkin, Y.C. Lin-Lee, M.P. Mims, A. Hughes, C.D. Montgomery, J.D. Roberts, T.S. Parker, D.M. Levine, and S.L.C. Woo. In vivo gene therapy for hyperlipidemia: phenotypic correction in Watanabe rabbits by hepatic delivery of the rabbit LDL receptor gene. J. Clin. Invest., 95:768–773, 1995.
48. Starzl, T.E., H.T. Bahnson, R.L. Hardesty, S. Iwatsuki, J.C. Gartner, D.W. Bilheimer, B.W. Shaw Jr, B.P Griffith, B.J. Zitelli, J.J. Malatack, and A.H. Urbach. Heart-liver transplantation in a patient with familial hypercholesterolemia. Lancet, 1:1382–1383, 1984.
49. Bilheimer, D.W., J.L. Goldstein, S.M. Grundy, T.E. Starzl, and M.S. Brown. Liver-retransplantation to provide low-density-lipoprotein receptors and lower plasma-cholesterol in a child with homozygous familial hypercholesterolemia. N. Engl. J. Med., 311:1658–1664, 1984.
50. Hoeg, J.M., T.E. Starzl, and H.B. Brewer. Liver transplantation for treatment of cardiovascular disease: comparison with medication and plasma exchange in homozygous familial hypercholesterolemia. Am. J. Cardiol., 39: 705–707, 1987.
51. Kozarsky, K., D.R. McKinley, L.L. Austin, S.E. Rapert, L.D. Stratford-Perricaudet, and J.M. Wilson. In vivo correction of low density lipoprotein receptor deficiency in

the Watanabe heritable hyperlipidemic rabbit with recombinant adenoviruses. J. Biol. Chem., 269:13695–13702, 1994.

52. Grossman, M., S.E. Raper, K. Kozarsky, E.A. Stein, J.F. Engelhardt, D. Muller, P.J. Lupien, and J.M. Wilson. Successful ex vivo gene therapy directed to liver in a patient with familial hypercholesterolemia. Nature Genet., 6:335–341, 1994.

53. Kobayashi, K., K. Oka, T. Forte, B. Ishida, B. Teng, K. Ishimura-Oka, M. Nakamuta, and L. Chan. Reversal of hypercholesterolemia in low density lipoprotein receptor knockout mice by adenovirus-mediated gene transfer of the very low density lipoprotein receptor. J. Biol. Chem., 271:6852–6860, 1996.

54. Spady, D.K., J.A. Cuthbert, M.N. Willard, and R.S. Meidell. Adenovirus-mediated transfer of a gene encoding cholesterol 7a-hydroxylase into hamsters increases hepatic enzyme activity and reduces plasma total and low density lipoprotein cholesterol. J. Clin. Invest., 96:700–709, 1995.

55. Soonpaa, M.H., G.Y. Koh, M.G. Klug, and L.J. Field. Formation of nascent intercalated discs between grafted fetal cardiomyocytes and host myocardium. Science, 264:98–101, 1994.

56. Koh, G.Y., M.H. Soonpaa, M.G. Klug, H.P. Pride, D.P. Zipes, B.J. Cooper, and L.J. Field. Stable fetal cardiomyocyte grafts in the hearts of dystrophic mice and dogs. J. Clin. Invest., 96:2034–2042, 1995.

57. Klug, M.G., M.H. Soonpaa, G.Y. Koh, and L.J. Field. Genetically selected cardiomyocytes from differentiating embryonic stem cells form stable intracardiac grafts. J. Clin. Invest., 98:216–224, 1996.

58. Li, R.K., D.A.B. Mickle, R.D. Weisel, J. Zhang, and M.K Mohabeer. In vivo survival and function of transplanted rat cardiomyocytes. Circ. Res., 78:283–288, 1996.

59. Zibaitis, A., D. Greentree, F. Ma, D. Marelli, M. Duong, and R.C.J. Chiu. Myocardial regeneration with satellite cell implantation. Transplant Proc., 26:3294, 1994.

60. Yoon, P.D., R.L. Kao, and G.J. Magoveru. Myocardial regeneration: transplanting satellite cells into damaged myocardium. Tex. Heart Inst. J., 22:119–125, 1995.

61. Koh, G.Y., M.G. Klug, M.H. Soonpaa, and L.J. Field. Differentiation and long-term survival of C2C12 myoblast grafts in heart. J. Clin. Invest., 92:1548–1554, 1993.

62. Koh, G.Y., M.H. Soonpaa, M.G. Klug, and L.J. Field. Long-term survival of AT-1 cardiomyocyte grafts in syngenic myocardium. Am. J. Physiol., 264 (Heart Circ. Phisol. 33): H1727–H1733, 1993.

63. Leor, J., H. Prentice, V. Sartorelli, M.J. Quinones, M. Patterson, L.K. Kedes, and R.A. Kloner. Gene transfer and cell transplant: an experimental approach to repair a "broken heart." Cardiovasc. Res., 35:431–441, 1997.

64. Murry, C.E. M.A. Kay, T. Bartosak, S.D. Hauschka, and S.M. Schwartz. Muscle differentiation during repair of myocardial necrosis in rats via gene transfer with MyoD. J. Clin. Invest., 98:2209–2217, 1996.

65. Chiu, R.C.J., A. Zibaitis, and R.L. Kao. Cellular cardiomyoplasty: myocardial regeneration with satellite cell implantation. Ann. Thorac., 60:12–18, 1995.

66. Report of the 1995 World Health Organization/International Society and Federation of Cardiology Task Force on the Definition and Classification of Cardiomyopathies. Circulation, 93:841–842, 1996.

67. Vulpian, A. Contribution a l'etude des retrecissements de l'orifice ventriculo-aortique. Archiv. Physiol., 3:220–222, 1868.

68. Wigle, E.D., A. Sasson, M.A. Henderson, T.D. Ruddy, J. Fulop, H. Rakowski, and W.G. Williams. Hypertrophic cardiomyopathy. The importance of the site and the extent of hypertrophy. A review. Prog. Cardiovasc. Dis., 28:1–83, 1985.

69. Schwartz, K., L. Carrier, P. Guicheney, and M. Komajda. Molecular basis of familial cardiomyopathies. Circulation, 91:532–540, 1995.

70. Peotter, K., H. Jiang, S. Hassanzadeh, S.R. Master, A. Chang, M.C. Dalakas, I. Rayment, J.R. Sellers, L. Fananapazir, and N.D. Epstein. Mutation in either the essential

or regulatory light chains of myosin are associated with a rare myopathy in human heart and skeletal muscle. Nature Genet., 13:63–69, 1996.

71. Schiaffino, S., and C. Reggiani. Molecular diversity of myofibrillar proteins: gene regulation and functional significance. Physiol. Rev., 76:371–423, 1996.

72. Liew, C.C., M.J. Sole, K. Yamauchi-Takihar, B. Kellam, D.H. Anderson, L. Lin, and J.C. Liew. Complete sequence and organization of the human cardiac b-myosin heavy chain gene. Nucl. Acid Res., 18:3647–3651, 1990.

73. Sata, M., and M. Ikebe. Functional analysis of the mutations in the human cardiac b-myosin that are responsible for familial hypertrophic cardiomyopathy. J. Clin. Invest., 98:2866–2873, 1997.

74. Vikstrom, K.L., and L.A. Leinwand. Contractile protein mutations and heart disease. Curr. Opini. Cell Biol. 8:97–105, 1996.

75. Arai, S., R. Matsuoka, K. Hirayama, H. Sakurai, M. Tamura, T. Ozawa, M. Kimura, S.I. Imamura, Y. Furutani, K. Joh-o, M.. Kawana, A. Takao, S. Hosoda, and K. Momma. Missense mutation of the b-cardiac myosin heavy-chain gene in hypertrophic cardiomyopathy. Am. J. Med. Genet., 58:267–276, 1995.

76. Moolman, J.C., P.A. Brink, and V.A. Corfield. Identification of a novel Ala797Thr mutation in exon 21 of the beta-myosin heavy chain gene in hypertrophic cardiomyopathy. Hum. Mutat., 6:197–198, 1995.

77. Makajima-Taniguchi, C., H. Matsui, N. Eguchi, S. Nagata, T. Kishimoto, and K. Yamauchi-Takihara. A novel deletion mutation in the b-myosin heavy chain gene found in Japanese patients with hypertrophic cardiomyopathy. J. Mol. Cell. Cardiol., 27:2607–2612, 1995.

78. Kuang, S.Q., J.D. Yu, L. Lu, L.M. He, L.S. Gong, S.J. Chen, and Z. Chen. Identification of a novel missense mutation in the cardiac b-myosin chain gene in a patient with sporadic hypertrophic cardiomyopathy. J. Mol. Cell. Cardiol., 28:1879–1883, 1996.

79. Charron, P., L. Carrier, O. Dubourg, F. Tesson, M. Desnos, P. Richard, G. Bonne, P. Guicheney, B. Hainque, J. Boubour, A. Mallet, J. Feingold, K. Schwartz, and M. Komajda. Penetrance of familial hypertrophic cardiomyopathy. Genetic Counseling, 8:107–114, 1997.

80. Rayment, I., H.M. Holden, J.R. Sellers, L. Fananapazir, and N.D. Epstein. Structural interpretation of the mutations in the b-cardiac myosin that have been implicated in familial hypertrophic cardiomyopathy. Proc. Natl. Acad. Sci. USA, 92:3864–3868, 1995.

81. Barton, P.J.R., A. Cohen, B. Robert, M.Y. Fiszman, F. Bonhomme, J.L. Guenet, D.P. Leader, and M.E. Buckingham. The myosin alkali light chains of mouse ventricular and slow skeletal muscle are indistinguishable and are encoded by the same gene. J. Biol. Chem., 260:8578–8584, 1985.

82. Lowey, S., G. Waller, and K. Trybus. Skeletal muscle myosin light chains are essential for physiological speeds of shortening. Nature, 365:454–456, 1993.

83. Rarick, H.M., T.J. Opgenorth, T.W. von Geldern, J.R. Wu-Wong, and R.J. Solaro. An essential myosin light chain peptide induces supramaximal stimulation of cardiac myofibrillar ATPase activity. J. Biol. Chem., 271:27039–27043, 1996.

84. Gulick, J., T.E. Hewett, R. Klevitsky, S.H. Buck, R.L. Moss, and J. Robbins. Transgenic remodeling of the regulatory myosin light chains in the mammalian heart. Circ. Res., 80:655–664, 1997.

85. Flavigny, J., P. Richard, R. Isnard, L. Carrier, P. Charron, G. Bonne, J.F. Forissier, M. Desnos, O. Dubourg, M. Komajda, K. Schwartz, and B. Hainque. Identification of two novel mutations in the ventricular regulatory myosin light chain gene (MYL2) associated with familial and classical forms of hypertrophic cardiomyopathy. J. Mol. Med., 76:208–214, 1998.

86. Akiyama, K., A. Akopian, M.P. Jinadasa, T. Gluckman, and R.J. Bing. Myocardial infarction and regulatory light chain myosin. J. Mol. Cell Cardiol., 29:2641–2652, 1997.

87. Geisterfer-Lowrance, A.A.T., M. Christe, D.A. Conner, J.S. Ingwall, F.J. Schoen, C.E. Seidman, and J.G. Seidman. A mouse model of familial hypertrophic cardiomyopathy. Science, 272:731–734, 1996.

88. Vikstrom, K.L., S.M. Factor, and L.A. Leinwand. Mice expressing mutant mysoin heavy chains are a model for familial hypertrophic cardiomyopathy. Mol. Med., 2:556–567, 1996.

89. Cuda, G., L. Fananapazier, W.S. Zhu, J.R. Seller, and N.E. Epstein. Skeletal muscle expression and abnormal function of b-myosin in hypertrophic cardiomyopathy. J. Clin. Invest., 91:2861–2865, 1993.

90. Sweeney, H.L., A.J. Straceski, L.A. Leinwand, B.A. Tikunov, and L. Faust. Heterologous expression of a cardiomyopathic myosin that is defective in its actin interaction. J. Biol. Chem., 269:1603–1605, 1994.

91. Lankford, E.B., N.D. Epstein, L. Fananapazier, and H.L. Sweeney. Abnormal contractile properties of muscle fibers expressing b-myosin heavy chain gene mutations in patients with hypertrophic cardiomyopathy. J. Clin. Invest., 95:1409–1414, 1995.

92. Cuda, G., L. Fananapazier, N.D. Epstein, and J.R. Sellers. The in vitro motility activity of b-cardiac myosin depends on the nature of the b-myosin heavy chain gene mutation in hypertrophic cardiomyopathy. J. Muscle Res. Cell Motil., 18:275–283, 1997.

93. Spirito, P., C.E. Seidman, W.J. McKenna, and B.J. Maron. The management of hypertrophic cardiomyopathy. N. Engl. J. Med., 336:775–785, 1997.

94. Wigle, E.D., H. Rakowski, B.P. Kimball, and W.G. Williams. Hypertrophic cardiomyopathy: clinical spectrum and treatment. Circulation, 92:1680–1692, 1995.

95. McKenna, W.J., D. England, Y.L. Doi, J.E. Deanfield, C.M. Oakley, and J.F. Goodwin. Arrhythmia in hypertrophic cardiomyopathy. I. Influence on prognosis. Br. Heart J., 46:168–172, 1981.

96. McIntosh, C.L., and B.J. Maron. Current operative treatment of obstructive hypertrophic cardiomyopathy. Circulation, 78:487–495, 1988.

97. Slade, A.K.B, N. Sadoul, L. Shapiro, et al. DDD pacing in hypertrophic cardiomyopathy: a multicentre clinical experience. Heart, 75:44–9, 1996.

98. Marain, A.J., and R. Roberts. Recent advances in the molecular genetics of hypertrophic cardiomyopathy. Circulation, 92:1336–1347, 1995.

99. Watkins, H., A. Rosenzweig, D-S. Hwang, et al. Characteristics and prognostic implications of myosin missense mutations in familial hypertrophic cardiomyopathy. N. Engl. J. Med., 326:1108–1114, 1992.

100. Watkins, H., W.J. McKenna, L. Thierfelder, et al. Mutations in the genes for cardiac troponin T and a-tropomyosin in hypertrophic cardiomyopathy. N. Engl. J. Med., 332:1058–1064, 1995.

101. Lederberg, J. Biological future of man. In: Man and His Future. Boston, Little, Brown, 1963.

Chapter 14

Electrophysiology

B. LÜDERITZ
H. HELLERSTEIN†
A. SENNING
R.J. BING

Cardiac Arrhythmia, Cardiac Resuscitation, Pacemakers

The Beginnings

As in all fields of science, chance has played an important role in the development of electrophysiology. Chance was particularly influential in Galvani's discovery of bioelectricity.

Electricity had become the popular topic of the day for hypotheses and speculation when Luigi Galvani (1737–98) performed the first of his classic experiments. Galvani's career was a mixture of triumph and frustration (1). His initial great discoveries were followed by years of tumultuous controversy during which he tried in vain to uphold a mistaken hypothesis. Born in Bologna in September 1737, he became a doctor and soon after married the daughter of Professor Galeazzi. He had great success in comparative anatomy, made ninety dissections of birds, and published an article on the urinary apparatus of birds (1). Appointed a lecturer at the University of Bologna at the age of twenty-five, he was later appointed professor of anatomy.

Interest in electrical phenomena was based on knowledge derived from four sources: the electric ray or torpedo fish, rubbed amber, the lodestone, and terrestrial lightning (2–6). The interrelationships among these sources were established over a total period of nearly two hundred years. One of the sciences created out of this conjunction was electrophysiology.

Interest in animal electricity was widespread in the early part of the eighteenth century; electricity and electrical experiments were the fashion of the day. The numbing power of the torpedo fish had begun to arouse the interest of experimenters at the end of the seventeenth century. Bancroft in 1676 suggested that the active discharge of the torpedo fish might be electrical in origin. Almost one hundred years later, John Walsh reported that the shock of the torpedoes was due to the release of compressed electrical fluid. At the same time, John Hunter confirmed Walsh's anatomic and physiologic findings. Catastrophic effects on animal tissue of powerful electrical discharges from electric machines (friction) and Leyden jars (condensers) had been noted. The uses of electricity were manifold— for example, to kill small animals, to shock large numbers of persons connected to one another by wire, and so on. In one notable case, lightning was lethal to Professor Richmann in St. Petersburg Russia, when he repeated Benjamin Franklin's famous kite experiment, unfortunately, with an improperly insulated rod. In 1756 Leopoldo Caldani, a former student of Morgagni, demonstrated excitation of an isolated nerve and muscle by discharge from a Leyden jar. Luigi Galvani was a student of Caldani at that time.

Electricity had also become fascinating for clinical practitioners and anatomists. Electricity was not only in the air; it was also fashionable. The identity of lightning and electricity had been established. Leyden jars, electric machines (friction machines), and other machines were the fashion in science. This vogue flourished because of the considerable number of scholars, students, and experimentalists who were receptive to new and attractive ideas. It was not unusual that an obstetrician, an eminent practitioner, and professor of anatomy at the University of Bologna, Luigi Galvani should possess electrical machines and use them in scientific investigations. These experiments are now listed in the annals of history. The following is a quotation from Galvani, as translated by Foley in 1953 (7, 8):

> The course of the work has progressed in the following way. I dissected a frog and prepared it. . . . Having in mind other things, I placed the frog on the same table as the electrical machine . . . so that the animal was completely separated from and removed at a considerable distance from the machine's conductor. When one of my assistants by chance lightly applied the point of a scalpel to the inner crural nerve of the frog, suddenly all the muscles from the limbs were seen so to contract that they appeared to have fallen into violent tonic convulsions, Another assistant observed that this phenomenon occurred when a spark was discharged from the conductor of the electrical machine. . . . Marvelling at this, he immediately brought the unusual phenomenon to my attention when I was completely engrossed in contemplating other things. Hereupon, I became extremely enthusiastic and eager to repeat the experiment so to clarify the obscure phenomenon and make it known. I, myself, therefore, applied the point of the scalpel first to one and then to the other crural nerve, while at the same time some of the assistants produced a spark. The phenomenon repeated itself in precisely the same

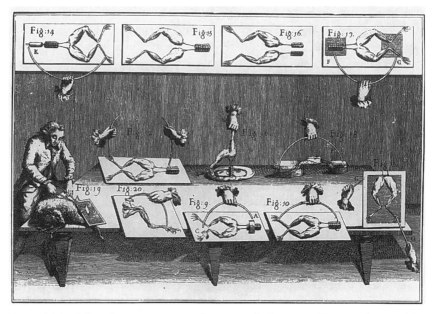

Figure 14.1. Galvani's experiments to show animal electricity. (*Private collection of Dr. Richard Bing, with permission*)

manner as before. Violent contractions were induced in the individual muscles of the limbs, and the prepared animal reacted just as though it were seized with tetanus at the very moment when the spark were discharged.

This fortuitous observation of twitching of frog legs under the action of electric current, together with an alert, communicative assistant, was the beginning of many experiments by which Galvani tried to prove the importance of electricity in physiological phenomena (Fig. 14.1). A somewhat different account of this event was presented by Cohen (7) as follows:

One evening, Galvani was in his laboratory doing some experiments with some friends and with one of his nephews, Camille, of whom he was particularly fond. By chance, some skinned frogs out of which they were going to make soup had been placed on a table where there was an electric machine: the frogs were separated from the conductor by a certain space. One of the men who was helping in the experiment put, by accident, the point of a scalpel close to the internal crural nerve of one of the animals; immediately, all the muscles of the members underwent strong convulsions. Galvani's wife was present: she was struck with the novelty of the phenomenon: she believed that she noticed that it coincided with the release of the electric spark. She ran to tell her husband who decided immediately to verify this extraordinary fact. Having as a consequence brought the point of the scalpel a second time close to the crural nerves of the frog while a spark from the electric machine was released, the contractions began to take place. They could be attributed simply to the contact of the scalpel which served as a stimulus rather than to the release of the spark. To clarify this doubt, Galvani touched the same nerves on other frogs while the electric machine was inactive; then, the contraction did not take place: the experiment was repeated often and was constantly followed by the same results. (*Doubts have been raised whether the good Luigi would have been preparing this delicacy in the laboratory rather than in the kitchen. The fact remains, however, that his wife was ill, and she died one year before the publication of his manuscript.*)

Influenced by Franklin, Galvani hoped to demonstrate that lightning flashes acted upon the limbs in an identical fashion when similar electrical connections were made for it. The next experiment proved also to be the source of the great Galvani–Volta controversy. One day, presumably on November 6, 1786 (or September 20, 1786, according to Garrison), being interested in testing the influence of atmospheric electricity on the muscles of frogs, Galvani hung up a number of skinned frogs, possibly with their legs on the balcony of a terrace of his home (iron lattice in his garden). He

hooked the hind legs to the iron of the balcony by a copper wire which passed under the lumbar (crural) nerves. Galvani noted with surprise that every time the feet touched the balcony, the frogs' limbs contracted even though at that moment there were no signs of a stormy cloud and, therefore, no particular influence of the atmosphere. At first, he thought this was due to the escape to the earth of some atmospheric electricity accumulated in the frog. Stimulation occurred when both metals (copper and iron) were in contact with some part of the body. Galvani pursued this new line of investigation with vigor and enthusiasm. He repeated the same conditions indoors. Placing the frog on an iron plate and pressing a brass hook against it produced similar muscular contractions. Other combinations of metal or even a circuit through his own body or homogenous wire, with which he made a conducting arc between nerve and muscle, had the same effects, but insulators did not.

Thus, Galvani believed that there was a cumulative electricity inside a muscle that could be discharged by the dissimilar metals and, thereby, cause electrical stimulation. The influence of contemporary science is shown by the comparison Galvani made between muscular contraction in frogs and other animals and the commotions produced by the discharge of a Leyden jar. Galvani's classic monograph in 1791, *De Viribus Electricitatus in Motu Musculari Commentarius* (8), was his only major communication.

Alessandro Volta (1745–1827), then professor of natural physiology at Pavia, at first accepted Galvani's own explanation and hailed these discoveries as being of epochal value, equivalent to those of Franklin. However, within a year he uncovered facts that forced him to differ from Galvani. Volta proved there was a contact between dissimilar metals that produced electricity, one of the metals being charged with positive and the other with negative electrification. These charges combined to traverse the muscle and nerve. Volta, thus, showed that the behavior of muscle described by Galvani was not caused by animal electricity but, rather, by the action of physical electricity between two different metals.

Galvani was spurred on by Volta's objections, and with further experiments he was able to produce, in 1794, contractions without metals (9). Subsequently, he studied the nature of the electrical circuits more carefully and found that some metals were less effective in the conducting arc; liquids could be used; and a single conductor was less effective than one side of two metals. Galvani was unimpressed by the importance of the bimetallic circuit because convulsions were obtained with a single conductor. He was convinced that the conducting arc was an ordinary conductor of electricity since he had earlier excluded Leyden jars, electric machines, thunderstorms, and other familiar sources of electricity as stimuli in his experiments. Since it appeared that mere metal connection of the nerve and muscle was able to produce the same contraction as the application of electrical stimulus, he assumed that the stimulus given by a nerve to a muscle was electrical.

He postulated that the electricity was prepared in the brain and distributed by the nerves; and that the principal reservoirs of this electricity are the muscles, each fiber of which may be considered as having two surfaces and therefore two types of electricity, positive and negative, each of them representing a small Leyden jar, of which the nerves are the conductors. The animal electricity entered the muscles and caused them to contract. Galvani postulated his theory of animal electricity on the basis of many meticulous experiments repeated over and over again in the next five years. His complete theory was summarized by DuBois-Reymond in a later generation (10):

1. Animals have electricity peculiar to themselves which is called Animal Electricity.
2. The organs to which this Animal Electricity has the greatest affinity, and [to] which it is distributed, are the nerves, and the most important organ of its secretion is the brain.

The principal value of Galvani's work was the interest generated by the discovery of bioelectricity. It led to the proper explanation of his experiments, development of the battery, electrometers, and eventually demonstration of bioelectricity.

In 1797 von Humboldt demonstrated bioelectricity when he bridged the freshly cut section of a muscle and its undamaged surface with the sciatic nerve and caused contraction. Von Humboldt repeated the experiments of Galvani and of Volta and recognized that both had discovered real phenomena. After numerous experiments, he concluded that Galvani had made two genuine discoveries (11). Galvani had not discovered a new example of animal electricity but had "invented" a new electrical instrument and a source of electricity in motion—the bimetallic conductor of his later experiments.

Electricity emerged as a science from phenomena originally studied for their physiologic significance, then reinterpreted by physicists, and finally analyzed by chemists. For the next twenty years, the chemical manifestation of electricity dominated research with the work of Oersted (12) and Faraday, when the mechanical effects of current electricity, provided by the voltaic battery, attracted attention. All this was the fruit of one crucial invention of the voltaic pile, the battery to which Volta was led systematically from the first chance observations of Galvani. Volta, as the inventor, gave electrical experiments a constant source of current of nonbiologic origin for the first time.

The development of batteries led to new concepts, such as electromagnetism. With the development of more sensitive galvanometers, the electric phenomena of muscle, nerve, and other tissues including the heart could be identified and measured.

Understanding the electrophysiology of the heart was facilitated by development of the mercury capillary electrometer of Lippmann (13), its use by Waller in intact animals and man (14), the development of the string galvanometer by Ader (1897) (15), its improvement by Einthoven in 1903 (16), and its application as a diagnostic and investigative tool. With the development of the practical usable galvanometer for recording electrocardiograms and with the advances in knowledge of the anatomy of the conducting system, a great outburst of work in electrocardiography developed, which has continued to the present.

Electrocardiography

The era of modern electrocardiography was opened by Ader who, in 1897, invented a new type of galvanometer known as the string galvanometer. This galvanometer works on the principle that a current generates a magnetic field acting at right angles to its course, which varies with the strength of the current and which may, thus, exert a varying attraction or repulsion upon a second magnetic field in its vicinity. William Einthoven, professor of physiology at the University of Leiden and founder of modern electrocardiology, recognized the potential value of Ader's new, elegant galvanometer. Einthoven's construction of an improved and more sensitive galvanometer superseded all others throughout the scientific world at that time (for example, the clinical polygraph, the capillary electrometer) and provided a practical tool for electrocardiography. Einthoven recognized the vast potential importance of the electrocardiogram as a diagnostic and investigative tool.

The fact that the heart lies within the animal body, which is in essence a three-dimensional solid conductor, was known to Waller in 1889 (14) and a subject of theoretical analysis by Einthoven. "In such a solid conductor, an electrical field can be envisioned, and the electrical currents created by the heart can be considered as fluctuating vectorial force subject to mathematical analysis" (17).

The heart vector may be defined as a manifest potential difference in the medium surrounding the heart resulting from its electrical activity. Drastic changes have occurred in the concept and manner of measuring the magnitude and direction of this vector quality, following Waller's original presentation in 1887 and 1889 (14, 18).

The laws governing the distribution of potential differences within solid conductors were evidently known to Waller in 1889. Waller was aware that the entire mass of ventricles did not contract simultaneously. He believed that the wave of excitation began at the apex and lasted longer at the bases. He was convinced that the ventricular muscle could be considered electrically as a single unit. He represented the isopotential surface as if the apex of the heart could be treated as the negative pole and the base as the positive pole, the source of the potential differences produced by the ventricles. Waller used this diagram to present "the current axis of the heart" in order to explain why some leads yielded favorable larger deflection and others did not. He recognized the relationship of the position of the heart in the body to the mode of distribution of its potential and presented his findings in a human subject with situs inversus viscerum (14) with the heart tilted to the right. Thus, he was also aware of the influence of the position of the human heart on the form of the electrocardiogram. Waller noted that the dog heart has an electrical medium position behind the sternum (vertical in modern terminology). He used lead combinations to reflect the vertical, horizontal, and sagittal (front to back of the chest) components of the heart vectors. For clinical studies, he later presented the electrical field as a four-sided figure, a "tetrahedron," his own term, formed by the mouth, right arm, left arm, and left leg, from which he obtained five leads. He decried the omission of leads from the mouth, since he considered they afforded the most convenient demonstration of the difference between the right and left sides and, in certain cases, information not obtained from observations of the right and left lateral leads.

In 1913 Einthoven, Fahr, and DeWaert (17) made a seminal contribution to the new science of electrocardiography when they described their methods of determining the direction and the "manifest value" of the potential difference produced by the heartbeat at any given instant in the cardiac cycle. This contribution has been the source of inspiration, controversy, misunderstanding, and misinterpretation. Einthoven and associates were concerned with the effect of the position of the heart on the form of the electrocardiogram. "One understands easily that if, by a change of position of this organ, an alteration in the form of the curve has been produced, difficulty would be encountered in deciding about the activity of the heart by means of this form. This difficulty can be best resolved if one has previously learned to recognize exactly the influence of position" (17). Being thoroughly familiar with electric therapy and with mathematical physics, but apparently not with the reciprocity theorem of Helmholtz (19), Einthoven made several assumptions in order to establish certain relationships between leads based on the assumed geometry of the body. In answering the question, "How, from the tracings taken in the three leads, is one to determine the actual direction of the potential difference in the body?" Einthoven stated that one obtains the goal in the simplest way by schematizing the human body. In his schema the body was represented as a flat, homogenous plate in the form of an equilateral triangle. Current was led off to the galvanometer from the corners, R representing the right arm, L to the left arm, and F representing the potential of both feet. A lead from R and L corresponded, therefore, to lead I, from R to F to lead II, and from L to F to lead III. A small spot, H, in the middle of the triangle, represented the heart. The difference of potential between the two points on the surface of the heart was proportional to the cosine of the angle formed by the line of derivation of the adis of the electrical force. The value of the potential of each lead at a given moment was represented by the geometric projection of the assumed heart vector on the corresponding side of the triangle (20).

Einthoven and associates made the assumption that the heart lies as a material point in a homogenous mass and that the distance of the heart from the three leads and also the resistances concerned are equally great and that the three leads form the equilateral triangle. They assumed that the electromotive forces of the heart in the frontal plane may be represented as a single vector in the center of an equilateral triangle (20).

For the third of a century following the postulation of Einthoven's triangle and his assumptions, students of electrocardiography were confronted by a barrage of publications expanding theory based on their validity and often disputing or confirming the validity of these postulates.

Wilson, in the 1930s, gave a needed introduction to the complication of volume conductors to which Helmholtz, Einthoven, and others had contributed for the benefits of electrocardiography. Wilson and his associates described the laws that govern the distribution of electromotive forces in solid conductors, assuming the conductor to be infinite and homogenous, and the source to be a single, fixed dipole, and showed that these laws pertaining to the flow of current in volume conductors applied to electrocardiography (21). These findings were confirmatory of Craib's studies employing strips of cardiac and skeletal muscle and medullated nerve fibers (22, 23). These laws were considered to be important for the scientific analysis of chest leads in which one electrode is placed near the heart and the others in the analysis occurring by direct leads.

From these theoretic extensions based on Einthoven's postulates, V leads and, later, augmented unipolar leads (the so-called unipolar limb leads), and the central terminal with a resistive network were developed and received widespread clinical acceptance. It was believed possible to determine the potential variations produced by the heart beat at any point of the body and on or near the heart, free from the influence exerted by potential variations at the distant, supposedly indifferent electrode. These laws were applied to the distribution of the currents of action and myocardial injury.

Cardiac Arrhythmias

The diagnosis and treatment of cardiac arrhythmias including cardioversion and defibrillation, has a long and fascinating history (24–33). From earliest times, an irregular heart beat was recognized by patients and physicians. In fact, Ludwig van Beethoven set his own cardiac rhythm disturbance to music (piano sonata opus 81a, "Les adieux") long before Einthoven graphically documented the electrical expression of regular and irregular cardiac activity in the form of an electrocardiogram. Although ancient Chinese pulse theory laid the foundation for the study of arrhythmias in the fifth century B.C., the most significant breakthrough in the identification and treatment of cardiac arrhythmias first occurred in this century. In the last decades, our knowledge of pharmacology and electrophysiology has increased exponentially and the clinical significance of cardiac rhythm disturbances has favored these advances. Patients live longer and thus are more likely to experience arrhythmias and circulatory problems of the cardiac vessels. Arrhythmias are the main complication of ischemic heart disease, and have been directly linked to the frequently arrhythmogenic sudden death syndrome, which is now presumed to be an avoidable "electrical accident" of the heart.

In the majority of cases, the diagnosis of cardiac rhythm disorders relies on noninvasive examinations in addition to the clinical analysis of symptoms. Vague or broadly defined symptoms may require invasive diagnostic techniques. Electrocardiography, including resting, exercise, and esophageal ECG, and Holter monitoring are noninvasive techniques. For bradycardias, provocative testing may also be used (carotid sinus massage, atropine) (34). Electrocardiography, the basic tool for noninvasive arrhythmia diagnosis and prerequisite of antiarrhythmic therapy, translates each cardiac action into a potential variation over time. In the beginning, studies were confined to the anatomy and physiology of the heart and also to analysis of the pulse (Fig. 14.2). The analysis of the pulse as a

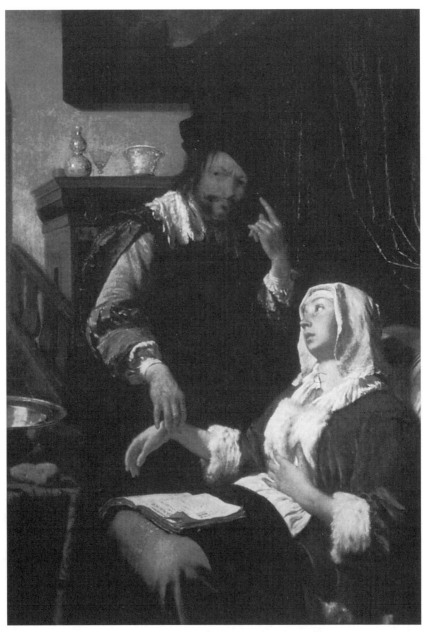

Figure 14.2. Physician's visit. Oil painting by Frans van Mieris (1635–81). *(Courtesy of Dr. Berndt Luderitz)*

mechanical expression of heart activity goes back several millennia. In China, in the year 280, Wang Shu Ho wrote a classic treatise about the pulse. The Greeks called the pulse "sphygmos," and sphygmology deals with the theory of this natural occurrence. In Roman times, Galen interpreted the various types of pulse according to the concept of the times, that each organ has its own pulse pattern depending on the nature of the disease.

Therapy for cardiac rhythm disturbances may be divided into general measures (such as bed rest, sedation, possibly vagal stimulation, etc.), pharmacological therapy, electrotherapy (especially cardioversion and defibrillation), and, in some cases, antiarrhythmic surgical interventions. By definition, a causative therapy works on the cause of the underlying condition, for instance, therapy of coronary heart disease or myocarditis, elimination of glycoside toxicity or electrolyte imbalance, normalization of hyperthyroidism, or replacement of a defective pacemaker. Yet in cases of dangerous arrhythmias, it is often necessary to eliminate the arrhythmia regardless of the underlying disease; in such instances pharmacological treatment or, sometimes, electrical devices including the implantable cardioverter/defibrillator must be considered. The history of electrophysiology of cardiac arrhythmias is shown below.

Historical Perspectives on Electrophysiology of Cardiac Arrhythmias

The History of Electrotherapy from the sixteenth to the twentieth centuries is summarized by Luderitz (35).

1580	Mercuriale, G. (1530–1606): *Ubi pulsus sit rarus semper expectanda est syncope* (36)
1717	Gerbezius, M. (1658–1718): *Constitutio Anni 1717 A.D. Marco Gerbezio Labaco 10. Decem. descripta. Miscellanea-Emphemerides Academiae Naturae Curiosorum. Cent. VII, VIII. 1718: in Appendice* (37)
1761	Morgagni, G.B. (1682–1771): *De sedibus et causis morborum per anatomen indagatis* (38)
1791	Galvani, L. (1737–98): *De viribus electricitatis in motu musculari commentarius* (8)
1800	Bichat, M.F.X. (1771–1802): *Recherches physiologiques sur la vie et la mort* [Physiologic study on life and death] (39)
1804	Aldini, G. (1762–1834): *Essai theorique et experimental sur le galvanisme, avec une serie d'experiences faites en presence des commissaires de l'institut national de France, et en divers amphitheatres de Londres* [Theoretical and experimental essay on galvanism with a series of experiments conducted in the presence of representatives of the National Institute of France at various amphitheaters in London] (40)
1827/1846	Adams, R. (1791–1875); Stokes, W. (1804–78): *Cases of diseases of the heart accompanied with pathological observations: Observations of some cases of permanently slow pulse* (41, 42)
1872	Duchenne de Bologne, G.B.A. (1806–75): *De l'ectrisation localisée et de son application à la pathologie et à la thérapeutique par courants induits et par*

courants galvaniques interrompus et continues [On localized electrical stimulation and its pathological and therapeutic application by induced and galvanized current, both interrupted and continuous] (43)

1882   von Ziemssen, H. (1829–1902): *Studien über die Bewegungsvorgänge am menschlichen Herzen sowie über die mechanische und elektrische Erregbarkeit des Herzens und des Nervus phrenicus, angestellt an dem freiliegenden Herzen der Catharina Serafin* [Studies on the motions of the human heart as well as the mechanical and electrical excitability of the heart and phrenic nerve, observed in the case of the exposed heart of *Catharina Serafin*] (44)

1890   Huchard, H.: *La maladie de Adams–Stokes* [Adams Stokes Syndrome]

1932   Hyman, A.S.: *Resuscitation of the stopped heart by intracardial therapy. II. Experimental use of an artificial pacemaker* (45)

1952   Zoll, P.M.: *Resuscitation of heart in ventricular standstill by external electrical stimulation* (46)

1958   Elmquist, R.; Senning, A: *An implantable pacemaker for the heart* (47)

1958   Furman, S.; Robinson, G.: *The use of an intracardiac pacemaker in the correction of total heart block* (48)

1961   Bouvrain, Y.; Zacouto, F.: *L'entrainement électrosystolique du coeur* [Electrical capture of the heart] (49)

1962   Lown, B., et al.: *New method for terminating cardiac arrhythmias* (50)

1962   Nathan, D.A., et al.: *An implantable synchronous pacemaker for the long-term correction of complete heart block* (51)

1969   Berkovits, B.V., et al.: *Bifocal demand pacing* (52)

1969   Scherlag, B.J., et al.: *Catheter technique for recording His bundle activity in man* (53)

1972   Wellens, H.J.J., et al.: *Electrical stimulation of the heart in patients with ventricular tachycardia* (54)

1975   Zipes, D.P., et al.: *Termination of ventricular fibrillation in dogs by depolarizing a critical amount of myocardium* (55)

1978   Josephson, M.E., et al.: *Recurrent sustained ventricular tachycardia* (56)

1980   Mirowski, M., et al.: *Termination of malignant ventricular arrhythmias with an implanted automatic defibrillation in human beings* (57)

1982   Gallagher, J.J., et al.: *Catheter technique for closed-chest ablation of the atrioventricular conduction system: A therapeutic alternative for the treatment of refractory supraventricular tachycardia* (58)

1982   Scheinman, M.M., et al.: *Transvenous catheter technique for induction of damage to the atrioventricular junction in man* (59)

1982   Lüderitz, B., et al.: *Therapeutic pacing in tachyarrhythmias by implanted pacemakers* (60)

1985   Manz, M., et al.: *Antitachycardia pacemaker (Tachylog) and automatic implantable defibrillator (AID): Combined use in ventricular tachyarrhythmias* (61)

1987   Borggrefe, M., et al.: *High frequency alternating current ablation of an accessory pathway in humans* (62)

1988   Saksena, S.; Parsonnet, V.: *Implantation of a cardioverter-defibrillator without thoracotomy using a triple electrode system* (63)

1991   Jackman, W.M., et al.: *Catheter ablation of accessory atrioventricular pathways (Wolff-Parkinson-White Syndrome) by radiofrequency currentt* (64)

1991   Kuck, K.H., et al.: *Radiofrequency current catheter ablation of accessory atrioventricular pathways* (65)

1995   Lau, C.P., et al.: *Implantable atrial defibrillator* (66).

1997   Jung W., et al.: *First worldwide implantation of an arrhythmia management system* (67).

Pacing/Cardioversion

In treating tachyarrhythmias (such as tachycardia caused by premature contractions, atrial flutter, supraventricular or ventricular tachycardia), temporary or permanent pacing is used once it has been determined that the rhythm disorder is drug refractory. In the 1970s and 1980s various pacing methods to terminate tachycardia have been reported, such as overdrive pacing, dual-chamber pacing (68), high-rate pacing, programmed (competitive) stimulation with or without extrastimuli (68, 69), and scanning stimulation (35, 70). Currently, overdrive pacing, programmed stimulation, and high-rate pacing are used.

Overdrive pacing, which prevents as well as terminates tachyarrhythmias, is defined as supraventricular or ventricular pacing in which the pacemaker elevates the heart rate over the intrinsic rhythm, thus suppressing ectopic tachyarrhythmias. Programmed stimulation, used mainly to terminate supraventricular or ventricular reentry tachycardias, involves delivering one or more output pulses to the heart at precisely timed points in the cardiac cycle. This depolarizes the myocardium prematurely and, in so doing, interrupts the circus movement (71). High-rate pacing is used to terminate supraventricular tachycardia. For atrial flutter induced by digitalis toxicity, atrial high-rate pacing is the therapy of choice. Sinus rhythm is usually restored via induction of atrial fibrillation.

CATHETER ABLATION

Noninvasive catheter ablation of the bundle of His, AV node, or accessory pathways has become an available method for treating symptomatic, drug-resistant supraventricular tachycardias.

BUNDLE OF HIS ABLATION

In 1981 Gonzales et al. (72) reported the first AV block induced by an electrode catheter. A patient was undergoing an electrophysiologic study following defibrillation when the defibrillating electrode accidentally came into contact with an electrode catheter in the bundle of His. This accidental discovery became the basis of the work of Gallagher et al. (58), as well as Scheinman et al. (59, 73), on patients with drug-refractory supraventricular tachycardia. In these patients, a noninvasive percutaneous excision and coagulation of the bundle of His was performed using direct current shock via a catheter. This method necessitates an initial electrophysiological study for diagnostic purposes, followed by an electrode catheter inserted in the bundle of His. An electrical shock is delivered from an external defibrillator. Generally, this leads to coagulation necrosis. Throughout this procedure, an external pacemaker provides ventricular pacing support (74). Percutaneous His bundle ablation represents a new and very promising method of treating drug-resistant supraventricular tachycardia.

ACCESSORY PATHWAYS

In 1983 Weber and Schmitz (75) reported the first treatment of Type B Wolff-Parkinson-White syndrome using catheter ablation. The accessory pathway was interrupted by positioning a tripolar electrode in the right atrium. Based on the studies by Kuck et al. (65) and Jackman et al. (64), invasive, but not operative catheter ablation is the therapy of choice for symptomatic preexcitation syndromes (76). In contrast to high-frequency catheter ablation (64, 77, 78, 79, 80), another technique known as laser photo ablation (81, 82) uses a more controllable energy to remove accessory AV pathways and therefore the source of ventricular tachycardia. However, laser photo ablation is not used at the present time.

High-frequency energy was first used in 1986 in catheter ablation by Borggrefe et al. to interrupt an AV bypass tract (62). This group also performed the first high-frequency ablation in a patient with ventricular tachycardia. In these early procedures, the energy discharged (up to 50 W) was also applied to direct current ablation; a unipolar electrode catheter and a large-surface reference electrode placed on the chest were used. Unlike in direct current ablation, energy was applied for longer periods (ten to ninety seconds). Because the energy applied can be precisely controlled, high-energy catheter ablation carries with it less risk of complications than the direct current approach (83).

IMPLANTABLE CARDIOVERTER/DEFIBRILLATOR

After many years of animal experimentation, Bouvrain and Zacouto (49) published a report in 1961 that described a combination of devices they called a "resuscitation device," consisting of a heart monitor, a defibrillator, and a pacemaker. This was the first time individual pieces of equipment had been combined to work together in the case of ventricular fibrillation. Although implantable pacemakers have been available since the late 1950s, it took two more decades before implantable defibrillators were routinely used. Essentially developed by Mirowski (84, 85, 86), the AID/AICD system consists of an abdominally implanted device with a lead system for arrhythmia detection and a system for delivery of defibrillatory or cardioverting shock (Fig. 14.3). An implantable cardioverter/defibrillator is indicated in patients with life-threatening conditions when drug-refractory ventricular tachycardia or ventricular fibrillation has been documented and when an antiarrhythmic cardiological surgical intervention is not suitable or appropriate.

Another important step in the development of electrotherapy for tachyarrhythmia is the combined application of antitachycardia pacemakers and automatic cardioverter/defibrillators, first described in 1985 (61; Fig. 14.4). This method has been well documented by a series of investigations (35, 61, 87, 88). Modern implantable cardioverter/defibrillator systems now combine bradycardia

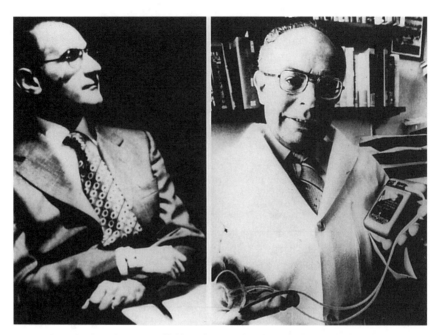

Figure 14.3. Fred Isaac Zacouto (left) and Lieczyslaw ("Michel") Mirowski (right). *(Courtesy of Dr. Berndt Luderitz)*

and antitachycardia pacing and defibrillatory options in a single device. An important development was the implantation of a transvenous defibrillator with a three-electrode system (63). A summary of electrical device therapy was published in 1994 (89).

An automatic, implantable pharmacologic defibrillator is currently being tested by Cammilli et al. (90, 91). This device combines electrical therapy with pharmacological treatment. It represents an alternative course in the treatment of refractory ventricular tachycardias, providing it can be refined and tested.

IMPLANTABLE ATRIAL DEFIBRILLATORS

The implantable atrial defibrillator is the logical extension of intraatrial defibrillation for treating symptomatic atrial fibrillation. This new form of electrical therapy is currently under clinical evaluation (92). Considered candidates for an implantable atrial defibrillator are patients with intermittent, drug-refractory atrial fibrillation that occurs at a frequency of from once a week to once every three months. After sufficient experience, when atrial fibrillation occurs, the patient can activate the implantable atrial defibrillator with a magnet or the device may respond automatically. To identify atrial fibrillation, the system uses a variety of algorithms with a high specificity for atrial fibrillation. Once the

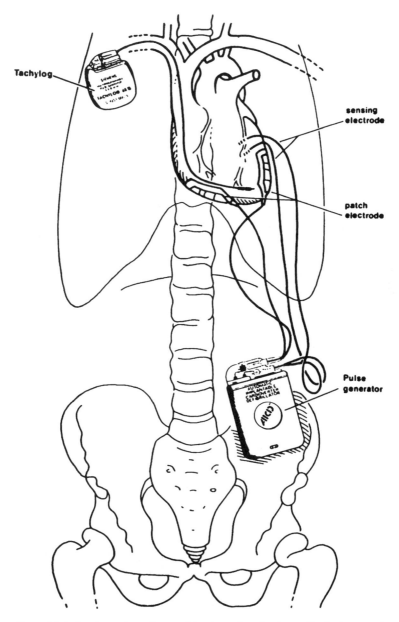

Figure 14.4. Implantation of a combination of antitachycardia devices: anti-tachycardia pacemaker (Tachylog) with transvenous, intracardiac, right ventricular leads, plus an automatic, implantable cardioverter/defibrillator with two path leads and a bipolar control lead. *(Courtesy of Dr. Berndt Luderitz)*

defibrillator system has detected and confirmed atrial fibrillation, the defibrillator's capacitors charge and a low-energy shock at a programmed energy level is delivered to terminate the arrhythmia. The clinical utility of the implantable atrial defibrillator remains to be seen, as there are still some open issues with respect to this innovative new electrical therapy, for instance, the potential risk of inducing a life-threatening cardiac rhythm disorder as well as patient acceptance of a device that delivers repeated shocks. Furthermore, it has not yet been determined if an anticoagulant is needed to prevent thromboembolism.

Patients with frequent episodes must be excluded as candidates for implantation of an atrial defibrillator because of too frequent discharges, causing patient discomfort, and because of rapid battery depletion. Similarly, patients with episodes of short duration and spontaneous termination are poor candidates. Selected patients with infrequent, symptomatic attacks of long-lasting episodes of AF despite antiarrhythmic drug therapy may benefit from an implantable atrial defibrillator.

A recent innovation in the electrical management of cardiac rhythm disorders is the implantable atrioventricular defibrillator (model 7250, Medtronic Inc.) The first such device was implanted on January 10, 1997. The system combines two therapeutic principles in one device: it automatically detects atrial and ventricular signals and delivers electrical therapy in the appropriate chamber to terminate the arrhythmia (67).

The implantable cardioverter-defibrillator has established a permanent place as a secondary line of defense in patients with malignant ventricular tachyarrhythmias. The Multicenter Automatic Defibrillator Implantation Trial (MADIT) study came to the conclusion that for patients with a previous myocardial infarction and increased risk for ventricular tachyarrhythmia, there was a better survival rate with an implanted defibrillator than with conventional drug therapy (93). Preliminary results of the AVID study were released on April 14, 1997, when the National Heart Lung and Blood Institute announced that the trial was to be halted eighteen months early because the defibrillator treatment was clearly superior. Implantable cardiac defibrillators are significantly better at preventing death from ventricular arrhythmias than antiarrhythmic drugs such as amiodaroneor sotalol. This was the first large randomized trial to show that implantable defibrillators improve survival. The findings of the AVID trial do not mean that the drug therapy is no longer useful. Drug therapy remains an important part of treatment (94, 95, 96).

Cardiopulmonary Resuscitation

The most informative and detailed report on the effect of electricity on the heart has been published in a book by Schechter on the origins and developments of electrical cardiac stimulation to the present (97). Schechter relates that Harvey in his book, *De Motu Cordis*, described experiments on pigeons in which the heart had wholly ceased to pulsate. Harvey wetted his fingers with saliva and placed them for a short time on the heart, observing that "under the influence of this procedure the heart recovered new strength and life, so that both ventricles and auricles (atria) pulsated, contracting and relaxing alternately, recalled as it were from death to life" (98). In 1791 Galvani applied a live torpedo fish to the nerves, muscle, and heart of a dead frog. Convulsive contractions occurred, and ceased after withdrawal of the fish (8). In 1797 von Humboldt experimented on the heart of a carp (11). When the heart was touched with the solution of "protosulphide of potassium" the number of beats declined.

Execution by guillotine turned out to be a bonanza for the study of the effect of electrical stimulation on the human body. Early experiments were summarized by Schechter (97). Bichat, who worked during the French Revolution, would avail himself of the bodies of guillotine victims to experiment on the effect of electricity. They were at his disposal thirty or forty minutes after the execution (39). He stated that he could not produce motion in the hearts of these executed victims through the spinal marrow or the heart nerves. "However, mechanical excitants directly applied to the flesh fibers produced contractions in them." In 1802 Nysten, working on a guillotined criminal under dramatic conditions in a Parisian cemetery, found that the contractility of the left ventricle was extinguished soon after death and always before that of other muscle organs, that the right ventricle could be made to contract more than one hour after death, that both atria continued to contract under Galvanic influence long after movement was totally abolished in other muscles, that the contractile faculty of the right atrium was always preserved much more than that of any other part of the heart, that a portion of the superior vena cava adjacent to the right atrium had contractile capacity almost equal to that of the right atrium, and, finally, that the aorta was unresponsive to electrical stimulation (99). Schechter also describes the activity of a physicians' club in Mainz, Germany, engaged in assessing the effects of different kinds of electricity on the body. "A physician's club—received a windfall of study material when on November 21, 1803 there was a mass execution of 20 marauding brigands (100). A hut was erected at 150 feet from the scaffold, so that the corpses could be delivered as quickly as possible to the eager scientists. The bandits were decapitated faster than the experiments could be done, however, so that only a few of the bodies could be examined, at 4 and 22 minutes for the first two, and a couple of hours after death for the other two." Schechter also mentions the observation by Carpne, who wrote an article on Galvanic experiments on a hanged man (101). On a corpse which he obtained, he introduced air into the trachea while massaging the chest and passing current from a voltaic pile to the intercostal nerves and the vagi, the phrenic nerves, and the rectum during ten-minute intervals. Apparently, the cadaver's face began to lighten, and when Carpne connected his battery to the pericardium and diaphragm, the pectoral muscles began to move as well as the atria of the heart, but not the ventricles (101).

The background of clinical cardiac electrostimulation is also comprehensively described by Schechter (97). He quotes an article published by Kite on "The Recovery of the Apparently Dead" published in London in 1788, which described electric shock for resuscitation (102). The apparatus consisted of pieces of brass-wire enclosed in glass tubes with knobs at one end, which were to be applied to "those parts between which we intend the electric fluid to pass. . . . In this manner, shocks may be sent through any part of the body: and their direction constantly varied, without a probability of the resistance receiving any inconvenience" (102). In 1862 Walshe suggested that irregular movements arising out of "mechanical difficulties and modified innervation of the hearts contractility, impairment and unsteadiness of the nervous force presiding over its tenacity, may be possibly contribute a share of feeble, wavering non-rhythmical motion." He suggested that successive electrical impulses which can succeed each other at appreciable intervals of time, may be a treatment of "fluttering palpitation" (103).

In 1869 the famous French physician Duchenne treated a patient with

> smallness and extreme rapidity of the pulse (136 to 140 pulsations) with such irregularity and intermittences that often 6 or 8 successive pulsations missed; impossible to distinguish the rhythm of valvar sounds on auscultation of the heart; . . . however it being urgent to act, I wished to try to modify the morbid condition of the center giving rise to the to nerves of the heart and lungs by electrocutaneous excitation of the region related to that nervous center (43).

It is likely that the patient had diphtheria and myocarditis.

The effect of electrocution on the heart was also thoroughly explored by Prevost and Battelli toward the end of the nineteenth century. They quantitatively demonstrated that fibrillary contraction induced by electricity could be abolished by another powerful discharge of either alternating or direct current—a visionary look into the future (104). Direct stimulation of the beating heart was first carried out by Ziemssen (44). Ziemssen had the advantage of observing a forty-two-year-old woman who had a huge defect on the anterior left thoracic wall consequent to resection of a chest wall tumor. In this patient the heart covered only by skin was visible and palpable. Ziemssen performed detailed studies, most of them electrical, on this conveniently exposed normal heart and reported his findings in 1882. The results of these experiments prompted Ziemssen to use electric currents in patients with intact thorax. His main conclusion was that currents of sufficient intensity and frequency were required to modify the action of the heart (44).

Schechter quoted the work of MacWilliams, published from 1887 to 1914, in which the treatment of Adams-Stokes attacks was considered (105).

> But, on the other hand, in certain of forms of cardiac arrest there appears to be a possibility of restoring by artificial means the rhythmic beat and tiding over a sudden and temporary danger—. Now we know that when the mammalian heart has been inhibited through the vagus nerve it is quite possible to excite an immediate renewal of the rhythmic action by direct stimulation of the organ. No doubt it is very possible, as I have already suggested in a former paper, that the fate of the heart may be sealed in cases of fatal inhibitory arrest by the supervention of fibrillar contraction or heart-delirium in the ventricles.

In 1904 Andrew Smith mailed this suggestion to the editor of the *Medical Records,* as quoted by Schechter: "Sir: As a possible successful means of resuscitation in sudden heart-failure I would suggest laying bare the pericardium over the left ventricle and applying electricity at the bottom of the wound" (97). Even more direct was the approach of Robinovitch, who in 1907 resuscitated a patient by means of rhythmic electrostimulation (106). The patient as quoted in the book by Schechter was a young woman, a chronic morphine user. The patient apparently had a cardiac arrest and became

> black in the face and none of those present expected any good results from the application of rhythmic electric excitations. We practiced rhythmic excitations during a period of about 30 seconds; the duration of the closure of the circuit was about 1/2 of a second and the period of the opening of the circuit was about 1 second. We shortened the period of the opening of the circuit—as against our own indications and our papers on the subject of resuscitation, because the patient seemed to be thoroughly asphyxiated—as we judged her condition from the color of her face. As the rhythmic excitations were being repeated, it was astonishing to see the accompanying change of color in the patient's face; the dark blue color changed to pale, then to almost natural color; at the end of the 30 seconds of rhythmic excitations, the patient took a long spontaneous breath, opened her eyes and said: "Oh I feel so cold in my back." The cold she felt was the wet cotton of the electrodes. But the interesting point is that the patient felt no other inconvenience during the rhythmic excitations—while she was in profound syncope (106).

In 1926 Consolidated Electric Company of New York City, concerned by the increasing number of electric shock accidents and deaths, sought advice from the consultants of the Rockefeller Institute. Five working groups were established, and one chaired by Professor Howell was given the task of studying the effects of electric shock on physiological parameters (107). In 1928 the Consolidated Edison, a New York power company, gave Johns Hopkins University a $10,000 grant to investigate the effects of electricity in the body, because many linemen were dying from electrical shock. W.H. Howell elected a number of scientists, among them Kouwenhoven, to begin these studies (108). The increasing mortality rate from accidental electrocution by faulty electric appliances had led to a conference on electric shock and to the appointment of a Committee on Physiology for its study. Carl J. Wiggers was in a receptive frame of mind to go into a new direction of research when Howell invited him in 1929 to join with Donald R. Hooker to research possible ways of resuscitating hearts from fibrillation induced by electric currents (109).

The invitation in 1929 from Howell to join with Hooker and others in research to resuscitate hearts from ventricular fibrillation was unexpected but most opportune and welcome. Howell had taken an interest in Wiggers' career and had stimulated his interest in physiology by recommending his membership in the American Physiologic Society in 1907, by "kindly providing comments on his presentation of papers, and by mentioning 'my minor contributions' in his textbooks" (109). Howell had successively become professor of physiology and histology at the University of Michigan from 1889 to 1892, associate professor of physiology at Harvard in 1892–93, professor of physiology in the Medical School at Johns Hopkins University from 1893 to 1917, and later in the School of Hygiene at Johns Hopkins from 1917 to 1931, remaining professor emeritus from 1931 to 1945 (the year he died).

Interest in defibrillation by countershock was stimulated by Howell in 1930 when he suggested to the investigators at both institutions that they reinvestigate the claims of Prevost and Battelli, who in 1899 (110) reported that strong currents do not produce ventricular fibrillation but may even abrogate it when it does exist. They described a technique for defibrillating the heart of a dog using a charged capacitor. Wiggers stated, "The idea seemed so fantastic that I read their reports in a biased and unfriendly frame of mind and concluded that their experimental evidence fell short of their claims. At any event, I did not deem a reinvestigation of their claims worthy of the time, effort or expense it would involve" (109).

Hooker, in association with Kouwenhoven and Langworthy, did accept the challenge to test the countershock method for fibrillation. A preliminary report of its success was made in 1932 and a more detailed paper appeared a year later (111). Wiggers and his associates then repeated the procedure and confirmed its effectiveness. In the meantime, Ferris and his associates confirmed the observation that a single strong shock applied during the vulnerable period induced ventricular fibrillation and that this can be abolished by immediate application of a strong current to the chest wall (112).

Research efforts of the two groups, at Western Reserve University and at Johns Hopkins, followed different roads but ultimately came together on the exposed heart and the Johns Hopkins group on the closed chest, the latter because of their commitment to solve the problem of defibrillation of linemen exposed to high tension (107, 109).

Countershock directly to the heart or to the intact chest was found by both groups to be effective in restoring normal heart beats only when applied within two or three minutes after induction of fibrillation (113, 114). This period was so short that countershock proved a useful defibrillating method in animal experiments only when electrodes had been applied to the heart previous to the onset of ventricular fibrillation and when the equipment for furnishing shocks of appropriate strength was immediately available. Consequently, efforts were made to extend the period of revival during which countershock would be effective after the development of fibrillation. The inability to restore normal action of the heart by applying countershock after more than five minutes was usually not due to failure to abrogate it but rather the failure of the ventricles to develop vigorous beats.

Wiggers and associates recognized that the fibrillating ventricles lose their power of effective contraction after two to three minutes because they are deprived of a supply of oxygenated blood. Two approaches were developed to restore the vigor of myocardial contraction after countershock: Wiggers used cardiac massage, and Hooker and associates used central carotid injections of saline with adrenaline and calcium (107, 115).

It was apparent to Wiggers that the remedy needed was a supply of oxygen for the myocardium before application of countershock. If oxygen were provided, muscular contractions would become vigorous the moment incoordination was abolished by countershock (115). In 1936 Wiggers recommended that cardiac massage be started as quickly as possible and continued (115). Wiggers described a method of cardiac massage as consisting of "gentle manual compression of the ventricles about 40 times per minute, thereby raising aortic pressure to 50 or 60 mm Hg. This pressure proved sufficient to supply the heart with oxygenated blood, restore vigorous fibrillatory movements, and incidentally maintained the viability of the center nervous system. An electric shock applied after this procedure usually resulted in prompt redevelopment of the coordinated ventricular beats" (115). Wiggers reported, "I have personally witnessed over 1,000 revivals in all kinds of fibrillation in dogs weighing up to 18 kg through use of this method" (109). Wiggers' major contribution to the problem, which ultimately had clinical application by Claude Beck and others, was the development of experimental methods to extend the period of revival.

Defibrillation was occasionally difficult in dogs with large hearts because the current used was not strong enough to penetrate all parts of the myocardium.

Wiggers and associates developed a technique called serial defibrillations, consisting of three to five brief shocks at approximately two-second intervals, which was found to be effective in abolishing ventricular fibrillation (116). Beck and associates also occasionally encountered difficulty in successful defibrillation in the laboratory and sought a modification for use on the human heart "if it should be necessary at the time of operation" (117). Mautz, Beck's associate, demonstrated that procaine or metycaine applied directly to the fibrillating heart reduced the irritability of the myocardium and that electric shock would uniformly stop ventricular fibrillation (118). Soon, Mautz (119) adopted Wiggers' modification of the countershock method (massage, serial shocks if necessary) and found that injections of a small amount of procaine into the ventricular cavity prior to the use of massage and countershock was helpful in abolishing residual areas of fibrillation.

Open Chest Cardiac Resuscitation: Application to Humans

Wiggers produced ventricular fibrillation in animals with electrical currents as well as by ligating of the coronary arteries. He found that the coronary ligatures had to be removed before he could defibrillate a dog's heart (115). Because of this, he seriously questioned whether ventricular fibrillation could be corrected electronically after coronary thrombosis. "The normal dog's heart can rarely be revived unless the occlusion is removed, and this is impossible in man" (115).

Beck appeared to share a similar view in 1937, when he wrote, "I should like to make this statement, that any heart that stops beating in the operating room can be revived provided there is no intrinsic disease of the heart. Of course, a heart that is poisoned by bacterial toxin or a heart that is poorly vascularized because of coronary artery disease cannot be expected to recover. Patients who die suddenly and who have good hearts constitute a group that can be saved if we are trained to grasp the occasion as it arises" (120).

In 1937 and thereafter, with messianic zeal, Claude Beck disseminated widely, with lectures, articles, demonstrations, and motion pictures, his procedure for defibrillation of the ventricles in the operating room (121). Beck and Mautz presented a motion picture of fibrillation and defibrillation to the American Surgical Association in 1937. Unfortunately, the audience was not appreciative of the possible clinical application (121, 122, 123).

Beck's recommended procedure was as follows:

> Adequate aeration of the lungs. This is possible only through an intratracheal tube and intermittent insufflation with air and oxygen. This is the first step to be taken and requires preparation. Exposure of the heart and massage of the ventricles about 50 times per minute. This will raise arterial pressure to 40 to 60 mm of mercury. It must be so vigorous as to bruise the myocardium. The central nervous system is now being oxy-

genated and reflexes return. Restoration of circulation with oxygenated blood to the brain and to the myocardium is essential. As long as it is carried out, recovery is a possibility, even though the ventricles continue to fibrillate. It is possible to continue this artificial circulation over a period long enough to wash out an overdose of anesthetic and long enough for drug effect to disappear. . . . Before the next step is taken two things must be accomplished by the massage. First, the dilated heart must have a good color. A cyanotic heart is also prone to keep on fibrillating. When both of these objects are accomplished by aeration and massage, the heart will show slow and coarse fibrillatory movements. An electrode, preferably of silver, measuring about 25 square centimeters in area, is placed on each side of the heart and an electric current is sent through the ventricles. The electrodes need not be padded to prevent burning if there is a large area of contact with the heart. The current is an ordinary alternating current of 60 cycles and 1 to 1.5 amperes. The duration of the current is short, from 0.5 to about two seconds.

If the shock fails to stop fibrillation, the use of procaine is indicated. Two cubic centimeters of 5 percent solution are dripped upon the auricles and the ventricles. Massage as before until dilation disappears. Electric shock is usually successful in stopping fibrillation. If it is not, 2 cc. of procaine in 10 cc. of physiologic solution of sodium chloride are injected into the right ventricular cavity. Massage until dilation disappears. Electric shock now will stop the fibrillation routinely in dogs.

Every vestige of fibrillatory movement must disappear before there is any hope of success. After fibrillation has been abolished and the heart is at a standstill, massage is used. This usually starts a coordinated rhythm. At this place in the procedure, epinephrine may be useful.

After using procaine or metycaine upon the heart, ventricular fibrillation may be converted into ventricular standstill by the current without restoration of any signs of contractibility. In this event massage is continued, and a solution of calcium chloride is injected into the right ventricle. . . .

It is needless to say that throughout the entire procedure, massage of the ventricles is absolutely necessary to preserve the viability of the brain and the myocardium. We have succeeded in reviving hearts that were in ventricular fibrillation or standstill for periods as long as 30 minutes. During this entire period an arterial pressure was maintained by massage of the heart. . . .

Defibrillators were placed by Beck and his associates in the emergency room and various operating rooms of the university hospitals of Cleveland. Lectures and laboratory demonstrations were frequently made. The staff was alerted. Beck defibrillated a human heart in 1938 and another in 1939, but these patients died sometime later from damage to the brain (117).

Resuscitation Procedures

Resuscitation was started on a patient who fibrillated while in bed in her room in a medical area in 1956. "The chest was opened by the medical resident; the heart was pumped by hand, and the lungs were oxygenated. This consumed 15 minutes. The oxygen-system was maintained in transit to the operating room and this consumed 10 minutes. The chest was draped. The heart was defibrillated. The patient made an uneventful recovery" (124).

As a result of the successful recovery of a patient in 1947, Beck renewed his efforts to spread the "gospel" of "Hearts Too Good to Die" (117) with the development of a policy statement for the Veterans Administration and with the establishment of postgraduate courses for nurses and physicians on the prevention and management of cardiac arrest. He dared to recommend that the procedure be done on victims who had "fatal" heart attack outside the hospital. This involved opening the chest. The dean of the Medical School of Western Reserve University stated that Beck "was not a safe man to have on the faculty" (117). Nevertheless, the concept of "Hearts Too Good to Die" was disseminated with hands-on experience in Beck's surgical laboratory and qualification of the medical students of Western Reserve University School of Medicine, of the resident physicians in training, and of over 3,500 physicians and nurses in two-day courses of instruction each month from 1950 to 1965 (117, 125, 126). Some participants of the latter group came from Britain, France, Sweden, and other countries. Soon reports of successful open chest resuscitation outside of the hospital appeared in a great variety of venues, in the hallways of hospitals, darkrooms, in the offices of physicians and dentists, on the golf course, at athletic contests.

In 1950 Beck provided the Veterans Administration Technical Bulletin TB 10-65, on the treatment of cardiac arrest (126). This became policy throughout the Veterans Administration. There was emphasis on the restoration of the oxygen system, restoration of the heart beat, methods of application of drugs in asystole and ventricular fibrillation, and closure of the chest.

The birth and development of the coronary care ward was another byproduct of the concept of "Hearts Too Good to Die." "At the University Hospitals of Cleveland in 1958 Doctor David Leighninger (Doctor Beck's associate) gave round-the-clock care to a patient stricken with coronary occlusion" (117). The patient was a professor of pediatrics who had developed cardiac standstill while rushing up several flights of stairs. Blows to the precardium by a medical resident initiated a heartbeat. The patient was transported to a private hospital room and connected to a direct writing electrocardiograph for continuous motoring. Leighninger slept in an adjacent room and was made available over a period of seven days. In 1962 Hughes A. Day established a physical unit to provide this specialized care to the coronary patient (see Chapter 7). A letter to Beck from Day, Bethany Hospital in Kansas City, Kansas, September 12, 1969, follows:

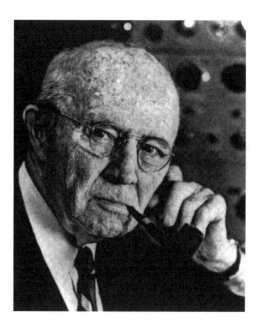

Figure 14.5. Photograph of William B. Kouwenhoven in 1973 when he received the Albert and Mary Lasker Foundation Award for Clinical Medical Research. *(Courtesy of the Lasker Foundation, New York)*

During the six years I served a Director of the Unit from 1962 to 1968, a total of 530 proven myocardial infarcts were treated. There were 98 deaths. Ventricular fibrillation occurred in 59. Of these, 44 were resuscitated for a salvage rate of 74 percent. Similar results are occurring in other coronary care units across the country. My first two articles were published in *Lancet*, 1962 and 1963. They were published in *Lancet* for tne simple reason that I could not get any national journal to publish them. One editor wrote me that "the article on Cardiac Resuscitation was nothing new and everything had been written about cardiac resuscitation that was worthwhile" (127).

Development of Closed Chest Cardiac Massage and Defibrillation

The driving force for closed chest resuscitation at the Johns Hopkins Hospital was William Bennett Kouwenhoven (Fig. 14.5). He and his Johns Hopkins group, because of contractual interest, focused on closed chest defibrillation and developed a simple electrical apparatus for closed chest ventricular defibrillation of humans (107, 114). Survival depended on the termination of ventricular fibrillation within one or two minutes of its onset. Wiggers had established that cardiac massage with restoration of some coronary perfusion was essential *before* countershock (115), and Kouwenhoven and his group continued to be unable to produce recovery with restoration despite successful closed chest defibrillation (abrogation of ventricular fibrillation) unless it were applied within one or two minutes of onset (114); after a longer period of time, although the heart could be defibrillated, even central carotid artery infusion with epinephrine and other materials was not successful (114). This approach had limited application clinically and in the field. In the meantime, the investigators at the Johns Hopkins University continued to conduct research on closed chest defibrillation and, unlike Wiggers and Beck, had been able to restore animals and humans after the development of ventricular fibrillation when closed chest electrical shock alone was provided unless after one or two minutes. In 1956 Zoll and associates successfully terminated ventricular fibrillation of several patients in an intensive care monitoring area. They externally applied electrical stimulation without external chest cardiac massage (128).

Kouwenhoven recalled that as a result of Wiggers' demonstration of the importance of restoring coronary flow with cardiac massage *before* countershock, it was no longer necessary to defibrillate within two or three minutes, the limitation of the Johns Hopkins closed chest approach. Beck's first successful defibrillation of a human heart on December 7, 1938, did not result in survival because of brain damage (123).

Kouwenhoven was concerned at the time with methods of providing circulation without resorting to thoracotomy:

> It was clearly recognized that time was the most important factor and that time as measured in seconds, literally. The first method tried was to insert needles through the chest into the myocardium and apply pacemaker shocks to the fibrillating heart. These proved to be ineffective and the method was abandoned (107).
>
> A series of experiments was conducted in which a brief AC defibrillating shock of one tenth or less seconds was applied to the chest at the rate of a shock per second. In these applications only three dogs were saved in a large group. Many times it was impossible to defibrillate the heart when the stimuli had been applied for several minutes. This scheme was also abandoned (107).

The potential solution to providing circulation during ventricular fibrillation was initiated by a "misadventure" during open chest cardiac resuscitation at Johns Hopkins, supposedly an indirect result of the influence of Beck's concept of "Hearts Too Good to Die." Kouwenhoven recalled that a young medical officer physician when working in the Johns Hopkins Hospital emergency room applied "Claude Beck's approach" to cardiac resuscitation, that is, emergency thoracotomy, manual massage of the fibrillating heart, and successful defibrillation, with survival. This case was presented enthusiastically at grand rounds. Several months later, another case with ventricular fibrillation was presented. Another house officer had performed an emergency thoracotomy on a patient with ventricular fibrillation. Unfortunately, in the course of making an incision in the left chest, he had inadvertently cut the heart, almost transecting it, of course, with an unfavorable outcome.

According to Kouwenhoven, at the grand rounds presentation of this case of near-transection of the heart, he stated he was struck by the absurdity of the open chest cardiac massage technique. This misadventure provoked his interest in exploring an earlier chance observation that should provide an alternative to open chest cardiac massage. The idea of closed chest resuscitation originated when Kouwenhoven recalled that when Mine Safety electrodes were pressed on an animal's chest, there was a slight rise in blood pressure before a shock was applied. Chance favors the prepared mind! In 1958 his assistant, Guy Knickerbocker, a twenty-four-year-old graduate student of electrical engineering who had joined Kouwenhoven to participate in the program of the Edison project in 1954, also noticed this phenomenon (107). When interviewed in July 1991, Knickerbocker said that with the passage of many years, he presently was not sure who made the observation initially, whether it was he who had made the observation or that he and Kouwenhoven made it together. He did recall looking at the Sanborn record pressure curve, which showed a definite rise in the intraarterial femoral pressure. He and Kouwenhoven

> were proceeding with their studies in closed-chest defibrillation when they observed that there was a rise in intra-arterial pressure when the heart defibrillator electrodes were applied to the chest wall of the dog with ventricular fibrillation. A relaxation and push caused additional increase in arterial pressure. They considered that the rhythmic application of pressure to the chest wall might cause the heart to empty and provide circulation. These observations and ideas were discussed with the staff of the Johns Hopkins Hospital, but they were assured that pressing on the animal's chest was like pressing on a balloon: when the pressure was relaxed, the chest expanded and the pressure returned to normal; the rise was not sufficient indication of circulation (107).

Inadequate consideration was given to the concepts of the production of an artificial circulation by external cardiac compression, because others previously had condemned this technique. Pike and colleagues in 1908 had attempted massage without success.

> They noted that rhythmic manual compression of the thorax of a cat over the heart gave fairly good results in certain stages of heart stoppage, but the time when massage was effective was much too limited to make the method a sure one. They questioned whether, in fact, the loss of the pulse was associated with the heart ceasing to beat. . . . [Electrocardiograms were not in common use at that time.] Furthermore, they noted

that rhythmic compression of the thorax of a large dog could not be kept for a sufficiently long time (129).

George Crile's report of resuscitation by chest compression was similarly rejected.

In 1908, Crile, Cleveland, Ohio, had been successful in animals with arterial perfusion and squeezing the unopened chest. He demonstrated that latter before the Cleveland Academy of Medicine in 1908. As he stated, "This led naturally to the use of adrenaline saline solution intravascularly, combined with rhythmic pressure on the chest as a means of resuscitation." This furnishes an external pseudocardiac reaction. Direct massage is, therefore, not essential (130).

During the first decade of the twentieth century, three patients had been successfully resuscitated. Crile's patient, a twelve-year-old girl, was one. At one time he referred to this incident as death and resurrection. The medical profession marveled for a short time, but they were not ready to accept cardiac resuscitation. Acceptance was extended to the Pulmotor, a mechanical device (130).

Earlier, in 1878, Boehm reported treatment of the arrested heart with a closed chest method of resuscitation. "Working with cats, he grasped the chest in his hand at the area of greatest expansion and applied rhythmic pressure. His results were quite striking in some series of tests." Tournade and his co-workers reported that compression of the thorax of a dog in a cardiac arrest could produce blood pressure of 60 or 100 mm. There were no survival data. In 1933, Killick and Eve reported that the rocking technique of artificial respiration by which a patient is tilted about 60° in each direction from the horizontal plane will produce a change in the blood pressure at the atrium from 38 to 76 mm Hg. Eve hypothesized that this change will produce sufficient blood flow to nourish the heart and the brain" (131).

At the time (1957) when Knickerbocker and Kouwenhoven were developing their technique for external cardiac massage, they first became aware of the 1947 publication of N.L. Gurvich and G.S. Yuniev (132), who approximately ten years earlier had found that a capacitor discharge, sent through the chest of a dog, would be followed by resumption of cardiac function if applied not later than one or one and one-half minutes after the onset of induced ventricular fibrillation, and that this time limitation might be extended to as long as eight minutes by rhythmical application of pressure on the thorax by squeezing both sides of the chest in the region of the heart. In tests that lasted ten to fifteen minutes, nineteen animals survived and seventeen died (132). These authors, however, gave no specific information as to the method of application of the pressure. Their method had not been applied to a patient. According to Knickerbocker in 1958, a Russian delegation of clinicians visited the Johns Hopkins University, and when asked whether any practical use of Gurvich's technique had ever been used in Russia, they indicated that that had not been the case but certainly upon re-

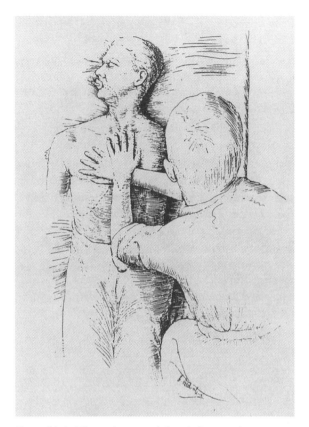

Figure 14.6. The technique of closed chest cardiac massage in 1960, from the landmark article on closed chest cardiac massage. (*Courtesy of the* Journal of the American Medical Association, *173:1064–1067, copyright 1960*)

turn to Russia they would spread the gospel and, of course, give priority to a fellow Russian! The next day after the Russians left, Kouwenhoven made a hasty visit to Blalock, head of the Department of Surgery and informed him that it was entirely likely that the Russians would claim closed chest cardiac massage as a Russian invention, as they had also made claims of priority in the development of other advances such as the airplane, the automobile, and so on. Blalock called the editor of the *Journal of the American Medical Association* and urged that early publication of the article, which had been already submitted in February 1960, be facilitated. Indeed, the article did appear in July 1960, possibly expedited in order to establish firmly the appropriate priority of this technique to the Johns Hopkins group. Three years later, when Knickerbocker visited Gurvich and Negovshy's Institute in the U.S.S.R., he was pleased to find that an enlarged photograph of the technique of closed chest massage (Fig. 14.6) was prominently displayed.

Kouwenhoven's group began "an extensive series of experiments in which pressure was applied not only to the sternum but also on the sides of the chest" (108). In these experiments, it was the practice to give an anesthetized dog a fibrillating shock and wait one minute before starting to press on the sternum and the chest. After applying pressure for a few minutes, a defibrillating shock could be given and attempts made to save the animal. A number of these animals were autopsied and broken costal junctions and ribs and other injuries were observed. The blood pressure, however, was 40 percent of the normal.

Henry T. Bahnson joined Kouwenhoven's group, and when it was found that a dog could be maintained viable for a period of ten minutes by the application of rhythmic pressure on the lower third of the sternum with a force of eighty to one hundred pounds at the rate of one per second, Bahnson was eager to apply the technique to a patient. His opportunity arrived on the night of February 15, 1958, when he resuscitated a two-year-old child whose heart was in ventricular fibrillation with the new combined method—external cardiac compression and closed chest defibrillation. The next day Blalock directed that external cardiac massage be applied to children where indicated. James Jude returned from Army service in July 1958, was appointed resident surgeon, and was assigned to work with Kouwenhoven. Systematically, they developed a technique of external cardiac compression. They were able to demonstrate that the compression of the chest was sufficient to augment the arterial blood pressure to a point that adequate coronary artery perfusion took place. Later in 1958, external cardiac massage was applied to an obese woman in her forties who experienced ventricular fibrillation while undergoing anesthesia. The cardiopulmonary resuscitation was successful (107, 131).

A report of the method of closed chest cardiac massage and the results were published on July 9, 1961, in the *Journal of the American Medical Association*. This was a landmark article (133). Longmire reports in his biography of Alfred Blalock that Blalock, discussing a paper by Jude, Kouwenhoven, and Knickerbocker presented before the American Surgical Association in 1961, stated that "There are two things of great interest to me in this project; first, it proves that a man over three score and ten years can still have original ideas, and second, that most really significant contributions are relatively simple in concept" (134).

The new concept of external cardiac compression in association with artificial ventilation as the primary step in the management of a patient with cardiac arrest received wide acceptance and was successful. It is almost a quarter of a century since the publication of "Closed-Chest Cardiac Massage" in JAMA. During this period, thousands and thousands of persons across the whole world have owed their lives to those who were able to show that without special equipment, and using only the two hands, anyone with training can save a life. Only a few years before his death, Kouwenhoven, at the age of eighty-three, said that the discovery and development of cardiopulmonary resuscitation made the closed chest de-fibrillator a useful and effective device for depolarizing fibrillating human hearts. "Many lives have been saved and I thank the Lord for the opportunity that has been granted to me" (131).

Cardiac Pacemakers

The first electrical pacing was used in an attempt to resuscitate a patient. Lidwill and Booth (135) succeeded in reviving a stillborn baby with their electric "pace-maker" after "everything else had been tried." The pacing stimulus was supplied to the heart by an insulated needle with a bare tip. Hyman constructed a machine with a magnetic generator in 1932 (45).

Design of an effective method for defibrillation was an important step in the introduction of the pacemaker. Many of these developments have been de-scribed in an earlier chapter. The Swiss physiologists Prevost and Battelli (104) in 1900 published a method to defibrillate hearts by means of capacitor dis-charge.

Already in 1804 Vasalli (136) had pointed out the necessity to ventilate the lungs during resuscitation; Wiggers stressed the importance of supplying the myocardium with oxygenated blood by cardiac massage before applying a coun-tershock. This technique was crowned with the first successful intraoperative de-fibrillation by Beck (123) in 1947. Beck subsequently installed defibrillators in operating and emergency rooms. He was not able to interest his colleagues in this technique. The defibrillator was not accepted as standard equipment in the op-erating room and intensive care units until fifteen to twenty years later.

Senning's group in Stockholm first used electrically induced ventricular fib-rillation (137) in order to avoid air embolism during open heart surgery with ex-perimentally unclamped aortas in 1952 (Fig. 14.7). After a period of three to four hours of ventricular fibrillation, using 380 Volt/20ms AC countershock, defibril-lation was always successful. However, sometimes asystole followed, and pacing for one to two minutes was required.

Late in the sixteenth century Geronimo of Padua had first described typical Adams-Stokes attacks (138). Subsequently, many others reported the typical symptoms with syncope and slow pulse. Cardiac pacing during Adams-Stokes attacks was first introduced 370 years later by Zoll in 1952 (146), using external thoracic electrodes. Thus the era of cardiac pacing had begun. In 1951 Callaghan and Bigelow (139) described an electrical pacemaker with transvenous electrodes, which they used to pace hypothermic animals in asystole. In patients, however, this method was unsuccessful. The tip of the intravenous electrode was intro-duced into the auricle, "two inches too short" (139).

In 1957 Weirich, Gott, and Lillehei (140) reported the use of myocardial

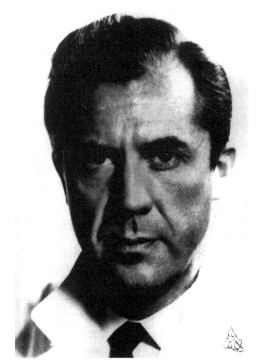

Figure 14.7. Ake Senning. *(With permission)*

electrodes to pace hearts with iatrogenic AV block after closure of a ventricular septal defect.

In the late 1950s the treatment of Adams-Stokes syndrome with percutaneous electric stimulation was frequently performed. For this purpose, pacemakers for external use were built by Medtronic in the United States and Elema in Sweden. Unfortunately, infection frequently caused abscesses, sepsis, and death. Only implantation of the total pacer assembly solved this problem. Transistors became available in 1956, allowing construction of smaller implantable electrical pacemakers. In 1957 the first experiments on implantation were started in Stockholm. Electrical parameters for clinical cardiac pacing were defined on patients with Adams-Stokes syndrome, who carried external pacemakers. On the basis of these data an artificial pacemaker was constructed together with Elmquist (137). On October 8, 1958, the unit was implanted in a patient with a total AV block resulting from a viral myocarditis. During the last weeks the patient had twenty to thirty cardiac arrests a day. In order to avoid publicity, the implantation was carried out in the evening when the operating rooms were empty. The first pacemaker functioned only eight hours. The second was implanted with better success.

The energy source of the first pacemakers was a rechargeable battery, which was charged once a month by induction from a radio-frequency generator. The energy source was later changed to mercury batteries. In 1960 Chardack (141) implanted pacemakers, which were constructed by Greatbatch (142). Now the doors had opened for the pacemaker industry, with Medtronic in the United States and Elema in Europe leading the way. The early years were full of troubles: rapid threshold rises, electrode displacements, lead and insulation breaks, fast battery depletion, and especially a negative attitude on the part of most cardiologists. The first implanted pacemakers were so short-lived that our first patient is now equipped with his twenty-fourth pacemaker.

Infections fortunately have disappeared. With the use of improved leads and inert platinum electrodes with lithium iodine batteries and metallic housing (142), the pacemaker became a durable and reliable instrument for treating bradycardic arrhythmias.

The first pacemakers had a fixed stimulation rate of 72 beats per minute. The fixed rate occasionally caused ventricular fibrillation, when the stimulus fell into the vulnerable phase of late systole of the patient's own heart beat. These accidents were avoided with the introduction in 1964 of on-demand pacemakers with R-wave inhibition (143) and R-wave triggering in 1966 (144). In 1969 Berkovits (52) reported on the bifocal demand pacing.

In the beginning, pacemaker electrodes were placed by thoracotomy either on or into the myocardium. In 1958 Furman and Schwedel (145) used the transvenous route in two patients; this already had been accomplished by Callaghan and Bigelow in 1951 (139).

Pacemaker implantation without thoracotomy was done in 1962 by Ekeström, Johansson, and Lagergren (146), who introduced the electrode transvenously with its tip in the right ventricle. In 1963 a trial triggered 100 ms delayed ventricular pacing without thoracotomy was introduced by the same investigators (147). They placed the sensing electrode on the atrium via a mediastinoscope and installed the ventricular electrode transvenously.

The transvenous route of electrode placement is used today in more than 98 percent of pacemaker implantations. Early reports of a high displacement rate and excessive threshold rise led to the development of electrodes with various types of active and passive fixation mechanism for atrial and ventricular position. Improvement in inert pacemaker electrode designs has reduced the acute and chronic threshold. A lower threshold allows greater patient safety margins and increases the pacemaker's battery life. A new steroid-loaded pacing electrode, which was developed by Medtronic, elutes a minimal amount of a steroid compound into cardiac tissue, in order to reduce tissue reaction and thus maintain a low threshold.

With the progress in electronics, the circuits changed from discrete to hybrid to integrated circuits, and finally to microprocessors. Programmability progressed from the simple invasive change of rate and voltage (Medtronic, 1960) to external noninvasive radio-frequency adjustments of all pacing parameters. The ultimate universal pacing system could be achieved in the dual chamber "physiologic" pacing system; it is the ideal treatment of high degree AV block, reestablishing AV synchrony. At present, the introduction of rate-responsive sensor-controlled pacemakers allows patients with chronotropic incompetence or atrial fibrillation to increase their heart rate during exercise.

Development of the modern pacemaker has been the result of teamwork among cardiologists, electrophysiologists, electronic engineers, and the industry. Today's technique can respond to most cardiac rhythm disturbances. Hopefully the practice at the bedside can keep up with the rapid technical developments.

References

1. Sue, P. Histoire du galvanisme et analyse des differens ouvrages publiés sur cette decouverte depuis son origine jusqu a ce jour. Paris, Bernard, 1802.
2. Amberson, W.R. The influence of fashion in the development of knowledge concerning electricity and magnetism. Am. Sci., 46:33–50, 1958.
3. Fleming, J.A. s.v. ("Electricity"). Encyclopedia Britannica, 11th ed.
4. Bidwell, S. s.v. ("Magnetism"). Encyclopedia Britannica, 11th ed.
5. Franklin, B. Experiments and Observations on Electricity made at Philadelphia in America. London, 1769.
6. Schecter, D.C. Exploring the Origins of Electrical Cardiac Stimulation. Minneapolis, MN, Medtronics, 1983.
7. Cohen, L.B. Introduction. In: Galvani, L. Commentary on the Effects of Electricity on Muscular Motion. Tr. M.G. Foley. Norwood, CT, Burndy Library, 1954.
8. Galvani, L. De viribus electritatis in motu musculari commentarius. De Bononiensi Scientarium et Artium. Instituto atque Academia Commentarii, 7:363, 1791.
9. Galvani, L. Dell'uso e dell'attivita dell'arco conduttore nelle contrazioni dei muscoli. Bologna, S. Tommaso d'Aquino, 1794.
10. Du Bois-Reymond, E. Untersuchungen ueber thierische Elektricitaet. Berlin, Reimer, 1848–84.
11. Humboldt, F.W.H.A. von. Versuche ueber die gereizte Muskel und Nervenfaser nebst Vermuthungen ueber den chemischen Process des Lebens in der Thierund Pflanzenwelt. Posen, Decker, 1797, Lettre de Humboldt à Loder sur les applications du Galvanisme, Bibl. Germanique 4:301 (1797); Lettre de Humboldt à Blumenbach, Ann. Chim., Paris, 64:1 (1797).
12. Oersted, H.C. Galvanic magnetism. Phil. Mag., 56:394, 1820.
13. Lippmann, G. Relations entre les phenomenes electriques et capillaires. Ann. Chim. (Phy.), ser. 5, 5:494, 1875.
14. Waller, A.D. On the electromotive changes connected with the mammalian heart, and of the human heart in particular. Phil. Trans. B., 180:169, 1889.
15. Ader, C. Sur un nouvel appareil enregistreur pour cables sousmarins. C.R. Acad. Sci. (Paris), 124:1440, 1897.
16. Einthoven, W. Die galvanometrische Registrierung des menschlichen Elektrokardiogramms, angleich eine Beurtheilung der Anwendung des Capillar-Elektrometers in der Physiologie. Pfluegers Arch. Physiol., 99:472–480, 1903.
17. Einthoven W., G. Fahr, and A. de Waart. Ueber die Richtung und die manifeste

Groesse der Potentialschwankungen im menschlichen Herzen and ueber den Einfluss der Herzlage auf die Form des Elektrokardiogramms. Pfluegers Arch. Physiol., 150: 275–315, 1913.

18. Waller, A.D., and E.W. Reid. On the action of the excised mammalian heart. Phil. Trans. B., 178:215, 1887.

19. Helmholtz, H. Ueber einige Gesetze der Verteilung elektrischer Stroeme in koerperlichen Leitern, mit Anwendung auf die thierisch elektrischen Versuche. Ann. Physik. Chem. (Ser. 2), 89:211, 1853.

20. Einthoven, W., G. Fahr, and A. de Waart. On the direction and manifest size of the variations of potential in the human heart and on the influence of the position of the heart on the form of the electrocardiogram. Tr. by H.E. Hoff and P. Sekelj. Am. Heart J., 40:163–211, 1950.

21. Wilson, F.N., A.G. Macleod, and P.S. Barker. The Distribution of the Currents of Action and of Injury Displayed by Heart Muscle and Other Excitable Tissues. Ann Arbor, University of Michigan Press, 1933.

22. Craib, W.H. A study of the electrical field surrounding active heart muscle. Heart, 14:71–109, 1927.

23. Craib, W.H. A study of the electrical field surrounding skeletal muscle. J. Physiol. (Lond.), 66:49–73, 1928.

24. Lüderitz, B. History of the Disorders of Cardiac Rhythm. Armonk, NY, Futura Publishing Co., 2nd ed., 1998.

25. Purkinje, J.E. Mikroskopisch-neurologische Beobachtungen. Arch. Anat. Physiol. Wiss. Med., II/III:281–295, 1845.

26. Paladino, G. Contribuzione all'anatomia, istologia e fisiologia del cuore. Napoli, Movim. Med. Chir., 1876.

27. His, W. Jr. Die Taetigkeit des embryonalen Herzens und deren Bedeutung fuer die Lehre von der Herzbewegung beim Erwachsenen. Arb. Med. Klin., 14–49, 1893.

28. Aschoff, L., and S. Tawara. Die heutige Lehre von den pathologisch-anatomischen Grundlagen der Herzschwaeche. Kritische Bemerkungen auf Grund eigener Untersuchungen. Jena, Fischer, 1906.

29. Wenckebach, K.F. Beitraege zur Kenntnis der menschlichen Herztaetigkeit. Arch. Anat. Physiol. (Physiol. Abt.), 297–354, 1906.

30. Keith, A., and M. Flack. The form and nature of the muscular connections between the primary divisons of the vertebrate heart. J. Anat. Physiol., 41:172–189, 1907.

31. Bachmann, G. The inter-auricular time interval. Am. J. Physiol., 41:309–320, 1916.

32. Mahaim, I. Kent fibers and the AV paraspecific conduction through the upper connections of the bundle of His-Tawara. Am. Heart J., 33:651, 1947.

33. James, T.N. Morphology of the human atrioventricular node, with remarks pertinent to its electrophysiology. Am. Heart J. 62:756–771, 1961.

34. Lüderitz, B. Herzrhythmusstoerungen. Diagnostik und Therapie. 5. Berlin Heidelberg New York, Tokyo, Aufl. Springer, 1998.

35. Lüderitz, B. Historical aspects of device therapy for cardiac arrhythmias. In: Interventional Electrophysiology, Lüderitz, B. and S. Saksena (eds). Mount Kisco, NY, Futura Publishing, 1991, pp. 333–352.

36. Hirsch, A. (Hrsg). Biographisches Lexikon der hervorragenden Aerzte aller Zeiten und Völker. 3. Aufl. Bd. IV. München, Berlin, Urban & Schwarzenberg, 1929.

37. Volavsek, B. (ed). Marko Gerbec. Marcus Gerbezius 1658–1718. Syndroma Gerbezius-Morgagni-Adams-Stokes. Ljubljana, 1977.

38. Cammilli, L., and G.A. Feruglio. Breve cronistoria della cardiostimolazione elettrica date, uomini e fatti da ricordare. Publicazione Distribuita in Occasione del Secondo Simposio Europeo di Cardiostimolazione. Firenze, 3–6 Maggio, 1981.

39. Bichat, M.F.X. Recherches physiologiques sur la vie et la mort. Paris, Brosson, Gabon & Cie, 1800.

40. Aldini, G. Essai theorique et experimental sur le galvanisme, avec une serie d'experiences faites en presence des commissaires de l'institut national de France, et en divers amphitheatres de Londres. Paris, Fournier, 1804.

41. Adams, R. Cases of diseases of the heart, accompanied with pathological observations. Dublin Hosp. Rep., 4:353–453, 1827.

42. Stokes, W. Observations on some cases of permanently slow pulse. Dublin Quart. J. Med. Sci., 2:73–85, 1846.

43. Duchenne de Boulogne, G.B.A. De l'ectrisation localisée et de son application à la pathologie et à la therapeutique par courants induits et par courants galvaniques interrompus et continues. Paris, Bailliere, 1872.

44. Ziemssen, H. von. Studien ueber die Bewegungsvorgaenge am menschlichen Herzen sowie ueber die mechanische und elektrische Erregbarkeit des Herzens und des Nervus phrenicus, angestellt an dem freiliegenden Herzen der Catharina Serafin. Arch. Klin. Med., 30:270–303, 1882.

45. Hyman, A.S. Resuscitation of the stopped heart by intracardial therapy. II. Experimental use of an artificial pacemaker. Arch. Intern. Med., 50:283–305, 1932.

46. Zoll, P.M. Resuscitation of heart in ventricular standstill by external electric stimulation. N. Engl. J. Med., 247:768–771, 1952.

47. Elmquist, R., and A. Senning. An implantable pacemaker for the heart. In: Medical Electronics, Proceedings of the Second International Conference on Medical Electronics, Smyth, C.N. (ed.). Paris, 1959. London, Iliffe & Sons, 1960.

48. Furman, S., and G. Robinson. The use of an intercardiac pacemaker in the correction of total heart block. Surg. Forum., 9:245–248, 1958.

49. Bouvrain, Y., and F. Zacouto. L'entrainement electrosystolique de Coeur. Utilisation medicale. Presse Med., 69:525–528, 1961.

50. Lown, R., Z. Amarasingham, and J. Neumann. New method for terminating cardiac arrhythmias. Use of synchronized capacitor discharge. JAMA, 182:548–555, 1962.

51. Nathan, D.A., S. Center, C.Y. Wu, and W. Keller. An implantable synchronous pacemaker for the long-term correction of complete heart block. Circulation, 27:682–685, 1963.

52. Berkovits, B.V., A. Castellanos Jr., and L. Lemberg. Bifocal demand pacing. Circulation [Suppl.], 40:III–44, 1969.

53. Scherlag, B.J., S.H. Lau, R.H. Helfant, W.D. Berkowitz, E. Stein, and A.N. Damato. Catheter technique for recording His bundle activity in man. Circulation, 39:13–18, 1969.

54. Wellens, H.J.J. Electrical Stimulation of the Heart in the Study and Treatment of Tachycardias. Leiden, Kroese, 1971.

55. Zipes, D.P., J. Fischer, R.M. King, A.D.B. Nicoll, and W.W. Jolly. Termination of ventricular fibrillation in dogs by depolarizing a critical amount of myocardium. Am. J. Cardiol., 36:37–44, 1975.

56. Josephson, M.E., L.N. Horowitz, A. Farshidi, and J.A. Kastor. Recurrent sustained ventricular tachycardia. Circulation, 57:431–440, 1978.

57. Mirowski, M., P.R. Reid, M.M. Mower, L. Watkins, V.L. Gott, J.F. Schauble, A. Langer, M.S. Heilman, S.A. Kolenik, R.E. Fischell, and M.L. Weisfeldt. Termination of malignant ventricular arrhythmias with an implanted automatic defibrillator in human beings. N. Engl. J. Med., 303:322–324, 1980.

58. Gallagher, J.J., R.H. Svenson, J.H. Kasell, L.D. German, G.H. Bardy, A. Broughton, and G. Critelli. Catheter technique for closed-chest ablation of the atrio-ventricular conduction system: A therapeutic alternative for the treatment of refractory supraventricular tachycardia. N. Engl. J. Med., 306:194–200, 1982.

59. Scheinman, M.M., F. Morady, D.S. Hess, and R. Gonzales. Transvenous catheter technique for induction of damage to the atrioventricular junction in man. Am. J. Cardiol., 49: 1013, 1982.

60. Lüderitz, B., N. d'Alnoncourt, G. Steinbeck, and J. Beyer. Therapeutic pacing in tachyarrhythmias by implanted pacemakers. PACE, 5:366–371, 1982.

61. Manz, M., U. Gerckens, and B. Lüderitz. Antitachycardia pacemaker (Tachylog) and automatic implantable defibrillator (AID): Combined use in ventricular tachyarrhythmias. Circulation [Suppl.], 72:III–383, 1985.

62. Borggrefe, M., T. Budde, A. Podczeck, and G. Breithardt. High frequency alternating current ablation of an accessory pathway in humans. J. Am. Coll. Cardiol., 10:576–582, 1987.

63. Saksena, S., and V. Parsonnet. Implantation of a cardioverter-defibrillator without thoracotomy using a triple electrode system. JAMA, 259:69–72, 1988.

64. Jackman, W.M., X. Wang, K.J. Friday, C.A. Roman, K.P. Moulton, K.J. Beckman, J.H. McClelland, N. Twidale, H.A. Hazlitt, M.I. Prior, P.D. Margolis, J.D. Calame, E.O. Overholt, and R. Lazzara. Catheter ablation of accessory atrioventricular pathways (Wolff-Parkinson-White Syndrome) by radiofrequency current. N. Engl. J. Med., 324:1605–1611, 1961.

65. Kuck, K.H., M. Schlüter, M. Geiger, J. Siebels, and W. Duckeck. Radiofrequency current catheter ablation of accessory atrioventricular pathways. Lancet, 337:1557–1561, 1991.

66. Lau, C.P., H.F. Tse, K. Lee, N.S. Lok, D.W.S. Ho, M. Soffer, and A.J. Camm. Initial clinical experience of an human implantable atrial defibrillator. PACE, 19:625, 1996.

67. Jung, W., and B. Lüderitz. Implantation of an arrhythmia management system for ventricular and supraventricular tachyarrhythmias. Lancet, 349:853–854, 1997.

68. Krikler, D., P. Curry, and J. Buffet. Dual-demand pacing for reciprocating atrioventricular tachycardia. Br. Med. J., 1:1114–1116, 1976.

69. Ryan, G.F., R.M. Easley, L.I. Zaroff, and S. Goldstein. Paradoxical use of a demand pacemaker in treatment of supraventricular tachycardia due to the Wolff-Parkinson-White-Syndrome. Observation on termination of reciprocal rhythm. Circulation, 38:1037–1043, 1968.

70. Mandel, W.J., M.M. Laks, I. Yamaguchi, J. Fields, and B. Berkovits. Recurrent reciprocating tachycardias in the Wolff-Parkinson-White syndrome: control by use of a scanning pacemaker. Chest, 69:769–774, 1976.

71. Barold, S.S. Therapeutic uses of cardiac pacing in tachyarrhythmias. In: His Bundle Electrocardiography and Clinical Electrophysiology, Narula, O.S. (ed.). Philadelphia, Davis, 1975, pp. 407–433.

72. Gonzales, R., M.M. Scheinman, W. Margaretten, and M. Rubinstein. Closed-chest electrode-catheter technique for His bundle ablation in dogs. Am. J. Physiol., 241:H 283–287, 1981.

73. Scheinman, M.M., F. Morady, D.S. Hess, and R. Gonzales. Catheter-induced ablation of the atrioventricular junction to control refractory supraventricular arrhythmias. JAMA, 248:851–855, 1982.

74. Manz, M., G. Steinbeck, and B. Lüderitz. His-Buendel Ablation. Eine neue Methode zur Therapie bedrohlicher supraventrikulaerer Herzrhythmusstoerungen. Internist, 24:95–98, 1983.

75. Weber, H., and L. Schmitz. Catheter technique for closed-chest ablation of an accessory pathway. N. Engl. J. Med., 308:653–654, 1983.

76. Pfeiffer, D., J. Tebbenjohanns, B. Schumacher, H. Omran, W. Fehske, and B. Lüderitz. Radiofrequency catheter ablation of septal accessory pathways. J. Intervent. Cardiol., 7:69–76, 1994.

77. An, H., S. Saksena, M. Janssen, and P. Osypka. Radiofrequency ablation of ventricular myocardium using active fixation and passive contact catheter delivery systems. Am. Heart J., 118:69–77, 1989.

78. Huang, S.K.S., S. Bharati, A.R. Graham, M. Lev, F.I. Marcus, and R.C. Odell. Closed

chest catheter desiccation of the atrioventricular junction using radiofrequency energy. A new method of catheter ablation. J. Am. Coll. Cardiol., 9:349–358, 1987.

79. Huang, S.K.S. Radio-frequency catheter ablation of cardiac arrhythmias: appraisal of an evolving therapeutic modality. Am. Heart J., 118:1317–1323, 1989.

80. Huang, S.K.S. Advances in applications of radiofrequency current to catheter ablation therapy. PACE, 14:28–42, 1991.

81. Narula, N.S., B.K. Boveja, D.M. Cohern, J.T. Narula, and P.P. Tarjan. Laser catheter-induced atrioventricular nodal delays and atrioventricular block in dogs. J. Am. Coll. Cardiol., 5:259–267, 1985.

82. Weber, H., S. Hessel, L. Ruprecht, and E. Unsöld. A new electrode quartz fiber catheter for electrically guided percutaneous Nd-YAG laser photocoagulation of the subendocardium. PACE, 10:411, 1987.

83. Hindricks, G., M. Borggrefe, W. Haverkamp, U. Karbenn, X. Chen, T. Budde, M. Shenasa, and G. Breithardt. Short- and long-term complications of catheter ablation using radiofrequency energy—observations in 192 consecutive patients. J. Am. Coll. Cardiol., 19:184A (abstr.), 1992.

84. Mirowski, M., M.M. Mower, W.S. Staeven, B. Tabatznik, and A.I. Mendelhoff. Standby automatic defibrillator: an approach to prevention of sudden coronary death. Arch. Intern. Med., 126:158–161, 1970.

85. Mirowski, M., M.M. Mower, W.S. Staeven, R.H. Denniston, and A.I. Mendelhoff. The development of the transvenous automatic defibrillator. Arch. Intern. Med., 129:773–779, 1972.

86. Mirowski, M., M.M. Mower, A. Langer, M.S. Heilman, and J. Schreibmann. A chronically implanted system for automatic defibrillation in conscious dogs. Experimental model for treatment of sudden death from ventricular fibrillation. Circulation, 58: 90–94, 1978.

87. Lüderitz, B., U. Gerckens, and M. Manz. Automatic implantable cardioverter/defibrillator (AICD) and antitachycardia pacemaker (Tachylog): combined use in ventricular tachyarrhythmias. PACE, 9:1356–1360, 1986.

88. Manz, M., U. Gerckens, H.D. Funke, P.G. Kirchhoff, and B. Lüderitz. Combination of antitachycardia pacemaker and automatic implantable cardioverter/defibrillator for ventricular tachycardia. PACE, 9:676–684, 1986.

89. Lüderitz, B., and S. Saksena (eds). Electrical device therapy for cardiac arrhythmias: new concepts, problems, and alternatives. Proceedings of a symposium. Am. Heart J., 127:969–1200, 1994.

90. Cammilli, L., L. Alcidi, G. Grassi, G. Melissano, C. Massimo, G. Montesi, G. Menegazzo, V. Silvestri, and A. Mugelli. Automatic implantable pharmacological defibrillator (AIPhD). Preliminary investigations in animals. New Trends Arrhyth., 6:1131–1140, 1990.

91. Cammilli, L., A. Mugelli, G. Grassi, L. Alcidi, G. Melissano, G. Menegazza, and V. Silvestro. Implantable pharmacological defibrillator (AIPhD): preliminary investigations in animals. PACE, 14:381–386, 1991.

92. Jung, W., and B. Lüderitz. Intraatrial defibrillation of atrial fibrillation. Z. Kardiol., 85(6):75–81, 1996.

93. Moss, A.J., J.W. Hall, D.S. Cannom, J.P. Daubert, S.L. Higgins, H. Klein, J.H. Levine, S. Saksena, A.L. Waldo, D. Wilber, M.W. Brown, and M. Heo. Improved survival with an implanted defibrillation in patients with coronary disease at high risk for ventricular arrhythmia. N. Engl. J. Med., 335:1933–1940, 1996.

94. McCarthy, M. Implantable cardiac defibrillators cut deaths. Lancet, 349: 1225, 1997.

95. The Antiarrhythmics versus Implantable Defibrillators (AVID) Investigators. A comparison of antiarrhythmic-drug therapy with implantable defibrillators in patients resuscitated from near-fatal ventricular arrhythmias. N. Engl. J. Med., 337:1576–1583, 1997.

96. Lüderitz, B. Clinical and interventional electrophysiology: a personal historical perspective. J. Intervent. Cardiac Electrophysiology, 1:243–254, 1997.

97. Schechter, D.C. Exploring the origins of electrical cardiac stimulation. Selected works on the history of electrotherapy presented at the Seventh World Symposium in Cardiac Pacing. Vienna, Austria, 1983, Minneapolis, MN, Medtronic, 1983.

98. Harvey, W. The Circulation of the Blood. London, J.M. Dent & Sons Ltd., 1907.

99. Nysten, P.J. Expériences sur le Coeur et les autres Parties d'un Homme Decapité le 14 Brumaire, An XI. Paris, Levrault, 1802.

100. Vassali-Eandi, Julio, and Rossi. Rapport sue des expériences galvaniques faites sur les têtes et les troncs de trois hommes, peu de temps après leur decapitation, Rep. Acad. of Turin, 1803; Societe de Médicins, Etablis à Mayence: Expériences galvaniques Hommes et des Animaux, Frankfurt, 1804.

101. Carpne. Galvanic experiments on a hanged man, Phil. Magazine, Bible. Brit., 270:373, 1803.

102. Kite, C. The Recovery of the Apparently Dead. London, C. Dilly, 1788.

103. Walshe, W.H. A Practical Treatise on the Diseases of the Heart and Great Vessels. Philadelphia, Blanchard & Lea, 1862.

104. Prevost, J.L., and F. Battelli. Quelques effects des charges électriques sur le coeur des mammifieres. J. Physiol. Path. Gen., 2:40–41, 1900.

105. MacWilliams, J.A. Electrical stimulation of the heart in man. Br. Med. J., 1:348, 1889.

106. Robinovitch, L.G. Resuscitation of a woman in profound syncope caused by chronic morphine poisoning; means used: rhythmic excitations with an induction current; the author's method and model of coil. J. Ment. Path., 8:180, 1907.

107. Kouwenhoven, W.B., and O.R. Langworthy. Cardiopulmonary resuscitation. An account of forty-five years of research. JAMA, 226:877–886, 1973.

108. Kouwenhoven, W.B., W.R. Milnor, G.G. Knickerbocker, and W.R. Chesnut. Closed chest defibrillation of the heart. Surgery, 42:550–561, 1957.

109. Wiggers, C.J. Reminiscences and Adventures in Circulation Research. New York, Grune & Stratton, 1958.

110. Prevost, J.L., and F. Battelli. Sur quelques effets des echarges électriques sur le coeur des mammiferes. C.R. Acad. Sci., 129:1267, 1899.

111. Hooker, D.R., W.B. Kouwenhoven, and O.R. Langworthy. The effect of alternating currents on the heart. Am. J. Physiol., 103:444–454, 1933.

112. Ferris, L.P., B.G. King, P.W. Spence, et al. Effect of electric shock on the heart. Electrical Engineering, May 1936.

113. Wiggers, C.J. Revival of the heart from ventricular fibrillation by successive use of potassium and sodium salts. Am. J. Physiol., 92:223–239, 1930.

114. Kouwenhoven, W.B., D.R. Hooker, and O.R. Langworthy. Recovery of the electrically fibrillated dog heart by electric countershock. Am. J. Physiol., 101:65, 1932.

115. Wiggers, C.J. Cardiac massage followed by countershock in revival of mammalian ventricles from fibrillation due to coronary occlusion. Am. J. Physiol., 116:161–162, 1936.

116. Wiggers, C.J. The physiological basis for cardiac resuscitation from ventricular fibrillation-method for serial defibrillation. Am. Heart J., 20:413–422, 1940.

117. Beck, C.S. Reminiscences of cardiac resuscitation. Rev. Surg., 27:76–86, 1970.

118. Mautz, F.R. Reduction of cardiac instability of the epicardial and systemic administration of drugs as a protection in cardiac surgery. J. Thoracic Surg., 5:612–628, 1936.

119. Mautz, F.R. Resuscitation of the heart from ventricular fibrillation with drugs combined with electric shock. Proc. Soc. Exper. Biol. Med., 36:634–636, 1937.

120. Beck, C.S. Resuscitation for cardiac standstill and ventricular fibrillation occurring during operation. Am. J. Surg., 54:273–279, 1941.

121. Beck, C.S., and F.R. Mautz. The control of the heartbeat by surgeon: with special reference to ventricular fibrillation occurring during operation. Ann. Surg., 106:525–537, 1937.

122. Beck, C.S., W.H. Pritchard, and H.S. Feil. Ventricular fibrillation of long duration abolished by electric shock. JAMA, 135:985–986, 1947.

123. Beck, C.S. Historical communication. My life in heart surgery, 1923–1969. Geriatrics, 26:84–99, 1971.

124. Mozen, H., R. Katzman, and J. Martin. Successful defibrillation of heart. Resuscitative procedure started on medical ward and completed in operating room. JAMA, 161:111, 1955.

125. Beck, C.S. Surgery of the heart. Proceedings of the California Academy of Medicine 1937–1938 (address delivered February 20, 1937).

126. Beck, C.S. Treatment of cardiac arrest. Veterans Administration Technical Bulletin TB 10—65, July 18, 1950, Washington, DC.

127. Day, H.A. Letter to Dr. Beck. September 12, 1969.

128. Zoll, P.M., A.J. Linenthal, W. Gibson, M.H. Paul, and L.R. Notman. Termination of ventricular fibrillation in man by externally applied electric countershock. N. Engl. J. Med., 254:727–732, 1956.

129. Pike, F.H., C.C. Guthrie, and G.N. Stewart. Studies of resuscitation: I. The general conditions affecting resuscitation, and the resuscitation of the blood and of the heart. J. Exp. Med., 10:371–418, 1908.

130. Crile, G. Demonstration of arterial perfusion and compression of unopened chest. Cleveland Academy of Medicine, 1908. Cited by Hosler, E.M.: A concise history of cardiac resuscitation, November 28, 1975 for Archives of the Cleveland Health Museum and Education Center.

131. Sladen, A. Closed-chest massage, Kouwenhoven, Jude, Knickerbocker. JAMA, 251:3137–3140, 1984.

132. Gurvich, H.L., and G.S. Yuniev. Restoration of heart rhythm during fibrillation by a condenser discharge. Am. Rev. Soviet Med., 4:252–256, 1947.

133. Kouwenhoven, W.B., J.R. Jude, and G.G. Knickerbocker. Cardiac arrest. Report of application of external cardiac massage on 118 patients. JAMA, 178:1064–1067, 1960.

134. Longmire, W. P., Jr. Alfred Blalock: His Life and Times. William Longmire Jr., Publisher, 1991.

135. Lidwill, M.D., H.G. Mond, G.J. Sloman, and R.H. Edwards. The first pacemaker. PACE, 5:278–281, 1982.

136. Vasalli. In: Aldini, J. (ed.) Essai théorique et expérimental sur la galvanisme avec une serie d'expériences. Paris: Fournier, 1804.

137. Senning, A. Ventricular fibrillation used as a method to facilitate intracardiac operations. Acta Chir. Scand., 172, 1952.

138. Mercuriale, G. (Praelectiones Patavinae). De Cognoscendis et curandis humani corporis affectibus (Venezia 1606), opera postuma, pp. 238–243.

139. Callaghan, J.C., and W.G. Bigelow. Electrical artificial pacemaker for standstill of the heart. Ann. Surg., 134:8–17, 1951.

140. Weirich, W.L., V.L. Gott, and C.W. Lillehei. The treatment of complete heart block by the combined use of a myocardial electrode and an artificial pacemaker. Surg. Forum, 8:360–363, 1957.

141. Chardack, W.M., A.E. Gage, and W. Greatbatch. A transistorized self-contained implantable pacemaker for long term correction of complete heart block. Surgery, 48:643–648, 1960.

142. Greatbatch, W., L.H. Lee, and W. Mathias. The solid-state lithium battery: a new improved chemical power source for implantable cardiac pacemakers. Trans. Biomed. Engin., 18:317, 1971.

143. Castellanos, Jr., A., L. Lemberg, and B.V. Berkovits. The "demand" cardiac pacemaker: a new instrument for the treatment of A-V conduction disturbances. Inter. Am. Coll. Cardiol. Meeting, Montreal, June 1964.
144. Neville, J.F., K. Millar, W. Keller, and J.A. Abildskov. An implantable demand pacemaker. Clin. Res., 14:256–258, 1966.
145. Furman, S., and J.B. Schwedel. An intracardiac pacemaker for Stokes-Adam seizures. N. Engl. J. Med., 261:943–948, 1959.
146. Ekeström, S., J. Johansson, and H. Lagergren. Behandling av Adam Stokes syndrom med intracardiell pacemakerelectrod. Opuscula Medica, 7:175–176, 1962.
147. Carlens, E., L. Johansson, I. Karlöf, and H. Lagergren. New method for arterial triggered pacemaker treatment without thoracotomy. J. Thorac. Cardiovasc. Surg., 50: 229–237, 1965.

Chapter 15

History of Cardiology at the Bedside

R.J. BING

UNTIL THE 1930s, when medicine and cardiology turned into a science and cardiology became a separate branch of medicine, medicine was based on Hippocratic principles and diagnosis depended on the patient's appearance. Physicians defined the Hippocratic Facies and Hippocratic Digits (clubbed fingers). Examinations also included the inspection of urine and feces and palpation, particularly of the abdomen (1). Palpation was not all diagnostic; the touch of the hands was also healing. Lewis Thomas reminds us that touching the patient is the oldest and most effective act of physicians (1). Today, much to the regret of many, bedside observations have lost some of their importance. Where once cardiologists participated in lengthy bedside discussions on physical findings such as apical impulse, opening snap, and split-second sound (discussions that frequently failed to provide a definite diagnosis), diagnostic considerations now include printouts of data from cardiac catheterization, echocardiography, and magnetic resonance.

Proof that medieval medicine was based entirely on bedside diagnosis is evident from the writings of physicians connected with the school of Salerno in southern Italy. During the fourth decade of the eleventh century, the school of Salerno became the center for a group of physicians who not only practiced medicine, but also documented their art. In Salerno, which recently had been conquered by the Normans, the Latin and Arabic cultures mingled. It is likely that in Salerno medicine owed its origin to an itinerant physician from Sicily, Constantine Africanus. It was he who translated the classical books of Arabic medicine into Latin. His pupils, young physicians of Salerno, read these translations and taught and practiced their medicine accordingly. George W. Corner describes the romance of discovery of some of the books written in Salerno (2). In 1837 in

Breslau, then Germany, a manuscript, referred to as the Codex Salernitanus, was found that was written about 1170 by two doctors of Salerno. Physicians from Salerno used dissection of an animal (in this case, a pig), accompanied by a brief lecture as a teaching exercise. One of the few therapeutic measures practiced in Salerno was phlebotomy, which was considered as essential therapy for all ailments. It was thought that it "strengthened the mind and memory, purged the bladder, dried out the brain, cleared the hearing, restrained tears, and did many other favorable things." Physicians in the eighteenth century, who practiced bleeding to dangerous levels, should have listened to their colleagues in Salerno who taught that phlebotomy should be done with caution. The Salerno physicians maintained that the amount of blood withdrawn should be adjusted to the strength and age of the patient and that the bleeding should not be allowed to "run until the patient was overtaken by a lassitude or weakness of the stomach" (2).

A rhyming collection of rules, the Schola Salernitana, gives us a rare insight into the bedside manner of physicians in the eleventh century, not all so different from today's (2). To quote a few portions: "at your entrance inquire of him who greets you what disease the sick man suffers and how his illness progresses; this is advisable in order that when you come to him you might not seem entirely uninformed to the illness—entering the sick-room you should have neither proud nor greedy countenance; you should repeat the greetings of those who rise as you enter, and with a gesture seat yourself when they sit down—support his arm with your left hand and observe the pulse for at least 100 beats in order to feel all its variations, and thus you will be able to satisfy the expectant bystanders with words which they are glad to hear—when examining the urine you should observe its color, substance, quantity, and content; after which you may promise the patient that with the help of God you will cure him. As you go away, however, you should say to his servants that he is in a very bad way, because if he recovers you will receive great credit and praise, and if he dies, they will remember that you despaired of his health from the beginning. Meanwhile I urge you not to turn a lingering eye upon his wife, his daughter, or his maid-servant, for this sort of thing blinds the eye of the doctor, averts the favor of God, and makes the doctor abhorrent to the patient and less confident of himself.—Do not criticize the food or drink, and when in the country do not show distaste for country food, for example millet bread, even though you can scarcely control your stomach."

The end of medicine in Salerno and its high standing came in 1194 when the town was sacked by Henry VI of Hohenstaufen. But at that time, as Corner stresses, the works of Aristotle, Avicenna, and Rhazes, the great Greek and Arabic writers, had been translated. Finally, the rise of Bologna as a great medical center began, and by the thirteenth century, Salerno was no longer foremost among the medical centers (2).

Prior to the advent of scientific medicine, there already existed textbooks describing in detail the clinical symptoms of disease but offering little specific discussion on treatment, except bleeding, cupping, and violent purging, and a very limited pharmacopoeia. Physicians of the late nineteenth and early twentieth centuries often made a virtue of their lack of knowledge, glorifying therapeutic nihilism as a badge of honor rather than a sign of ignorance. One gets a good idea of the abject status of therapy in the eighteenth century by reading of the treatment Mozart received prior to his death in 1780. Mozart may have suffered from rheumatic fever, rheumatic carditis, or renal disease, preceded by streptococcal throat infections. Regardless of the nature of his disease, he was treated by bleeding and purging (3). One of Mozart's physicians, Dr. Sallaba, wrote in 1791 about the importance of treatment by "thorough venesections of rheumatic diseases." He ordered seven to eight venesections, each withdrawing a quarter of a liter of blood (3). The immediate cause of the death of Mozart and many others may well have been hemorrhagic shock resulting from repeated blood lettings. Cardiological examination was almost exclusively restricted to the observation of the pulse. Innumerable variations of the pulse were described and the student was expected to recognize them at the bedside. But their relationship to specific diseases of the heart was unknown.

In 1908 Sir William Osler edited eight volumes on internal medicine (4). Volume 4, authored by a variety of physicians, is partially devoted to diseases of the circulatory system. For pericarditis, local applications of poultices to the precordial regions are indicated. In addition, various "revulsants" such as local bleeding, leeching, hot applications, and a series of small blisters, not very different from the treatment in Mozart's time, are recommended. The only medication for pericarditis mentioned is the use of salicylates (which, however, is considered of no benefit) (4). The authors suggest opium or morphine. Paracentesis of the pericardium first proposed by Riolan in 1649 and termed by the surgeon Billroth as "a prostitution of surgical skill" is also described (4). There is no special treatment for tuberculous pericarditis. A special chapter on "diseases resulting from derangements of cardiac nutrition" authored by Robert H. Babcock is included (4). He mentions acute and chronic myocardial degeneration, senile heart disease, and heart strain as well as heart disease due to "immoderate beer-drinking." A small paragraph is devoted to coronary sclerosis, which is "undoubtedly the one great intrinsic factor to which chronic changes of the myocardium are to be attributed." The treatment of all these conditions is minimal, but "if injurious effects resulting from the condition of modern life were considered, they could exert appreciable influence over those patients whose habits or constitutional tendencies are fraught with danger"; and in a subsequent paragraph, "the patient should be told not to run for trains, not to climb mountains, not to commit excesses in Bacho et Venere [a Victorian description of alcohol and sex], and not to overeat." If a woman is devoting herself strenuously to social functions, charitable cause, or club work, she must be told to limit them; women also should not wear tight-fitting clothes. Havana cigars "must be forbidden altogether, greatly reduced, or replaced by mild domestic cigars." As medication Babcock mentions nitroglycerine, sodium nitrite, and erythroltetranitrate. In case of "cardiac incompetence" (myocardial failure), he recommends rest and Bad-Nauheim baths, a form of hydrotherapy (4). The author, however, recommends digitalis, which has remained to this day an important therapeutic measure, although its importance has decreased in favor of other medications. Babcock had great faith in morphine and heroin, drugs that were readily available at the end of the nineteenth century: "There is no single remedy of more single benefit than either of these two therapeutic agents when properly used." In the late nineteenth century venesection was still recommended in certain cases. For endocarditis Osler recommends potassium iodide (4). It is interesting that in 1908 among the causes of cardiac hypertrophy, skiing is mentioned because in Laplanders cardiac hypertrophy was supposed to be frequent. Equally bicycling was mentioned as a cause of cardiac hypertrophy (4).

The volume includes a beautiful chapter on congenital heart disease by Maude Abbott. Not surprisingly, the treatment of congenital heart disease takes only half a page, which contains the curious statement: "The administration of oxygen has been suggested. . . . Gibson, however, reports a negative result from its use in several cases" (4).

In the eighteenth century, the Hippocratic approach to observation and palpation was considerably extended by the introduction of percussion and auscultation. Joseph Leopold Auenbrugger is remembered as the discoverer of percussion as a diagnostic technique (Fig. 15.1). Auenbrugger was born in Graz, Austria, in 1722, the son of an innkeeper, and died in Vienna in 1809 (5, 6, 7, 8). After his medical studies in Vienna under the celebrated Van Swieten, the founder of the Viennese School of Medicine and one of Mozart's sponsors and physicians who had come to Vienna from Leiden in the Netherlands, Auenbrugger worked in Vienna at the Spanish military hospital, where he developed the method of percussion of the chest in 1761, publishing it in his book, *Inventum Novum* (9). Like many physicians and scientists in an academic environment, then and now, he ran afoul of his colleagues' jealousy and intrigues and resigned as a physician to the Spanish hospital, which also meant resigning from the medical faculty (8). He then devoted the rest of his professional life to general practice in Vienna and became one of the most popular physicians in the city for treatment of diseases of the chest (8).

During Auenbrugger's lifetime Vienna was the home of great musicians: Mozart, Haydn, Beethoven, Schubert, and Salieri. Salieri taught composition to Beethoven, Schubert, and Liszt, and Beethoven dedicated three violin sonatas to him. Salieri was no friend of Mozart (3). He was even accused of having

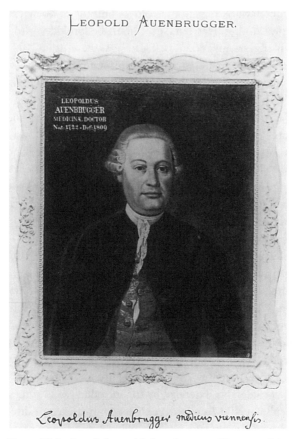

Figure 15.1. Joseph Leopold Auenbrugger. *(Courtesy of the New York Academy of Medicine)*

poisoned Mozart, an accusation without foundation (3). Auenbrugger's daughter, Marianna, was a pupil of Salieri and this relationship was probably responsible for Salieri's and Auenbrugger's collaboration on an opera, *The Chimney Sweep,* first performed in Vienna in 1781 (5). The opera was not very successful and its failure led to its replacement by Mozart's opera, *The Abduction from the Seraglio.* Mozart did not think much of the Salieri/Auenbrugger creation and wrote to his father in 1783, "As far as I can gather from your letter, you think it is an Italian Opera, but in fact it is a German Opera and a very bad one, which was written by Dr. Auenbrugger of Vienna" (5). It is very likely that Auenbrugger's feeling for music inspired his interest in percussion and enabled him to differentiate between the sounds elicited by the percussing finger.

In his book, Auenbrugger wrote, "I transmit to you, dear reader, a new design invented by me which is helpful in the recognition of the diseases of the chest. This design or procedure consists in a percussion of the human chest which permits one to obtain information of the condition of the chest cavity by different resonance of the tone thus produced" (9). Auenbrugger begins his book with the statement, "The thorax of a healthy man resounds when struck." He then describes the difference of the sound. He also experimented and proved his theory by injecting fluid into the pleural cavity of cadavers to see how the line of dullness corresponded to the level of the fluid (9). He was aware of the alteration of percussion tone over the compressed lung in hydrothorax, the change of resonance in pneumonia. In various chapters entitled "Observations," he described the findings in the healthy chest, the technique of percussion (the percussing hand should be covered with a glove or the chest should be covered with a shirt), the normal percussion sound, and the so-called thigh sound (the dullness that one would observe by tapping a thigh which is heard in consolidation of the lung). He also described changes noted in heart disease such as pericarditis (9).

Several informative articles on Auenbrugger have appeared in the English-language literature, among others by Bedford and Dock (7, 8). McKusick and Perloff also devote considerable space to Auenbrugger's work (10, 11). Bedford notes that Auenbrugger's treatise was republished twice in Latin, and that several French translations were published, including an important one by Corvisart. Percussion attracted little attention until publication of Laennec's book in 1819 in France after which physicians flocked to Paris to study physical diagnosis. Dock, in his welcome address at the opening exercises of the Department of Medicine in Ann Arbor, Michigan, in 1898, described the history of percussion, mentioning that percussion had always been performed by the potter, the mason, the carpenter, and others in some form (8). He also mentioned that percussion of the abdomen had been practiced at least since the time of Hippocrates and that the drumlike character of the sound had been noted, hence the term "percussion." According to Dock, Auenbrugger was remembered not only for his medical skill but also for his kindness, generosity, and charity (8).

Dock, both physician and historian, speculated how it came about that so important a discovery should have been neglected for so long (8). Auenbrugger himself predicted that his work was likely to meet obstacles because of envy, malice, detraction, and calumny, "for such is the fate of all who made discovery or improvements in art and science" (8). Dock explained the lack of interest in Auenbrugger because Auenbrugger's time was characterized by indolence and skepticism; "just the opposite is the case today [in 1898], with great restlessness and curiosity, with an exhaustible credulity" (8). He contrasted Auenbrugger's fate with that of medical discoverers of his own day such as Koller, the discoverer of the local anesthetic properties of cocaine, with the subsequent hundreds of clinical trials. Roentgen's announcement of the discovery of x-rays was followed immediately all over the world by physicists, clinicians, and investigators anxious to apply the marvelous technology. Dock felt that another reason for the neglect of Auenbrugger's discovery was that his method was not foolproof. "When experience, when it surely will, shows that the impossible has not happened, the subject is dismissed by the multitude with reproaches on those who introduced it." Dock advised the incoming medical students in 1898 to be critical. He wrote, "More than ever is it necessary to know as well as can be known, the right from the wrong, the genuine from the false in medicine." "The student," he advised, "should aim to learn principles rather than facts, the fixed rather than the transitory" (8). This is indeed good advice for the late nineteenth century as well as for our time. But today, sophisticated technical knowledge is needed to arrive at the truth.

After Auenbrugger's death, only a few references were made to auscultation in Vienna until the appearance of Skoda's book on percussion and auscultation (12). His chapters on percussion are concerned with "full and empty, bright and dull, tympanitic and non-tympanitic, high and deep and metallic sounds, and finally with the cracked pot sound." The percussion sound, which resembled a cracked pot, is found over a deep-lying pulmonary cavity, which contains air and communicates with the bronchial tree. In medical school in the late 1920s, my fellow students and I were required to know all about the cracked pot sound of percussion, but alas we never heard it.

It is obvious that Skoda was a man who liked details. He discussed the various techniques in percussion, referring to Auenbrugger, Corvisart, and Laennec (12). He mentioned that Piorry used percussion instruments made from ivory, Louis from rubber, Winterich from steel, and finally Burne from shoe leather (how similar these technical details are to today's discussions on different models of highly technical diagnostic equipment!) (12). Skoda then described the various percussion sounds and their origin. He mentioned that there is no difference in the sound over the liver, spleen, heart, lung, and stomach. It is quite astonishing how much he could read into these sounds. For example, he mentioned that in the presence of pulmonary exudates, sound over the lower portion of the lung is quite different as compared to the pulmonary apex, which has a tympanitic quality (12).

Aside from his work on auscultation, Skoda completely missed the connection between diseases of the coronary artery and angina pectoris (6). As he wrote, "The disease commences in old age and sometimes is very persistent. There have been physicians who attributed the pain to a disease of the coronary arteries. However this opinion is without any foundation, since autopsy, looking for changes in the coronary arteries, undertaken to relate them to the clinical history of angina pectoris, reveals complete absence of any relationship; just as sclerosis of the radial artery fails to cause pain in the hands, thus it is unlikely that coronary artery sclerosis causes pain in the heart; it is much more likely that an

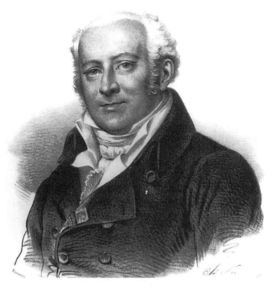

Figure 15.2. J.N. Corvisart. (*Courtesy of the New York Academy of Medicine*)

anomaly of innervation of the brachial plexus is responsible" (6). The severe anginal pain that was experienced and described in 1877 by the Viennese pathologist Rokitansky was characterized as "neuralgia." Rokitansky described his own attack of angina pectoris: "In addition there is the pain without equal, a neuralgic pain in the chest, a pain similar to that caused by a spike impaled in the sternum, originating in the back, contracting the esophagus and the larynx, spreading to the occipital region and the upper extremities, a pain which plays havoc with the muscles so that I would become unconscious unless I cease all activity" (6). A severe case of neuralgia indeed! Rokitansky is known for his description of the excessive deposition in the inner membrane of the vessels (see Chapter 6).

Stimulated by Corvisart's and Laennec's publication, Pierre Adolphe Piorry, who lived from 1794 to 1879, began to work on auscultation, his work culminating in his publication (13). Piorry's main innovation amounted to interposing a small plate between the skin and the percussing finger, which he called a plessimètre (plessimeter). He tried plates made from lead, leather, and cedar wood and finally settled on ivory (13). His main merit was to promote the teaching of bedside diagnosis. His contributions to physical diagnosis were minor, although during his lifetime his fame outshone that of the real pioneer, Auenbrugger.

In France in 1804, forty-seven years after Auenbrugger's publication, Corvisart published a French translation of *Inventum Novum*, adding 440 pages of commentary (14; Fig. 15.2). Dickinson Richards, humanist, clinician, writer, and pioneer in cardiac catheterization and winner of a Nobel prize for medicine in 1957, furnished the introduction to the translated version of Corvisart's book, *An Essay of the Organic Diseases and Lesions of the Heart and Great Vessels* (14).

Corvisart's original dedication of this book to Napoleon is worth quoting (14):

> To Napoleon I, Emperor of the French, and King of Italy,
>
> Sire: It is not for my feeble voice to pronounce eulogies, which could not measure up to the deeds with which you have astonished the world. I leave this immense effort to those who would dare attempt it. But, Sire, I have the ambition to ask the favor of placing your immortal Name before this work. Then, should I obtain this favor, I assure to my book a portion of the enduring fame which your Name guarantees to everything that bears it, I am with respect, Sire.
>
> To your majesty the most humble and most obedient servant and faithful subject, Corvisart (14).

Corvisart was born in 1755 in the small village of Dricourt, in the County of Champagne east of Rheims and died in 1821 (14). He first wanted to study law but soon turned to medicine. He became physician in La Charité in 1788 and professor of medicine in the College de France in 1797. He had an illustrious career as physician, friend, and confidant of Napoleon. Richards points out that, like all great teachers, he created a school of outstanding, bright stars of the succeeding generation such as the anatomist Cuvier, the surgeon Dupuytren, the clinicians Bayle and Bretonneau, and the great Laennec (14). Corvisart's book was not written by him personally but was assembled and published by one of his assistants, C.N. Horeau. Laennec himself notes that no one could do justice to Corvisart's greatness: "The uncertainty of the signs of disease, and the vagueness of descriptions of these, appear particularly striking to those who, like myself, were his pupils and habitual witnesses of the boldness and precision of his diagnostics. This defect [quality], no doubt, partly depends on the incommunicable tact of the physician, which forms so great a part of the art, and which Mr. Corvisart possessed in the highest degree." And Richards comments, "The incommunicable tact of the physicians. What an exquisite phrase!" (14).

The greatness of the Corvisart's contribution was to verify whenever possible clinical observation by autopsy findings. Horeau's introduction to the book points this out: "The point both difficult and important, the end truly useful, is to study on the living and diseased man, the characters peculiar to the different organs, to observe well their phenomena, and establish their symptoms, by observations sufficiently numerous, to prevent the possibility of misunderstanding them. Such a labor necessarily requires . . . a physician determined in his inquiries, never hesitating to inspect the morbid bodies of the dead" (14). Another great accomplishment of Corvisart was the inquiry into the mechanism of disease. By clinical and postmortem observations, he was able to focus on the essential connection between the morbid anatomy and clinical symptomology of heart failure (14).

Corvisart's book deals with diseases of the pericardium and the myocardium; he termed hypertrophy or dilatation of the heart as active and passive aneurysms (14). Richards relates that it was Laennec who changed the term "aneurysm" to "hypertrophy" or "dilatation." This chapter is followed by those dealing with valvular lesions and dilatation (aneurysms) of the aorta. Also included are interesting cases of congenital heart disease, such as "perforation of the partition of the ventricle," "the continuance of the foramen ovale in the adult man," and "the closing of the foramen ovale in the foetus." Of particular interest is the case history and pathology of a patient in whom the aorta arose from both ventricles. Corvisart describes the clinical picture first: "a child, having enjoyed good health during the first year of its life, when it began to deteriorate in the second year. The patient lived for twelve years, after that it fell a victim to a disease which, from its nature, seemed that it must have taken place much sooner." Corvisart (Horeau) describes that on dissection, the aorta, "instead of rising from the left ventricle only, had a mouth in each of the ventricles." In all likelihood, this was a case of tetralogy of Fallot, first reported by Stenson from Copenhagen (14) (see Chapter 4).

Corvisart also was concerned with congestive heart failure (14). He noted venous and jugular engorgement, abdominal fluid, and enlargement of the liver in these patients and ascribed the increased respiration and orthopnea to engorgement of the lung with blood. It is strange that he never mentioned angina pectoris or any changes in the coronary arteries at autopsy. This was an oversight for such a brilliant physician, particularly since a number of English physicians had mentioned angina pectoris, and some had connected it to diseases of the coronary arteries (see Chapter 7).

The introduction of percussion and auscultation in the eighteenth century was the first step on the long road to scientific cardiology. Indirect auscultation was introduced by Laennec in 1818 (15, 16). Others before him had thought of auscultation (17). Victor McKusick's book on cardiovascular sound contains an informative history of cardiovascular sound (10). It was customary during the Middle Ages for the physician to place the ear directly on the thorax (17). In the seventeenth century William Harvey had pointed to the importance of listening to the heart sounds (18). Laennec's teacher, Corvisart, as well as Bayle made use of direct auscultation by placing the ear directly on the chest of the patient, a method referred to as pectoral audition (18).

Aside from the English translation of Laennec's book, several biographies of Laennec have been published (16, 17). The biography by Webb is a delightful, informative description of Laennec's life and times (16).

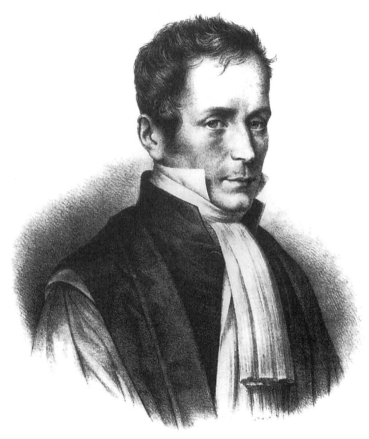

Figure 15.3. René Laennec. *(Courtesy of the New York Academy of Medicine)*

René Théophile Hyacinthe Laennec was born in 1781 in Quimper, Brittany (16; Fig. 15.3). His brief life spanned the French Revolution and the Napoleonic era. Laennec's love for his home in Brittany extended throughout his life and it was to Brittany that he retired and died. His mother died of tuberculosis and he was probably infected with the disease at an early age (16). His father, an unsuccessful lawyer, was somewhat of a gadfly, irresponsible in family matters, who fancied himself a poet and never assumed responsibility for the education of Théophile and his brother, Michaud. Their education was overseen by Théophile's uncle, Guillaume, an intelligent and generous physician who had moved to Nantes. He had graduated as a Doctor of Medicine from the University of Montpellier and further studied under Hunter in England. For three years Laennec and his brother, Michaud, were students in Nantes, where they experienced the

Terror of the French Revolution (16). Three thousand people met their death at Nantes during the Terror. When the guillotine proved of insufficient speed, the rabble tied naked men to naked women and flung them into the Loire River. Before he was fifteen years old, Laennec had seen fifty heads fall in the basket under the guillotine outside the window of his home and he had seen his uncle thrown into prison for six weeks on suspicion of not being in sympathy with the revolutionary government (16).

In 1807 Laennec began his studies in Paris under Corvisart. Dupuytren, a young surgeon, recognized his outstanding qualities and selected him for the Society of Medical Instruction, which represented the elite of the students. His first published work was an autopsy report in which he described ossification of the mitral valve with dilatation of the ventricle. During this time, Laennec was almost penniless and it was necessary for his uncle Guillaume to ask Théophile's father for support, mostly with no results (16). It was quite typical for his father to suggest that his son solicit his teacher for his [the father's] employment in Paris. Laennec answered that though he worked every day with Corvisart, the latter hardly recognized him. It is likely that at this time Laennec already suffered from tuberculosis and, like Pascal, he may have turned to the solace of religion (16). One of the classical quotations that Laennec used frequently was "gloria mundi peribit veritas Domini manet aeternum" (worldly glory passes, but God's truth lasts forever). Poverty made his career very difficult and his uncle tried to help by repeatedly begging Laennec's father to send him funds to allow him to finish his studies. But his father refused. It was at this time that Laennec pronounced his credo, "I profess medicine without bounds, I am not with the ancient nor with the modern, but I seek the truth in each and test everything by repeated trial" (16).

Laennec's career was not without political friction with his colleagues, especially Dupuytren. Dupuytren accused Laennec "as one who had learned everything from him without showing any gratitude." At the age of twenty-five Laennec had described peritonitis and melanotic tumors. He also identified phthisis with tuberculosis of the lungs; since that time, the term "pulmonary tuberculosis" has replaced the term "phthisis." During all this time Laennec continuously suffered from ill health; he wrote, "health is a treasure recognized only after it has eluded us" (16). In contrast to his teacher, Corvisart, Laennec was also interested in angina pectoris. In his writings he analyzed the ideas of Heberden and Jenner; the latter had clearly recognized the relationship of angina pectoris to lesions of the coronary artery (see Chapter 7). But like Skoda he was doubtful about the relationship between angina pectoris and coronary arteries because he rarely found lesions in the coronary artery in patients dying of angina pectoris; he, too, was inclined to attribute the pain to cardiac neuralgia (16).

Prior to Laennec it was customary for physicians to apply the ear directly to the chest. There were good reasons for avoiding direct contact with the patients, primarily for hygienic reasons. Laennec had an obese patient at Necker Hospital suffering from heart conditions. Walking through the gardens of the Louvre he noticed children scratching and tapping at the end of a wooden beam while others pressed the ear to the other end, listening to the transmitted sounds (16). Arriving at the hospital in the room of his patient, he seized a paper-covered book, rolled it into a tight cylinder, and placed one end of this crude instrument against the patient's heart while he applied his ear to the other end. Laennec himself described his discovery in a more scientific style: "then I remembered a well known acoustic fact, that if the ear be applied to one end of a plank it is easy to hear a pin's scratching on the other end. I conceived the possibility of employing this property of matter in the present case" (15). The instrument was called a *cornet de papier* in the records of the hospital. Later Laennec learned to use the lathe and made solid batons. With this instrument he could hear the heart sounds better but some of the signs that he could hear with the rolled paper were no longer audible. Therefore he constructed a central canal in his baton and from that moment on was able to improve transmission of the sounds. He now was able to hear pulmonary rales, a term he created. Laennec called his method "auscultation" from the word *auscultare* (to listen). He also named it *mediat* to indicate the use of the stethoscope (16).

He presented his discovery in 1818 before the Academy of Sciences. He experienced respect but not enthusiasm. In August 1819, he published his book (15). As typically the case after the introduction of new inventions and techniques there was skepticism; however, the majority of physicians quickly adopted the technique.

Laennec died in 1826. His private life was characterized by poverty, parental neglect, and sickness; he was a deeply religious man, compassionate toward his patients; his discoveries originated from his ability to see simple solutions for complicated problems, a true sign of greatness.

Further developments of the stethoscope are described in publications by Weinberg and Peck (19, 20). Weinberg describes attempts that were made to produce binaural stethoscopes as early as 1829; not until rubber was introduced in the middle of the nineteenth century was it possible to build a good model for the binaural stethoscope (19). Both Weinberg and Peck credited the invention of the binaural stethoscope to an American physician, Phillip Camman, who in 1853 published the specifications for this model, using ivory earpieces, a wooden chest piece, and a woven tubing held together by a broad rubber band (19, 20; Fig. 15.4). The well-known cardiologist Henry I. Bowditch praised this instrument as an intensifier to an extraordinary degree of every sound heard in auscultation (20). Camman, a graduate of Rutgers Medical College, became familiar with the stethoscope and the method of auscultation while in Paris. Possibly

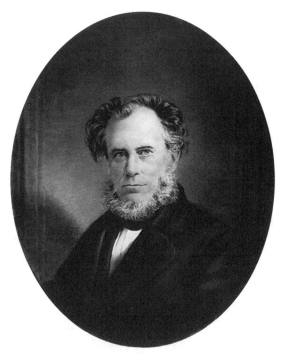

Figure 15.4. Phillip Camman. *(Courtesy of the New York Academy of Medicine)*

Camman's interest in cardiology stemmed from his own cardiac affliction, from which he died in 1863 in New York City. Camman's stethoscope, as described in pictures in the *New York Medical Times* in 1855, consisted of two tubes of German silver, with the objective end of ebony. Camman's modification of the stethoscope found universal praise, particularly from Austin Flint, who was referred to as "The American Laennec" (20).

As early as 1827, an "electronic" stethoscope was invented by Sir Charles Wheatstone, the inventor of the Wheatstone bridge. It consisted of two blades, one for each ear, with a curved rod or brass wire meeting in a single point; however, but it was considered as too complicated for use (20). In 1850 Landouzy of Paris built a polystethoscope having a bell-shaped chest piece with a number of elastic tubes by which several persons could listen at once. Arthus Leared of Ireland built a binaural stethoscope in 1851 which consisted of gutta-percha tubes attached to the chest piece at one extremity and at the other to the earpieces (20). The same year Marsh of Cincinnati patented a double stethoscope (20).

In 1941 the physical and acoustic principles of the stethoscope were explored

in great detail by Maurice Rappaport and Howard Sprague from the Massachusetts General Hospital in Boston (21). This article, while dwelling at great
length on the acoustic properties of the binaural stethoscope, also describes the
early electroacoustic devices, which operated on a principle similar to that of the
telephone, consisting of a carbon-granule microphone that modulated an electric current, and in turn excited a telephone receiver. One of those instruments
was designed by Einthoven, the discoverer of the electrocardiogram (21). Rappaport and Sprague investigated in great lengths such details as tubing length,
thickness of the tubing, comparisons of binaural with monaural effects, types of
heart sounds and murmurs, and energy output of cardiac vibrations (21). There
also was considerable discussion on the relative advances of the combination of
the bell and diaphram chest pieces for clinical examination. The article dealt in
great detail with threshold of hearing and feeling versus frequency, the importance of the decibel, the perceptible variations in intensity between frequency
limits, the minimum tonal perception time, and relative sensitivity curves of the
average normal human hearing mechanism. A thorough and comprehensive discussion of phonocardiography is contained in McKusick's book, which also deals
extensively with the development in this field (10).

Which bedside methods are still useful at the end of the twentieth century,
and how do they compare with objective, quantitative procedures? Perloff, in his
book on physical examination of the heart and circulation, selects several physical aspects, such as clinical appearance, arterial pulse, jugular pulse, movements
of the heart, and auscultation (11). He also stresses how much can be learned from
appearance of patients with isolated valvular pulmonary stenosis, supravalvular
aortic stenosis, infectious endocarditis, and several types of congenital heart disease. He extensively quotes Auenbrugger's work on percussion, but devotes only
one short paragraph to its clinical application, mainly concerned with the determination of the presence, degree, and localization of pleural effusion (11). Percussion of the chest is hardly practiced at present. Sixty-five years ago, while
studying at the medical school in Vienna, I was taught the importance of percussion, particularly the determination of heart size ("absolute and relative cardiac dullness"). In clinical examinations, my fellow students and I had to outline
the projection of the heart on the chest wall as determined by percussion. But
there were many cases in which both student and teacher missed cardiomegaly
as determined objectively by x rays, although the instructor never admitted his
mistake.

How do bedside observations compare to quantitative measurement of cardiac function, such as determination of ejection fraction or cardiac hemodynamics? What is the accuracy in assessing the severity of congestive heart failure
from bedside observations? A series of publications have reported such comparisons. In general, there is no agreement. For example, Badgett and colleagues

related patient history and examination of the jugular vein, third heart sound, presence of pulmonary rales, and type and severity to left-sided heart failure in adults (22). The authors conclude that the best method for detecting systolic dysfunction is the abnormal apical impulse. As related in the chapter on the cardiac catheterization, Chaveau and Marey had already graphically recorded the apex beat together with intracardiac pressure and found that ventricular systole and apical beat commence and terminate simultaneously (see Chapter 1). In 1971 the clinical characteristic of the apex beat was found by Conn to correlate well with muscular mass and volume of the left ventricle, as determined by quantitative angiography (23).

Gadsbøll et al. compared chest x ray, radionuclide ventriculography, and right-heart catheterization to physical signs at the bedside such as rales, apex beat, S_3-gallop, distended neck veins, and hepatomegaly (24). They found that S_3-gallop was associated with the most severe degree of cardiac dilatation and functional depression. In contrast, dyspnea, a displaced apex beat, and rales were of only limited value in differentiating between patients with and without pulmonary congestion or reduced ventricular function; one-third of patients in whom the apex beat was felt inside the midclavicular line had enlarged left ventricular diastolic volume; dyspnea was not always present when pulmonary capillary wedge pressure was elevated (24).

Reliability of bedside diagnostic tests was also examined by Butman and co-workers, who found that jugular venous distention more accurately predicted elevation of the pulmonary capillary wedge pressure than the presence of pulmonary rales (25). Furthermore, a positive abdominal jugular test identified patients with poor hemodynamic status whether or not there was evidence of jugular venous distention at rest (25). Accordingly, bedside clinical examination in chronic heart failure was considered to be extremely useful in predicting significant elevation of both left and right heart failure (25). Reliability of physical science as estimated by hemodynamics in chronic heart failure was also examined by Perloff, who related the third heart sound, pulmonary rales, an abnormal jugular venous pulse, and peripheral edema to hemodynamic measurements, primarily pulmonary capillary wedge pressure (11). Here, too, considerable discrepancies were found. Rales, edema, and elevated mean jugular venous pressure were absent in a number of patients with a pulmonary capillary wedge pressure greater than or equal to 22 mm Hg (11).

An ominous report on the prevailing auscultatory skills of medical students and physicians in training has recently been published (26). The authors describe a disturbing lack of skill in cardiac auscultation among generalists in training. Cardiac auscultation was chosen as paradigmatic for all bedside diagnostic skills. The deplorable lack of skill in cardiac auscultation may have been due to the current emphasis on highly technical procedures resulting in atrophy by disuse. Cardiac auscultation by a well-trained physician is certainly more cost-effective than examination by echocardiography or cardiac catheterization. Admittedly there are situations where auscultation is insufficient, such as in congenital heart disease. But, in some instances, examination by auscultation by an experienced physician needs little further confirmation.

The possibility of interpreting incorrectly bedside diagnostic signs is not surprising because of the differences in experience of the physician, variations of techniques, and lack of a homogeneous patient population. Neither surprising is the relative disparity between physical signs such as apical beat, rales, cardiac murmurs, venous pulse, and so on, and specific objective measurements such as pulmonary wedge pressure, ventricular end-diastolic pressures, and ejection fraction, now easily determined by echocardiography. But this by no means should relegate bedside physical examination and history to an inferior role. By inspection, physical examination, and a careful history, the physician sees the whole patient. Only thus is he or she able to evaluate the patient as a complete individual in need of care. The patient's history and physical examination at the bedside are an indispensable prelude to quantitative measurements.

References

1. Thomas, L. The Youngest Science, Notes of a Medicine Watcher. New York, Penguin Books, 1993.
2. Corner, G. The rise of medicine at Salerno in the twelfth century. Annals of Medical History, 3:13–15, 1931.
3. Neumayr, A. Music and Medicine. Bloomington, Medi-Ed Press, 1995.
4. Modern Medicine: Its Theory and Practice. William Osler (ed.), volume 4, Diseases of the Circulatory System—Diseases of the Blood—Diseases of the Spleen and Thymus and Lymph-glands. Philadelphia and New York, Lea & Febiger, 1908.
5. Sakula, A. Auenbrugger: Opus and opera. J. Roy. Coll. Phys., 12(2):180–188, 1978.
6. Wyklicky, H. Zur Geschichte der Kardiologie in Wien. Wien. Med. Wochenschr. 15/16:366–369, 1988.
7. Bedford, D.E. Auenbrugger's contribution to cardiology. History of percussion of the heart. Br. Heart J., 33:817–821, 1971.
8. Dock, G. Leopold Auenbrugger and the history of percussion. Michigan Alumnus, November 1898. Address at the Department of Medicine, University of Michigan, 27: 1–7, 1898.
9. Auenbrugger, L. Inventum novum ex percussione thoracis humani ut signo abstrusos interni pectoris morbis detegendi. Vindobonae, Typis Joannis Thomae Trattner, 1761.
10. McKusick, V.A. Cardiovascular Sound in Health and Disease. Baltimore, Williams & Wilkins Co., 1958.
11. Perloff, J. Physical Examination of the Heart and Circulation. Philadelphia, W.B. Saunders Co., 1982.
12. Skoda, J. Abhandlung uber Perkussion und Auskultation. 5th ed. Vienna, L.W. Seidel, 1854.
13. Sakula, A. Pierre Adolphe Piorry (1794–1879): Pioneer of percussion and pleximetry. Thorax, 34:575–581, 1979.
14. Corvisart, J.N. An Essay on the Organic Diseases and Lesions of the Heart and Great Vessels. Translated from the French with notes, by Jacob Gates, M.M.S.S. With an

introduction by Dr. Dickinson W. Richards. New York, published under the auspices of the Library of the New York Academy of Medicine by Hafner Publishing Company, 1962.

15. Laennec, R.T.H. A Treatise on the Diseases of the Chest. Translated from the French. New York Academy of Medicine, The History of Medicine Series, 1. New York, published under the auspices of the Library of the New York Academy of Medicine by Hafner Publishing Company, 1962.

16. Webb, G.B. René Théophile Hyacinthe Laennec, a Memoir. New York, Paul B. Hoeber, 1928.

17. Kervan, R. Laennec, His Life and Times. Translated from the French by D.C. Abrahams-Curiel. Oxford, London, New York, Paris, Pergamon Press, 1960.

18. Tutzke, D. Zur Geschichte der Auskultation. Medical Acta, Berlin, 4:286–287, 1978.

19. Weinberg, F. The history of the stethoscope. Canadian Family Physician, 39(10): 2223–2224, 1993.

20. Peck, P. Dr. Camman and the binaural stethoscope. J. Kansas Med. Society, 64:121–129, 1963.

21. Rappaport, M., and H. Sprague. Physiological and physical laws that govern auscultation and their clinical application. Am. Heart J., 21:257–318, 1941.

22. Badgett, R.G., C.R. Lucey, and C.D. Mulrow. The rational clinical examination. Can the clinical examination diagnose left-sided heart failure in adults? JAMA, 277(21): 1712–1719, 1997.

23. Conn, R.D., and J.S. Cole. The cardiac apex impulse. Clinical and angiographic correlations. Ann. Intern. Med., 75:185–191, 1971.

24. Gadsbøll, N., P.F. Høilund-Carlsen, G.G. Nielsen, J. Berning, N.E. Brunn, P. Stage, E. Hein, J. Marving, H. Løngborg-Jensen, and B.H. Jensen. Symptoms and signs of heart failure in patients with myocardial infarction: Reproducibility and relationship to chest x-ray, radionuclide ventriculography and right heart catheterization. European Heart Journal, 10:1017–1028, 1989.

25. Butman, S.M., G.A. Ewy, J.R. Standen, K.B. Kern, and E. Hahn. Bedside cardiovascular examination in patients with severe chronic heart failure: Importance of rest or inducible jugular venous distension. JACC, 22(4):968–974, 1993.

26. Mangione, S., and L.Z. Nieman, Cardiac auscultatory skills of internal medicine and family practice trainees. JAMA, 278:717–722, 1997.

Contributors

Dr. Walter Abelmann, Professor Emeritus of Medicine, Harvard Medical School, Boston, MA; Senior Physician, Beth Israel-Deaconess Medical Center, Boston, MA

Dr. Donald Baim, Chief Interventional Cardiology Section, Beth Israel-Deaconess Medical Center, Boston, MA; Professor of Medicine, Harvard Medical School, Boston, MA

Dr. John Baldwin, Vice President of Health Affairs, Dartsmouth College, Hanover, NH; Dean, Dartmouth Medical School, Hanover, NH

Dr. Richard J. Bing, Director of Experimental Cardiology, Huntington Medical Research Institutes; Visiting Associate in Chemistry, California Institute of Technology; Professor Emeritus of Medicine, USC, Pasadena, CA

Dr. Gisele Bonne, Institute of Myology, National Institute of Health and Medical Research, Paris, France

Dr. Tirone David, Professor of Surgery, University of Toronto, Canada; Head, Division of Cardiovascular Surgery, The Toronto Hospital, Canada

Dr. Richard DeWall, Professor Emeritus of Surgery, Wright State University School of Medicine, Dayton, OH

Dr. Pamela Douglas, Associate Professor of Medicine, Harvard Medical School, Boston, MA; Director of Noninvasive Cardiology, Beth Israel-Deaconess Medical Center, Boston, MA

Dr. Gerd Hasenfuss, Professor and Chairman, Department of Cardiology, University of Gottingen, Germany

Dr. Raymond Heimbecker, OC, Former Surgeon, Toronto General Hospital and University of Toronto, Canada; Former Chief, Cardiothoracic Surgery and Professor Emeritus of Surgery, University of Western Ontario, London, Canada; Honorary Surgeon, Bahama Out Islands

Dr. Herman Hellerstein,† Late Professor Emeritus of Medicine, Case Western Reserve University School of Medicine, Cleveland, OH; Attending Physician, University Hospitals of Cleveland, OH (deceased)

Dr. Arnold M. Katz, Professor of Medicine and Cardiology Division Chief Emeritus, School of Medicine, University of Connecticut, Farmington, CT

Dr. Scott A. LeMaire, Resident in Cardiothoracic Surgery, Baylor College of Medicine, TX

Dr. Berndt Luderitz, Professor of Medicine and Chairman, Department of Medicine and Cardiology, University of Bonn, Germany

Dr. Alexander Nadas, Emeritus Chief of Cardiology, Senior Associate in Cardiology, The Children's Hospital, Boston, MA; Professor Emeritus of Pediatrics, Harvard Medical School, Boston, MA

Dr. Oglesby Paul, Professor Emeritus of Medicine, Harvard Medical School, Boston, MA; Senior Physician Emeritus, Brigham and Women's Hospital, Boston, MA

Dr. Michael Reardon, Associate Professor of Cardiothoracic Surgery, Baylor College of Medicine, TX

Dr. Heinrich Schelbert, Professor of Radiological Sciences, Division of Nuclear Medicine and Biophysics, University of California, Los Angeles

Dr. Ketty Schwartz, Director of Research INSERM/CNRS, Institute of Myology, National Institute of Health and Medical Research, Paris, France

Dr. Ake Senning, Professor Emeritus of Surgery, University of Zurich, Switzerland

Appreciation of others who have been of immeasurable help:

Dr. Konrad Bloch, Higgins Professor Emeritus of Biochemistry, Department of Chemistry, Harvard University, Boston, MA; Nobelist

Dr. Edward B. Lewis, Professor of Biology, California Institute of Technology, Pasadena, CA; Nobelist

Dr. Maclyn McCarty, Professor Emeritus, Rockefeller University, NY

Dr. Vittorio Sartorelli, Assistant Professor, Institute for Genetic Medicine, Department of Biochemistry and Molecular Biology, University of Southern California School of Medicine, Los Angeles, CA

Dr. Leonard T. Skeggs Jr., Professor Emeritus of Biochemistry, Case Western Reserve University, Cleveland, OH

Index